Leadership and the Advanced Practice Nurse

The Future of a Changing Health-Care Environment

Leadership and the Advanced Practice Nurse

The Future of a Changing Health-Care Environment

Diane Whitehead, EdD, DNP, RN, ANEF
Core Faculty
DNP Program
Walden University
Minneapolis, MN

Patricia Welch Dittman, PhD, RN, CDE
Nurse Health Care Outcomes Coordinator
Florida Atlantic University Community Health Center
Adjunct Professor
Florida Atlantic University
Boca Raton, Florida

Denise McNulty, DNP, MSN, RN-BC, ARNP
Department Chair and Associate Professor, Nursing
Ave Maria University
Clinical Education Specialist
Lee Memorial Health System
Fort Myers, Florida

 F.A. Davis Company • Philadelphia

F. A. Davis Company
1915 Arch Street
Philadelphia, PA 19103
www.fadavis.com

Printed in the United States of America

Last digit indicates print number: 10 9 8 7 6 5 4 3 2 1

Senior Acquisitions Editor: Susan Rhyner
Developmental Editor: Kelly Horvath
Content Project Manager: Echo Gerhart
Electronic Project Editor: Kate Crowley
Design & Illustration Manager: Carolyn O'Brien

As new scientific information becomes available through basic and clinical research, recommended treatments and drug therapies undergo changes. The author(s) and publisher have done everything possible to make this book accurate, up to date, and in accord with accepted standards at the time of publication. The author(s), editors, and publisher are not responsible for errors or omissions or for consequences from application of the book, and make no warranty, expressed or implied, in regard to the contents of the book. Any practice described in this book should be applied by the reader in accordance with professional standards of care used in regard to the unique circumstances that may apply in each situation. The reader is advised always to check product information (package inserts) for changes and new information regarding dose and contraindications before administering any drug. Caution is especially urged when using new or infrequently ordered drugs.

Library of Congress Cataloging-in-Publication Data

Names: Whitehead, Diane K., 1945- author. | Dittman, Patricia, author. |
     McNulty, Denise, author.
Title: Leadership and the advanced practice nurse : the future of a changing
     health-care environment / Diane Whitehead, Patricia Dittman, Denise
     McNulty.
Description: Philadelphia : F.A. Davis Company, [2017] | Includes
     bibliographical references and index.
Identifiers: LCCN 2016052945 | ISBN 9780803640429 (alk. paper)
Subjects: | MESH: Advanced Practice Nursing—methods | Leadership | Power
     (Psychology) | Adaptation, Psychological
Classification: LCC RT62 | NLM WY 128 | DDC 610.7306/93—dc23
LC record available at https://lccn.loc.gov/2016052945

This book is dedicated to my wonderful husband, Steve. Thank you for believing in me and understanding the importance that nursing and nursing education have in my life. Your constant encouragement, support, and partnership enrich my life every day. Writing this book has brought many memories of the dedicated and caring nurses who have shared their continued education journey with me. You remind me on a daily basis how proud I am to share this profession with you.

DW

I dedicate this book to my family who are a constant encouraging source in my life. My husband, David, is my soul mate, confidante, and best friend. I could not have completed this book without his support. My son, David (D.J.), and daughter-in-law, Laura, were always there, ready to suggest creative ideas. Finally, I would like to thank the profession of nursing for its commitment to societal health.

PD

I would like to dedicate this book to all of the wonderful nurses and leaders I have had the honor of working with in Florida. Thank you for believing in my work on empowerment and for your support on this "journey." I would also like to thank Dr. Diane Whitehead for inviting me to serve as a coauthor for this book and my partner, Peter, and my parents for their unconditional love and support of my work with nurses, students, and patients.

DM

Epigraph

The greatest leader is not necessarily the one who does the greatest things. He is the one that gets the people to do the greatest things. —*Ronald Reagan*

If your actions inspire others to dream more, learn more, do more and become more, you are a leader. —*John Quincy Adams*

Preface

In 2008 the Robert Wood Johnson Foundation (RWJF) and the Institute of Medicine (IOM) partnered to assess and respond to the need to transform the nursing profession. With the establishment of the 2-year Initiative on the Future of Nursing, the committee reviewed the role of nurses in transforming the health-care system. One of the key messages from their report was the need for nursing to develop strong leaders from the bedside to the boardroom. The committee identified strong leadership as critical to the development and implementation of changes necessary to improve quality, access, value, and patient-centered care (IOM, 2011).

Although not all nurses begin their career understanding the importance of leadership, leadership competencies need to be embedded throughout all levels of nursing education and continued in practice mentoring programs. The American Association of Nurse Executives has developed core competencies for nurse leaders in a variety of practice settings and at different levels of responsibility. Both the Commission on Collegiate Nursing Education and the Accreditation Commission for Education in Nursing have developed leadership competencies for all levels of nursing education. The American Nurses Credentialing Center Magnet Standards support nursing practice through transformation leadership and structural empowerment. In addition, current research is focusing on the concept of staff nursing clinical leadership. Bohmer (2013) argues that the successful implementation of the RWJF and IOM initiatives is dependent on developing frontline clinical leaders.

Over the many years that the three of us have taught leadership courses, we have found that the majority of textbooks focus on formal leadership positions and the management functions within these positions. Our impetus for writing this book was our belief that leaders are those who exert influence over others, even if no formal authority has been given to them. We agree with our colleagues at RWJF and IOM that strong nursing leaders are needed at all levels regardless of the position held within the organization. Based on these assumptions, this textbook is about leadership at all practice levels and organizations.

Unit I explores the foundations of leadership, including theories, frameworks, workplace leadership challenges, and policy and regulation leadership issues. Unit II explores the leadership within the business of health care including economic and fiscal leadership, quality, safety, and leading with a nursing focus. Unit III focuses on the individual leadership development of self and helping others to develop as leaders. A unique feature of this textbook is the discussion of the Journey to Psychological Empowerment, a program developed and utilized by Dr. Denise McNulty. For more than 20 years, Dr. McNulty has used this approach in developing leaders at all levels within nursing organizations.

References

Bohmer, R. M. (2013). Leading clinicians and clinical leading. *New England Journal of Medicine, 268*(16), 1468–1470.

Institute of Medicine. (2011). *The future of nursing: Leading change, advancing health.* Washington, DC: National Academies Press.

Contributors

Julia W. Aucoin, DNS, RN-BC, CNE

Director of Practice, Quality & Research
UNC REX Healthcare
Raleigh, North Carolina

Deborah Saylor, MSN, RN, CMSRN

Retired Chief Nursing Officer
Titusville, Florida

Reviewers

Julia W. Aucoin, DNS, RN-BC, CNE

Nurse Research Scientist
Duke University Health System
Durham, North Carolina

Rebecca J. Bartlett Ellis, PhD, RN, ACNS-BC

Assistant Professor
Indiana University School of Nursing
Indianapolis, Indiana

Patricia Buchsel, RN, MSN, OCN, FAAN

Clinical Instructor
Seattle University College of Nursing
Seattle, Washington

Maureen Cluskey, PhD, RN, CNE

Associate Dean for Distance Learning
College of Education and Health
    Science
Bradley University
Peoria, Illinois

Sharyn Conrad, DNP, RN, APRN, FNP-BC

Adjunct Professor
Nova Southeastern University
Winston Salem, North Carolina

Gloria P. Craig, EdD, MSN, BSN, RN

Professor
South Dakota State University
Brookings, South Dakota

Ellen D'Errico, PhD, RN, NEA-BC

Associate Professor
Loma Linda University
Loma Linda, California

Sheila Grossman, PhD, APRN, FNP-BC, FAAN

Professor & Coordinator, FNP Track &
    Director, Evaluation, Faculty
    Scholarship and Mentoring
Fairfield University School of Nursing
Fairfield, Connecticut

Arlene N. Hayne, PhD, RN

Professor
Ida V. Moffett School of Nursing
Samford University
Birmingham, Alabama

Deborah Lessard, RN, BSN, MA, JD, CPHRM

Healthcare Consultant and Adjunct
    Faculty
Carlow University
Pittsburgh, Pennsylvania

Paula Maisano, PhD, RN

Assistant Professor
University of Oklahoma College of
    Nursing, Tulsa Campus
Tulsa, Oklahoma

Karen S. Neill, PhD, RN, SANE-A

Associate Director for Graduate Studies
Idaho State University
Pocatello, Idaho

Teresa Shellenbarger, PhD, RN, CNE, ANEF

Professor and Doctoral Nursing
    Program Coordinator
Indiana University of Pennsylvania
Indiana, Pennsylvania

Nashat Zuraikat, PhD, RN

Professor of Nursing and Master's
    Program Coordinator
Indiana University of Pennsylvania
Indiana, Pennsylvania

Acknowledgments

Our heartfelt thanks to our team at F. A. Davis: Susan Rhyner, Senior Acquisitions Editor; Echo Gerhart, Content Project Manager; and Kelly Horvath, our Developmental Editor. We are indebted to you for your patience and perseverance throughout this project.

Contents

Chapter 2

Workplace Leadership Opportunities   35

Chapter 3

Leading in Policy and Regulation   67

UNIT II

LEADING THE BUSINESS OF HEALTH CARE   93

Chapter 4
Economic and Fiscal Leadership   95

Chapter 5
Leading With a Culture of Quality and Safety   123

Chapter 6

UNIT III

LEADING SELF AND OTHERS   185

Chapter 7
Focusing on Self   187

Chapter 8
Empowering Nurses as Leaders   209

Chapter 9

Creating a Culture of Excellence   239

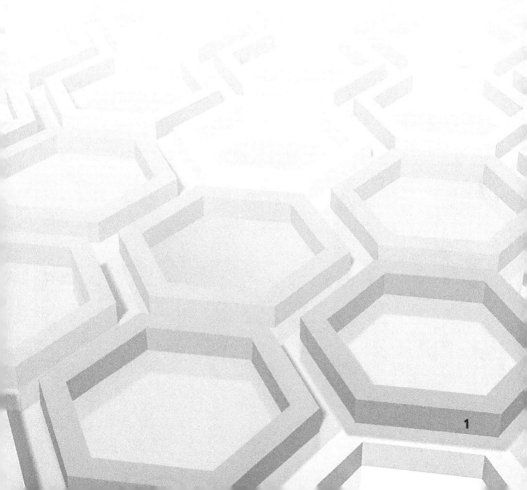

Laying a Foundation
for Leadership

Beginning the Leadership Journey

The literature is replete with books and articles on leadership. In 1990, Bass found more than 7,500 research studies, papers, and monographs published on the subject of leadership. A 2014 search of online databases using keywords "leadership" and "nursing" revealed more than 11,000 publications. With such an emphasis on the importance of leadership within the nursing profession, why then did Bulmer's 2013 study of registered nurses (RNs) find that fewer than 15% reported a desire to seek leadership positions at some time during their career? Research on nurse leaders in both practice and academia today shows that these leaders live in a world of chaos and uncertainly with high levels of responsibility and stress and often little respect and autonomy (Bulmer, 2013). Yet, those embarking on the leadership journey often believe that they bring special qualities to their organizations and that serving in leadership roles will bring them personal and professional satisfaction (Northouse, 2015) Research continues to explore what makes good leaders and how leadership influences job satisfaction, intent to stay in a position, and creation of an organizational culture that will move organizations forward (Cowden, Cummings, & McGrath, 2011; O'Neill, 2013).

This chapter explores the complex process of leadership. Beginning with a review of the historical approaches to leadership, the chapter follows with an exploration of the modern approaches that influence leaders today. It then looks at important influences on leadership today: change, innovation, complexity science, and the organization as a system. Box 1.1 includes questions upon which an emerging nurse leader might reflect.

LEADERSHIP DEFINED

Leadership and the search for a definition for it have been a topic of debate for more than a century. The definition of leadership has changed and evolved over time and has been influenced by world events, politics, culture research, and organizational change. Research in the 1990s and early 2000s identified leadership traits and actions from the perspective of other nurse leaders. These traits included a passion for nursing,

> BOX 1.1 **Personal Leadership Approaches**
>
> What approach or approaches resonate with my beliefs, personality, behaviors?
> What approach or approaches might I want to explore further as I develop my leadership abilities?
> What approach might work best in my organization now?

a sense of optimism, role modeling and mentorship, a set of moral principles, and an ability to form personal connections with staff (Aronson et al., 2014). When leadership is viewed as a trait, the broader context of the relationship of the leader to the followers is not taken into consideration. Today, research in nursing leadership emphasizes the importance of viewing leadership from a systems perspective, viewing the context and the relationships as a reciprocal process between the leader and the followers (Aronson et al., 2014).

Although numerous definitions of leadership exist, most contain one or more of the following themes (Summerfield, 2014):

- Democratic theme: The leader works to achieve a common goal.
- Collegial theme: Through a respectful and unifying approach, the leader influences rather than dictates the process.
- Enhancement theme: The results represent an improved current state.

For the purposes of this textbook, leadership is defined as "a process whereby an individual influences a group of individuals to achieve a common goal" (Northouse, 2015), and it has three key components. First, leadership is a *process*, an ongoing transaction between leaders and followers. Unlike the earlier definitions of leadership, the current definition does not include traits or characteristics of the leader as part of the definition, but recognizes an interactive, nonlinear, fluid relationship. Influence is the second key component, because without it, leadership cannot exist. Influence implies that the leader in some way affects the followers. Third, groups must be present for leadership to occur. These groups can be large or small; however, the leader must influence the group to meet common, mutually agreed-upon goals. This definition allows for anyone to emerge as a leader and does not imply that leaders are above or better than the followers—in fact, the same person may be a leader in one circumstance and a follower in another (Failla & Stichler, 2008; Markham, 2012; Northouse, 2015).

LEADERSHIP DESCRIBED

The following sections explore such concepts as how people become leaders, how power and leadership are related, and what distinguishes leadership from management.

Emergent Leadership

How does someone become a leader? A leadership position can be assigned, such as team leader, manager, department head, director, or administrator; however, being assigned a leadership position does not always mean that person becomes the "real" leader. Conversely, an individual perceived as one of the most influential people in a collaborative group is viewed as the *emergent leader*. No matter the title this person holds, he or she exhibits leadership through positive communication skills, positive self-efficacy, and social identification with the group (McMullen, Schneider, Firemark, Davis, & Spofford, 2013; Northouse, 2015).

Power and Leadership

French and Raven conducted the seminal work on power and leadership (1959). Their five bases of power are still widely referenced today. Power influenced by position is part of legitimate, reward, and coercive power, whereas personal power includes both referent and expert power (Table 1.1). Regardless of the power base, power is about the leader's capacity to influence followers (Box 1.2).

Leadership Versus Management

The study of management emerged in 1916 with Fayol's identification of management functions: planning, organizing, staffing, and controlling. Beginning in 1977 with Zaleznik, on the one hand scholars sought to define leadership and management as

TABLE 1.1 **Power Types and Bases**

Position Power	Personal Power
Legitimate: Formal position authority	Referent: Follower identifies or likes the leader
Reward: Ability to give rewards to others	Expert: Follower's perceptions of leader's competence
Coercive: Ability to penalize or punish others	

Adapted from: Northouse, P. (2015). *Leadership: Theory and practice* (7th ed.). Thousand Oaks, CA: Sage.

BOX 1.2 **Basis of Power**

After reviewing Table 1.1, identify people you know in leadership positions and people you describe as leaders. Where does their power come from? Is it power that is effective or benefits the followers and the organization? Why or why not?

totally different functions and constructs. The function of management produces order and consistency through planning, budgeting, organizing, staffing, controlling, and problem-solving. On the other hand, leadership is the function that produces change and movement of the organization by establishing direction, aligning people, motivating, and inspiring (Kotter, 1990). However, the relationship between these two constructs is complex and continues to be explored. Are managers and leaders different types of people? Is management focused on order and stability and leadership on adaptation and change? Regardless, both functions involve influencing a group toward attainment of a goal (Kotter, 1990; Northouse, 2015; Zaleznik, 1977).

EARLY APPROACHES TO LEADERSHIP

Earlier approaches to the study of leadership focused on the point of view of the leader or the follower and the context (Table 1.2). Those focusing on the leader emphasized traits, skills, or styles, whereas situational, contingency, and path-goal approaches focused on the follower and the context. Although these approaches have proved to be less than ideal, they give us historical perspective on leadership and are still taught in some leadership courses today. Importantly, they have also paved the way for the more current leadership approaches identified in today's research.

Trait Approach

Studies of leadership traits and leader characteristics first emerged in 1948. A century of research has identified common traits that individuals may wish to develop in order to be perceived as a leader: intelligence (including emotional intelligence [EI]), self-confidence, determination, integrity, sociability, and extraversion (Judge, Bono, Illies, & Gerhardt, 2002; Northouse, 2015; Shankman & Allen, 2008; Stone, 2011; Zaccaro, Kemp, & Bader, 2004).

> *Intelligence and emotional intelligence.* Theodore Roosevelt is quoted as saying, "No one cares how much you know until they know how much you care."

TABLE 1.2 **Early Leadership Theories**

Leader Focus	Follower and Context Focus
Trait approach	Situational
Skills approach	Contingency
Style approach	Path-Goal

Adapted from: Northouse, P.(2015). *Leadership: Theory and practice* (7th ed.). Thousand Oaks, CA: Sage.

Although leaders must demonstrate verbal ability, perceptual ability, and reasoning, emotionally intelligent leadership is showing a positive relationship to employee satisfaction, retention, and performance. EI has been widely studied during the past 20 years and is defined "as the ability to perceive and express emotions, to use emotions to facilitate thinking, to understand and reason with emotions, and to effectively manage emotions within oneself and with others" (Northouse, 2015). Emotionally intelligent leaders are effective listeners. They are able to understand and manage their own emotions as well as demonstrate an awareness of others' emotions. These leaders demonstrate an awareness of the emotional atmosphere of the work environment (Deutschendorf, 2014).

Self-confidence. If leadership involves influencing others, self-confidence involves believing in the ability to make a difference. Self-confident leaders display self-esteem and self-assurance.

Determination. Determination involves initiative, persistence, and drive.

Integrity. Integrity includes the qualities of honesty and trustworthiness. Leaders with integrity are loyal, dependable, and believable.

Sociability. Leaders demonstrate sociability by being friendly, outgoing, courteous, diplomatic, and sensitive to others' well-being.

Extraversion. The 2002 meta-analysis of leadership and personality studies (Judge et al., 2002) reviewed the relationship between five factors—neuroticism, extraversion, openness, agreeableness, and conscientiousness—and leadership and found that extraversion was the factor most strongly associated with leadership, whereas agreeableness was only weakly associated. Low neuroticism was also found to be a personality factor associated with leadership.

The trait approach focuses entirely on the leader. With extensive years of research to support findings, the trait approach gives us benchmarks for what to look for in leaders and how to develop ourselves as leaders. Although the list of traits leaders tend to share continues to emerge, none of them takes the situation into account.

Skills Approach

The skills approach also focuses on the leader, but on the leaders' skills and abilities rather than on personality characteristics. As early as 1955, Katz began dividing leadership skills into technical, human, and conceptual skills. Each level of management was viewed as needing various degrees of these three skills (Katz, 1955). The higher someone was in the organization, the more that person's position required conceptual rather than technical skills. In other words, the chief executive officer (CEO) would use conceptual skills the majority of the time, whereas the computer programmer would use technical skills. However, according to Katz, human skills are always required no matter the level or the position in the organization. This research continued to grow and resulted in a comprehensive skill-based model of leadership (Mumford, Zaccarro, Connelly, & Marks, 2000). Influenced by career experiences and the environment, the skill model of leadership focuses on the individual attributes of cognitive ability, motivation, and personality and the competencies of problem-solving skills, social-judgment skills, and knowledge resulting in effective problem-solving and performance.

Although this approach supports the premise that, with training, leadership is available to everyone, the skills model is really a combination of skills and traits. The model does not measure how these skills contribute to effective performance or positive outcomes.

Style Approach

Unlike the traits and skills approaches, the style approach emphasizes the behavior of the leader and the tasks assigned to the followers. The most widely used style approach was developed by Blake and Mouton (1985) and is shown in Table 1.3.

TABLE 1.3 Style Leadership Types

Description	Behavior
Country-club management	High concern for interpersonal relationships and low concern for tasks and production
Authority-compliance management	Heavy emphasis on task, viewing people as a tool for getting the job done
Middle-of-the-road management	Balancing both the task and the people, this leader avoids conflict giving up both the push for production and attention to follower needs
Team management	Emphasizing both tasks and relationships, the team leader stimulates participation, is open-minded, and sets priorities
Impoverished management	Lack of concern with both task and interpersonal relationships, demonstrating indifference, apathy, and little contact with followers
Maternalism/paternalism	The benevolent dictator treats the organization as a family, making most of the key decisions, rewarding loyalty, and punishing noncompliance
Opportunism	Using any combination of the first five styles for his or her personal advancement and personal gain

Adapted from: Blake, R.R., & Mouton, J.S. (1985). *The managerial grid III*. Houston, TX: Gulf.

The style approach is less a theory than it is a reminder that leader actions occur on both a task level and a relationship level. As the first approach that moved away from testing leadership as a personality trait, the style approach expanded research into what leadership actually did. This approach is useful in all organizations to prompt the leader to assess both the task and the leader's relationship with his or her followers.

Situational Approach

The situational approach to leadership developed by Hersey and Blanchard in the 1960s has undergone many refinements and is still used in leadership development programs today (Graeff, 1997). It is a time-tested, practical, flexible model. However, although it is widely used, critics of the model identify the lack of research supporting both the theoretical underpinnings and outcomes using this model.

The premise of this model is that leaders and followers move back and forth along a continuum based on the followers' abilities and the leader's style. Hersey and Blanchard see leadership as a composite of the behaviors of the person who attempts to influence others. These behaviors include both directive (tasks) behaviors and supportive (relationship) behaviors. Directive behaviors include giving directions, setting timelines, clarifying instructions, and setting priorities, whereas supportive behaviors include giving social and emotional support such as asking for input, offering praise, and sharing information about self. Table 1.4 summarizes behaviors related to situational leadership types.

TABLE 1.4 Situational Leadership Types

Behavior	Description
Low supportive, low directive	Delegating: Leader is involved in decision-making but leaves execution to followers.
High supportive, low directive	Supporting: Leader gives recognition and support to followers to bring out follower skills.
High directive, high supportive	Coaching: Leader makes the final decision on the goal, but offers strong supportive behaviors.
High directive, low supportive	Directing: Leader focuses on goal attainment; supervises carefully.

Adapted from: Graeff, C. L. (1997). Evolution of situational leadership theory: A critical review. *Leadership Quarterly, 8*(2), 153–170.

Contingency Approach

The contingency approach to leadership focuses on the leadership style and the situation. In the 1960s, Fiedler explored the most widely recognized contingency approach. Similar to the situational approach , the contingency approach focuses on tasks or relationships, matching the leader to the task. The effectiveness of the leader will depend on the leader's preferred leadership style, the task, and the position's power (the amount of authority a leader has to reward or punish followers). The strength of this approach is the recognition that a given leader may not be effective in all situations, but rather the leader's success depends on the match between leadership style and the situation. Although this theory approach is supported by strong empirical research, it is criticized for implying that the only alternative for a mismatch of leader orientation and an unfavorable situation is changing the leader. Nevertheless, contingency approach can be used to assess a leader's suitability for a task or to analyze why a leader is not successful in a given situation (Northouse, 2015).

Path-Goal Approach

The path-goal approach to leadership focuses on employee motivation, challenging the leader to behave in a manner that will enhance followers' goal attainment. This approach hypothesizes that leaders motivate by defining goals, clarifying processes, removing obstacles, and providing support. It looks at leadership behaviors, follower characteristics, and task characteristics. A practical model, the path-goal approach helps to illuminate the path that leaders need to take in order to guide and coach subordinates. The path-goal approach assumes that leaders are flexible and able to change their leadership style as situations require. The two variables, environment and follower characteristics, moderate the leader behavior–outcome relationship. This approach reminds leaders that their main responsibility is to help subordinates define and reach their goals in an efficient manner (Table 1.5).

TABLE 1.5 **Path-Goal Approach**

Leadership Behavior	Follower Characteristics	Task Characteristics
Directive	Dogmatic, authoritarian	Ambiguous, unclear, complex
Supportive	Unsatisfied	Repetitive, unchallenging
Participative	Autonomous, controlling	Unstructured, ambiguous
Achievement oriented	Need to excel	Challenging, complex

Adapted from: Northouse, P. (2015). *Leadership: Theory and practice* (7th ed.). Thousand Oaks, CA: Sage.

MODERN APPROACHES TO LEADERSHIP

Leadership as a Continuum

Transformational, transactional, and laissez-faire approaches to leadership are often viewed as a leadership continuum.

The transformational leadership approach, first described in the 1970s, gives more attention to the affective elements of a leader. Terms often used in describing transformational leadership include "charismatic" and "visionary." Unlike earlier leadership approaches that focused on the exchange between leaders and followers, transformational leadership is described as "an approach whereby a person engages with others and creates a connection that raises the level of motivation and morality in both the leader and the follower" (Northouse, 2015, p. 186).

The most current model of transformational leadership is often described as the opposite pole on a continuum to laissez-faire leadership, with transactional leadership in the middle (Table 1.6).

Transactional leaders focus on rewards and punishments, and the relationship between managers and subordinates is viewed as an exchange. When subordinates perform well, they receive a reward. When they perform poorly, they will be punished. Rules, procedures, and standards are essential in transactional leadership. Followers are not encouraged to be creative or to find new solutions to problems. Transactional leaders differ from transformational leaders in that the transactional leader does not focus on the personal development or the needs of followers, but exchanges things of value such as bonuses and additional time off. The far right side of the transformational–transactional continuum is the laissez-faire leader. These leaders give neither feedback nor encouragement to help others progress, abdicate responsibility, delay decisions, and have no long-range plans.

Transformational leaders embody the following behaviors (Northouse, 2015):

Idealized influence. This first leadership behavior is often described as charisma. Idealized influencers are strong role models and have high standards of moral and ethical conduct. They are usually highly respected and emulated by their followers, are trustworthy, and provide a sense of vision and mission to the organization and the people who work with them.

Inspirational motivation. Behavior two describes transformational leaders who communicate high expectations of others, inspiring and motivating them to share in the vision of the organization.

Intellectual stimulation. The third behavior is demonstrated as the transformational leader stimulates followers to be creative, questioning, and innovative.

Individualized considerations. The fourth behavior represents the supportive climate in which transformational leaders meet the individual needs of the followers.

Transactional leaders embody the following list of behaviors (Northouse, 2015):

Contingent reward. This fifth behavior is the first of the two transactional leadership factors. This is the exchange process whereby the effort of the followers is exchanged for a reward.

Management by exception. This transactional leadership behavior involves corrective criticism, negative feedback, and negative reinforcement and can take both active and passive forms.

TABLE 1.6 **Leadership Factors**

	Transformational Leadership	Transactional Leadership	Laissez-Faire Leadership
Factors			
1	Idealized influence Charisma		
2	Inspirational motivation		
3	Intellectual stimulation		
4	Individualized consideration		
5		Contingent reward Constructive transactions	
6		Management by exception Active and passive Corrective transactions	
7			Noninterference Nontransactional

Adapted from: Northouse, P. (2015). *Leadership: Theory and practice* (7th ed.). Thousand Oaks, CA: Sage.

Finally, laissez-fair leadership represents a very limited form of leadership.

A 2014 online literature search using the keywords "transformational leadership" and "nursing" revealed 177 peer-reviewed articles published during the previous 5 years. The idea of matching transformational leadership to the demands of nursing management was identified as early as 2002 (Wexford, 2002). Research supports the relationship between transformational leaders and employee performance, motivation, commitment, perceptions of fairness, trust, creativity, and patient safety outcomes (Bacha & Walker, 2013; Belle, 2013; Braun, Peus, Weisweiler, & Frey, 2012; Casida & Parker, 2011; Malloy & Penprase, 2010; McFadden, Henagan, & Gowen, 2009; Neilsen

& Daniels, 2012; Salanova, Lorente, Chambel, & Martinez, 2011; Tomlinson, 2012; Tremblay, 2010; Tse & Chiu, 2014; Walumbwa & Hartnell, 2011; Wang & Rode, 2010; Yang, Wu, Chang, & Chien, 2011;).

Recent research on the relationship of lateral violence in the workplace and leadership revealed that transformational and transactional leadership behaviors were associated with empowered teams and a decreased likelihood of lateral violence in the workplace (Curtis & O'Connell, 2011; Ertureten, Cemalcilar, & Aycan, 2013).

Contributing to the perceived overwhelming success of this approach is that it provides a broad set of generalizations and a general way of thinking about leadership. It does not provide a "how to" approach, but requires leaders to become aware of their own behavior and how these behaviors impact the employees and the organization. Transformational leaders:

- Create a culture where followers feel empowered to be creative and innovative;
- Have a strong sense of identify and moral values demonstrating confidence, competence, and strong ideals;
- Listen to others and are tolerant of opposing views;
- Create a vision from the collective views of individuals within the organizations, giving followers a sense of identity and self-efficacy;
- Immerse themselves in the culture of the organization and help shape shared meanings; and
- Effectively work with others to build trust and foster collaboration (Caldwell, Dixon, Floyd, Chaudoin, Post, & Cheokas, 2011; Hansbrough, 2012; Kaslow, Falender, & Grus, 2012; Kovjanic, Schuh, & Jonas, 2013; Mitra, 2013; Whittington, Coker, Goodwin, Ickes, & Murray, 2009).

The most widely used instrument to measure transformational leadership is the Multifactor Leadership Questionnaire (MLQ) developed by Bass and Avolio (Bass, Avolio, & Jung, 1999). The MLQ also assesses the individual's transactional and laissez-faire leadership behaviors. Box 1.3 contains links to the MLQ and other leadership measurement tools.

In their 2012 model of transformational leadership, Kouzes and Posner recommended five practices that have since been incorporated into the American

---

BOX 1.3 **Leadership Measurement Tools**

The Multifactor Leadership Questionnaire: Information on the MLQ can be found at www.mindgarden.com/products/mlqr.htm.

Authentic Leadership Questionnaire: Information on the ALQ can be found at www.mindgarden.com/products/alq.htm.

Servant Leadership Assessment Tools: See Liden, R., Wayne, S., Zhao, H., & Henderson, D. (2008). Servant leadership: Development of a multidimensional measure and multi-level assessment. *The Leadership Quarterly, 19*(2), 161–177.

Nurses Credentialing Center (ANCC) Magnet Recognition Program (Clavelle & Drenkard, 2012):

> *Model the way.* Find your voice, clarify your personal values, set an example, and align your actions with the shared values of your team and organization.
>
> *Inspire a shared vision.* Envision the future and enlist others in shared aspirations and a common vision.
>
> *Challenge the process.* Take risks, experiment, search for new opportunities, seek to change, and grow and learn from mistakes.
>
> *Enable others to act.* Promote collaboration, strengthen others by sharing power, and build trust and cooperation.
>
> *Encourage the heart.* Recognize individual contributions, show appreciation for excellence, celebrate achievements, and promote a spirit of community (Kouzes & Posner, 2012).

Accordingly, ANCC Executive Director Karen Drenkard tells us:

> Highly effective leaders have highly effective teams and a strong group culture. The leader does not have to be in charge of everything, but he or she must communicate the shared vision, encourage intellectual stimulation, consider individuals, and motivate the team to be innovative and take measured risks to improve. They must "set the table" where shared dialogue and shared problem solving can occur. (p. 57)

Authentic Approach

A second relatively new approach to leadership is authentic leadership. With a little more than a decade of research, authentic leadership has emerged as a complex phenomenon defined from intrapersonal, interpersonal, and developmental perspectives. These include self-awareness, ethical values and standards, convictions, emotions, and motives. Critical life events, values, and positive psychological capacities such as confidence, hope, optimism, and resilience also influence a person's ability to develop as an authentic leader (Sosik & Cameron, 2010; Walumbwa, Wang, Wang, Schaubroeck, & Avolio, 2010; Wong & Laschinger, 2013). The four major underlying components of authentic leadership, summarized in the following list, include self-awareness; unbiased, balanced information processing; authentic behaviors and actions; and relational transparency (Bamford, Wong, & Laschinger, 2013).

> *Self-awareness.* As part of an ongoing process of introspection, the authentic leader understands his or her values, beliefs, strengths, and talents. Aware of areas of improvement and sense of purpose, the authentic leader stays true to self and does not conform to the expectations of others.
>
> *Unbiased, balanced information processing.* Authentic leaders demonstrate this self-regulatory behavior when they analyze information objectively and explore others' opinions before making a decision. They remain unbiased and open.
>
> *Authentic behaviors and actions.* As the authentic leader remains consistent and acts in agreement with his or her values and convictions, authentic behavior is demonstrated. The authentic leader has no need to please others to attain recognition or status, but at the same time does not seek to avoid repercussions from contenders.
>
> *Relational transparency.* The authentic leader is open and honest in presenting his or her true self to others (Bamford et al., 2013; Murphy, 2012; Northouse, 2015).

Thus, the concept in authentic leadership that differentiates it from other approaches is the importance of self-awareness and self-regulation. "Being an authentic leader means being true to your values and doing what you say you are going to do, even if the outcome is not what the other person or group wants" (Buell, 2008). How does a leader demonstrate authenticity? Sosik and Cameron (2010) present a framework (Table 1.7) for understanding the universal virtues and character strengths for assessing and developing behavior consistent with authentic leadership.

Research on authentic leadership and nursing has demonstrated a positive relationship between this leadership style and RN work engagement, organizational citizenship behaviors, virtuous and committed team behaviors, new graduate favorable perceptions of interprofessional collaboration, staff retention, improved patient outcomes, and follower integrity and performance, as well as reduced workplace bullying and burnout (Bamford, Wong, & Laschinger, 2012; Laschinger & Smith, 2013;

TABLE 1.7 Universal Virtues and Character Strengths for Authentic Leadership

Universal Virtues	Character Strengths
Wisdom and knowledge: important antecedents are job knowledge and cognitive ability	Creativity, curiosity, open-mindedness, love of learning, and ability to have a wide perspective
Courage: emotional strength and will to accomplish goals in the face of adversity, uncertainty, and risk	Bravery, persistence, integrity, and vitality
Humanity: ability to reflect compassion, altruism, and social influences	Love, kindness, and emotional intelligence
Justice: encompass civic strengths that support a healthy community	Citizenship and fairness
Temperance: ability to protect against excesses and set limits on personal desires	Forgiveness, mercy, prudence, humility, modesty, self-regulation, and control
Transcendence: forging connections to the larger universe to provide meaning for self and others	Appreciation of beauty and excellence, gratitude, hope, humor, and spirituality

Adapted from: Sosik, J., & Cameron, J. (2010). Character and authentic transformational leadership behavior: Expanding the ascetic self toward others. *Consulting Psychology Journal: Practice and Research, 62*(4), 251–269.

Laschinger, Wong, & Grau, 2012; Leroy, Palanski, & Simons, 2012; Rego, Vitoria, Magalhaes, Ribeiro, & Cunha, 2013; Walumbwa et al., 2010; Wong & Giallonardo, 2013). Based on the positive research between authentic leadership, organizational culture, and healthy work environments (McSherry, Pearce, Grimwood, & McSherry, 2012; Shirey, 2009), the American Association of Critical Care Nurses includes authentic leadership as one of the six standards necessary for establishing and sustaining a healthy work environment (Kerfoot, 2006).

Although this approach is still in development, authentic leadership provides broad guidelines for becoming a trustworthy leader. Authentic leadership can be measured using a validated, theory-based instrument developed by Walumbwa and colleagues (2008). The Authentic Leadership Questionnaire (ALQ) measures the four components of self-awareness, relational transparency, ethical/moral behavior, and balanced processing (see Box 1.3).

Servant Approach

Servant leadership was originally introduced in the 1970s with the writings of Robert Greenleaf (1970). Until about 10 years ago, this leadership approach inspired little interest or empirical research. Similar to the skills and styles approaches described earlier in this chapter, servant leadership is an approach focusing on the leader and his or her behaviors. Servant leaders serve the followers first. They demonstrate strong moral behavior and emphasize follower development. The servant leader has a special responsibility to care for those less privileged by addressing social injustices and inequalities in the workplace. The 10 characteristics of a servant leader identified by Greenleaf make up the initial conceptualization of this approach:

1. Having the ability to listen
2. Being empathetic
3. Having the ability to heal
4. Being aware
5. Being persuasive
6. Having vision
7. Having foresight
8. Demonstrating stewardship
9. Being committed to the growth of individuals
10. Building community

As research has developed in this area, servant leadership is treated as a trait phenomenon by some and a behavioral process by others. In 2013 research on this approach, Liden, Panaccio, Meuser, Hu, and Wayne identified three main components: antecedent conditions, servant leader behavior, and leadership outcomes. Liden's team felt that three antecedent conditions affected the manner in which servant leadership occurred. The first of these was the organizational context and a particular culture. The second antecedent condition was the attributes of the leader, and the third was the receptivity of the followers. The servant leader characteristics validated by Liden et al. are provided in Table 1.8. Outcomes of these behaviors were identified to be follower performance and growth, organizational performance, and societal impact (Liden et al., 2013).

Servant leadership provides a philosophy and set of behaviors for teaching leadership skills and is used in employee training and development (e.g., at Starbucks,

TABLE 1.8 Key Characteristics of Servant Leadership

Authors	Characteristics
Laub (1999)	Developing people, sharing leadership, displaying authenticity, valuing people, providing leadership, building community
Dennis & Bocarnea (2005)	Empowerment, trust, humility, selfless love, vision
Barbuto & Wheeler (2006)	Altruistic calling, emotional healing, persuasive mapping, organizational stewardship, wisdom
Wong & Davey (2007)	Serving and developing others, consulting and involving others, humility and selflessness, modeling integrity and authenticity, inspiring and influencing others
Sendjaya, Sarros, & Santora (2008)	Transforming influence, voluntary subordination, authentic self, transcendental spirituality, responsible morality, covenantal relationship
Van Dierendonck & Nuijten (2011)	Empowerment, humility, standing back, authenticity, forgiveness, courage, accountability, stewardship
Linden, Panaccio, Hu, & Meuser (2013)	Conceptualizing, emotional healing, putting followers first, helping followers grow and succeed, behaving ethically, empowering, creating value for the community

Adapted from: Liden, R.C., Panaccio, A., Meuser, J. D., Hu, J., & Wayne, S. J. (2013). Servant leadership: Antecedents, processes, and outcomes. In *The Oxford handbook of leadership and organizations*. Oxford, England: Oxford University Press; Van Dierendonck, D. (2011). Servant leadership: A review and synthesis. *Journal of Management, 37*(4), 1228–1261.

AT&T, Southwest Airlines, Vanguard Group, Catholic Health). Research with health-care employees has demonstrated decreased turnover and increased collaboration, motivational autonomy, and well-being (Chen, Chen, & Li, 2013; Garber, Madigan, Click, & Fitzpatrick, 2009; Hunter et al., 2013; Mueller, 2011; Northouse, 2015; Waterman, 2011). Numerous questionnaires are available to measure servant leadership (see Box 1.3).

LEADERSHIP INFLUENCES

Having provided an overview of theoretical approaches to leadership, this chapter turns now to what influences leadership today, beginning with change and moving through complexity science, followership, and two of the more recent influences on leadership gaining popularity in research and in mainstream media—gender and culture.

Change

Any member of a health-care organization soon realizes that change is inevitable and ongoing. Planned change may include organizational goals and objectives. Unplanned change may be the result of sudden shifts in product or service demands, changes in the way services are delivered owing to technology or recent innovations, economic conditions, national disasters, or even a change in leadership (Table 1.9). Lippitt (1973, p. 3) states that "change is a very complex phenomenon involving the multiplicity of man's motivations in both micro and macro systems and that a man gets satisfied with his equilibrium and is resistant to changing his status quo." Leaders must be aware of the many challenges facing their organizations from the internal environment, industry, and society (Borkowski, 2011).

The most widely used model for change is Lewin's 1947 Theory of Planned Change (TPC). Viewing change as a series of forces working in different directions, the strength of the *driving* forces for change must be increased and the opposing *restraining* forces reduced or removed. Exploration of these factors is referred to as the force field analysis (FFA).

TABLE 1.9 **Leadership Challenges to Change**

Environment	Type of Change	Examples
Internal	Structure, process, procedures, resources	Institute of Medicine safety initiatives, The Joint Commission, Magnet designation
Industry	Shareholders, special interest groups, employees, customers, communities of interest, competitors	Managed care organizations, unions, Affordable Care Act, Health Insurance Portability and Accountability Act
Societal	Sociocultural, economic, political-legal, technology	Inflation, recession, Internet, stem cell research

Adapted from: Borkowski, N. (2011). *Organizational behavior in health care*. Sudbury, MA: Jones & Bartlett; Wheelen T. L., & Hunger, J. D. (1997). *Strategic management and business policy* (6th ed.). Upper Saddle River, NJ: Addison-Wesley.

The TPC describes the three phases of a change as unfreezing, moving, and refreezing. During unfreezing, identification of the FFA occurs. At this time, driving forces should be strengthened and restraining forces removed or weakened. During the second phase, the process of moving into action occurs. Coaching and clear communication are extremely important during this transition process, as participants often experience uncertainty and fear. During the final or third phase, refreezing, the change becomes embedded into the culture of the organization (Shirey, 2013). Table 1.10 provides an example of driving and restraining forces regarding acceptance of clinical practice guidelines (Borkowski, 2011).

To guide the leader to help the organization move toward a successful change, Kotter (1996) describes eight steps. Steps 1 through 4 take place during unfreezing:

1. Establish a sense of urgency. Discuss opportunities (e.g., increased revenue, decreased turnover, staff satisfaction) and examine the possible negative outcomes that could result without the proposed change (e.g., decreased revenue, poor patient satisfaction).
2. Create a powerful guiding coalition. Create a strong "cheerleading" group that includes members from all levels of the organization.
3. Develop a vision. Work with the coalition to create a vision and develop strategies for achieving it.
4. Communicate the vision. Use a variety of vehicles to communicate the vision including having the coalition teach new behaviors by example.

The moving phase comprises steps 5 through 7:

5. Empower others to act. Eliminate barriers to change and encourage creativity, innovation, and risk taking.

TABLE 1.10 Application of Lewin's Change Theory: Clinical Practice Guidelines

Driving Forces	Restraining Forces
Quality care delivery	Administrative cost control
Evidence-based practices	Legislative mandates
Effective use of resources	Financial penalties or incentives
Educational tool	Licensing/accreditation requirements
Excellent resource	Utilization review

Adapted from: Borkowski, N. (2011). *Organizational behavior in health care.* Sudbury, MA: Jones & Bartlett.

6. Plan for and create short-term wins. Recognize and reward visible improvements.
7. Consolidate improvements and produce more change. Use the success of the short-term wins to create more opportunities for change. Hire, promote, and develop employees who can articulate the vision and serve as change agents.

The final step occurs during refreezing:

8. Institutionalize new approaches. Reinforce change by pinpointing the connections between the change and organizational success.

Lewin's theory, although used extensively in planning change, has been criticized as being too simplistic and too linear for today's complex environment. Jacobs, van Witteloostuijn, and Christe-Zeyse (2013) warn us that most change initiatives increase costs while falling short on their goals. They contend that organizational change is more multifaceted than initial researchers such as Lewin described. However, the FFA approach to change forms a foundation for our understanding and approach to initiating the change process.

Complexity Science

The complexity of today's health-care organizations demands examining the best approach to serving as a leader and a change agent. Complexity science emerged in the early part of the 20th century. Through the work of Capra, a well-known physicist, other scientists in the field of computer science and meteorology began exploring this concept of nonlinear relationships as complex adaptive systems. A complex adaptive system is defined as

> a collection of individual agents with freedom to act in ways that are not always totally predictable, and whose actions are interconnected so that one agent's actions changes the context for other agents. Examples include the immune system, a colony of termites, the financial market, and just about any collection of humans, for example . . . a primary healthcare team. (Plsek & Greenhalgh, 2001, p. 625)

The following are major tenets of complexity theory (Holden, 2005; Sanger & Giddings, 2012; Wenberg, 2012; Wilson, 2009):

1. Complex systems consist of numerous subsystems interacting with each other through multiple, nonlinear, recurrent, feedback loops.
2. Complexity resides in the eye of the beholder—that is, individuals assess the complexity of a situation from their own views and experiences.
3. Health-care workers deal with some of the most complex systems imaginable.
4. Small changes in a complex system may have profound effects on the system over time—it is not possible to predict the effect.
5. Assessment of the complexity should be commensurate with the complexity of the system.
6. Complexity science offers an opportunity for nonlinear thinking, which can often lead to innovation.
7. Similar conditions can produce dissimilar results.

8. Just because an approach worked once does not guarantee that it will work again.
9. Complex systems are embedded in their own culture and history, which are often difficult to comprehend.

If the traditional framework of linear thinking, which consists of breaking a system into smaller pieces and studying them individually, is not working, what happens when no part of the system is constant, independent, or predictable? This is precisely what complexity science offers—a framework for viewing connections, organizational culture, diversity, and interactions. This framework allows us to answer the question, how do health-care organizations deliver high-quality health care and ensure optimal patient outcomes in this ever-changing health-care environment? Although adopting innovative strategies that increase the quality of interactions and solicit a variety of opinions would seem logical, many leaders revert to more traditional approaches during difficult times (Smith, 2011).

Nursing practice may use a complexity science framework in developing practice models. Nurse educators may use this framework to develop more effective instructional strategies that promote critical thinking and better decision making. Leaders must adjust their worldview to meet the emerging challenges of today and in the future. How does this process begin?

Several core realities are the basis of complexity leadership in health-care systems, recognizing that within a complex system the leader is only one agent among potentially many diverse, independent agents. The leader is not an external observer but part of the experience. Patterns emerge as the relationships intertwine, and, at the same time, new patterns emerge. As you focus on creating environments that foster relationships, which, in turn, create processes to transform organizations, review these seven core realities (Crowell, 2011).

1. *Who you are is how you lead.* To be an effective leader today, one needs a working knowledge of complexity science, a leadership style with a foundation in transformation leadership concepts, and an ability to perform self-reflection regularly. Ask yourself the following:
   • Can I mediate emotional issues without bias?
   • Can I remain relaxed during times of fear or desire to act?
   • Have I clarified my own inner conflicts?
   • Am I open and receptive regardless of the issue?
2. *You are not in control.* You are not in control of others, only of yourself. Recognize that there is no cause-and-effect pattern (I do this and you will do that), but only a pattern that is produced as each independent or system agent contributes to the process. Ask yourself the following:
   • Where can simple rules work more effectively than detailed instructions?
   • Who are the attractors in my organization that can motivate and empower others?
   • Can I let go and let others let go?
   • Can I detach and not overreact but just take action on an issue?
3. *There are no observers.* A key component of complexity science is the idea that we are all connected into one self-organizing system. We are part of an energy field that can be positive or negative. As leaders, we co-create the field

and influence the energy present. We must detach and stay centered in the field, not becoming influenced by the negative parts of the field. Ask yourself the following:
- How can I remain centered in this emotional field?
- What part have I played in this difficult situation?

4. *All organizations are complex adaptive systems.* During times of uncertainty and complexity, our first leadership impulse is often to be the fixer. Instead, we must encourage creativity, local interactions, and independence, allowing for a new or novel solution to emerge. Ask yourself the following:
- Do I seek diversity when assembling a workgroup? After assembling a diverse or multidisciplinary group can I trust their decisions?
- Can I demonstrate patience when a situation is disorganized and uncertain?
- Do I become directive during disagreements or uncertainty?

5. *Chaos and change are the order of the day.* In his 1998 book, *Who Moved My Cheese?*, Johnson states that stability is a myth. Trying to hold on to stability may even create disaster or cause opportunities to be missed. Taking small actions may have huge, systemwide consequences; conversely, making huge decisions may provide very few lasting results. Ask yourself the following:
- Am I holding on to a static, detailed strategic plan?
- Can I refrain from imposing a top-down change to fix a problem?
- Am I uncomfortable with disruption, conflict, and disorder?
- How can I gain the biggest result with the smallest expenditure?

6. *People in relationship with others will change the structure.* Wheatley (2006) describes organizations as self-organizing systems and asserts that the desired state is not equilibrium but being on the edge of chaos. Order is found in information that is abundant and open. "Self-organization is the ability of all living systems to organize themselves into patterns and structures without externally imposed plan or direction" (Wheatley, p. 13). Ask yourself the following:
- How can I create a relationship-rich, open atmosphere?

7. *Becoming a complexity leader is a journey.* As with any new journey, the first step is self-awareness and self-reflection. The following are some other actions to start your journey (Crowell, 2011, p. 210):
- Creating opportunities for people to form rich relationships.
- Deemphasizing hierarchy with a free flow of information and communication.
- Accepting that we live and work in a complex adaptive system and people do self-organize.
- Celebrating people's self-organizing creativity.
- Being willing to change and grow along with those you lead.

Complexity science shifts the worldview from a more traditional approach to an emergent worldview as outlined in Table 1.11.

Followership

Traditional leadership theories tend to focus on leaders as drivers of organizational performance, whereas followers are viewed as passive recipients. However, even in

TABLE 1.11 Traditional and Emerging Worldviews

Traditional Worldview	Emerging Worldview
Reductionism	Holism
Focus on parts	Focus on patterns
Focus on discrete entities	Focus on relationships
Linear causality	Mutual causality
Predictability	Unpredictability
Objective reality	Perspective reality
Observer outside the situation	Observer influences the situation
Systems adapt to stimuli	Systems self-organize
Logic	Paradox
Either/or thinking	Polarity thinking
Predictable	Understanding/analysis
Homogeneity	Diversity
Focus on outcomes	Focus on innovation

Adapted from: Dent, E. B. (2000). Complexity science: A worldview shift. *Emergence, 11*(4), 73–87.

the early years of leadership theory development (Fiedler, 1967; Vroom & Yetton, 1973) some researchers introduced the idea that followers were an integral part of leadership. Newer leadership theories influenced by complexity science recognize that leaders need to work collaboratively with followers (Grossman & Valiga, 2009). Although the notion of followership "appears" negative, demeaning, and unattractive in many textbooks, in reality, the follower role is a powerful one, because part of the responsibility for making the leader-follower relationship work obviously falls to the follower (Grossman & Valiga, 2009).

What does it mean to become a "good follower"? Following blindly, abdicating all responsibility for progress, or waiting passively for answers provided is not good followership. Followers need to be self-directing, active participants and trustworthy team members. Leaders, in return, need to support followers by seeking their input, encouraging them, and using their talents. A good follower must also know when and how to assume the role of a leader. No matter how high a leader climbs on the leadership ladder, a time will inevitably come when that leader must assume the role of the follower (Grossman & Valiga, 2009). Table 1.12 includes the relationship between the activities and qualities of exemplary leaders and followers.

While developing leadership, the leader must also be mindful of enhancing his or her ability to be an exemplary follower (Box 1.4).

Leaders are sometimes mistakenly treated as heroes or villains depending on how well their department or organization performs. Some leaders take credit for all successes and blame others for any failures. Effective leaders, by contrast, understand the importance of all members of the team to the success of the organization, supporting their own growth and that of others as both leaders and followers (Oc & Bashshur, 2013).

Gender

The popular press continues to take an interest in the topic of gender and leadership. Although women's ability to lead was once viewed as inferior to that of men, the question is no longer "Can women lead?" It has become "Are there differences in leadership style and efficacy between men and women?"

Northouse (2015) cautions that the differences between male and female leadership styles are influenced by what he calls the "leadership labyrinth," which describes the divergence of human capital, commitment, and bias that men and women experience (p. 355).

Human capital. Human capital refers to any stock of knowledge or characteristics the worker has (either innate or acquired) that contribute to his or her economic value or productivity. This includes knowledge, habits, and social and personality attributes. Although women obtain degrees at all levels at a rate greater than do men, they are still underrepresented in leadership positions. They have less work experience and employment continuity than do men, with more responsibility for child rearing and domestic duties. They appear to respond more to work–home conflicts by taking leave or assuming flexible positions in the workplace. Women also appear to have fewer work development opportunities such as encouragement, mentoring, and formal training than do men.

Commitment. Current research on leader emergence reveals that women are more likely to identify themselves as facilitators or organizers than as leaders. This

TABLE 1.12 **Activities of Exemplary Leaders and Followers**

Leaders	Followers
Study and create new ideas	Test new ideas
Make decisions	Challenge decisions as needed
Assign appropriate responsibilities	Know when to accept responsibility and do so
Create environments of trust, resulting in freedom	Use freedom responsibly
Take risks	Risk following
Are reliable	Are trustworthy and respectful
Are loyal to the followers	Are loyal to the leader
Are self-confident	Know themselves
Assume the leadership position	Follow when appropriate

Source: Grossman, S., & Valiga, S. (2009). *The new leadership challenge* (3rd ed.). Philadelphia, PA: F. A. Davis.

perceived lack of commitment to employment and motivation to lead has been cited as a barrier for women. However, research has shown that women demonstrate the same level of commitment and motivation as do men. Finally, the claim that men have more of the "traits" necessary for effective leadership than do women has not been supported by research.

Bias. The stereotype that leaders should be "masculine and tough" persists in some contexts, as does the idea that women should not be "manly." This double bias negatively affects perceptions and evaluations of females as leaders.

These barriers may also affect ethnic, racial, and sexual minorities. Creating equal opportunities for leadership can happen only by supporting a diverse pool of candidates in hiring and by promoting women and members of minority populations into

BOX 1.4 **Followership Characteristics**

- Being strong and independent
- Engaging in critical thinking
- Being willing to think for yourself
- Giving honest feedback and constructive criticism
- Being your own person
- Innovating and being creative
- Actively engaging in your organization
- Being cooperative and collaborative
- Being a self-starter
- Going above and beyond the call of duty
- Assuming ownership of your actions
- Taking initiative
- Having a positive sense of self-worth
- Being attentive to your surroundings
- Being energized by your work and your organization

Source: Grossman, S., & Valiga, T. (2009). *The new leadership challenge* (3rd ed., p. 45). Philadelphia, PA: F. A. Davis.

leadership positions. Although these gaps remain visible, evidence shows that they are starting to close. However, until the "leadership labyrinth" is addressed, identifying whether true differences in leadership styles exist between genders and minorities is impossible (Wang, Chiang, Tsai, Lin, & Cheng, 2013; Kark, Manor, & Shamir, 2012). Approaches to dealing with these barriers are discussed more fully in Chapter 2.

Culture

Chapter 2 explores diversity as a component within organizations. Here, the focus is on the relationship between leadership and culture. The increasing economic, social, technical, and political interdependence between nations presents both opportunities and challenges. This globalization creates the need for leaders to become culturally aware and skilled in creating transcultural vision and competencies. Effective leaders must examine themselves for *ethnocentrism* and *prejudice*. Ethnocentrism is the tendency for individuals to value their own ethnic, racial, or cultural group over those of others. Ethnocentrism is closely related to prejudice, the unsubstantiated, fixed attitude or belief about another individual or group. Leaders must address their own feelings of prejudice as well as the prejudices of followers.

As shown in Table 1.13, the 2004 research study from the GLOBE project, encompassing 17,000 participants from 62 countries, identified nine cultural dimensions addressing the relationship between culture and leadership (House et al., 2004). Table 1.14 lists the global leadership behaviors that emerged from this project (Grove, 2005).

TABLE 1.13 Cultural Dimensions of Leadership

Cultural Dimension	Definition
Uncertainty Avoidance	Degree to which the group relies on social norms, rituals, and procedures to avoid uncertainty
Power Distance	Degree to which the group expects and agrees that power should be shared unequally based on authority, prestige status, wealth, and material possessions
Institutional Collectivism	Degree to which the group encourages institutional or societal collective action rather than individual goals and accomplishments
In-Group Collectivism	Degree to which the group expresses pride, loyalty, and cohesiveness within the organization or family
Gender Egalitarianism	Degree to which the organization minimizes gender differences and promotes gender equality
Assertiveness	Degree to which the culture encourages people to be forceful, aggressive, and tough in social relationships
Future Orientation	Degree to which people engage in planning, investing in the future, and delaying gratification
Performance Orientation	Degree to which the group rewards group members for improved performance and excellence
Humane Orientation	Degree to which the group encourages and rewards members for being fair, altruistic, generous, caring, and kind

Adapted from: Northouse, P. (2014). *Leadership: Theory and practice* (6th ed.). Thousand Oaks, CA: Sage.

TABLE 1.14 **Global Leadership Behaviors**

Leadership Behavior	Description
Charismatic/ value based	Reflects the ability to inspire, to motivate, and to expect high performance from others based on strongly held core values
Team oriented	Emphasizes team building and a common purpose among team members
Participative	Reflects the degree to which leaders involve others in making and implementing decisions
Humane	Emphasizes being supportive, considerate, compassionate, and generous
Autonomous	Refers to independent and individualistic leadership, which includes being self-contained and unique
Self-protective	Reflects behaviors that ensure the safety and security of the leader and the group

Source: Grove, C. (2005). *Worldwide differences in business values and practices: Overview of GLOBE research findings.* Retrieved from http://www.grovewell.com/pub-GLOBE-dimensions.html

CONCLUSION

Leadership is a process that helps systems to function. It is not merely a position or a title. In 2010, Liz Wiseman, president of the Wiseman Group in Silicon Valley, was keynote speaker at the annual meeting of the American Organization of Nurse Executives. Her research with more than 150 leaders asked the question, "What are the vital few differences between intelligence diminishers and intelligence multipliers, and what impact do they have on organizations?"

Intelligence multipliers are genius makers. Everyone around them becomes smarter and more capable. They elicit each person's unique contribution and create an atmosphere of innovation, productive effort, and collective intelligence. *Intelligence diminishers* believe that really intelligent people are a rare breed. They think they are among a small set of very smart people and that other people could never figure anything out without them (Wiseman & McKeown, 2010).

The challenge today's leader faces is to become an intelligence multiplier. Leaders must also challenge themselves to continue expanding their leadership knowledge and skills. The evidenced-based approaches in this chapter provide a guidebook for the leadership journey.

One approach and influence might resonate perfectly with you. Perhaps a combination of approaches and influences seems more appealing. Regardless of what works for you, the importance of the leader's behavior, the needs of the followers, culture of the organization, and an understanding of complexity must be considered. Embarking on the leadership journey must start with self-reflection and asking the questions listed in Box 1.5 (Kouzes & Posner, 2012; Nicholson, 2013).

Although success is not guaranteed, those leaders who have proved successful counsel us to remain humble and human. Find something every day to make a difference. We may want to be part of organization-changing initiatives and grand visions, but true leadership is in the moment. Take those moments to make a difference. Remember that true leadership is not an affair of the head but of the heart—leaders love what they do and the progress they facilitate (Kouzes & Posner, 2012; Perkins, 2013).

BOX 1.5 Questions to Ask Yourself for Exemplary Leadership

Who am I and why am I here?

Who are we and what do we stand for?

Where are we going and why?

What are the values that should guide my decisions and actions?

What are my beliefs about how people ought to conduct the affairs of our organization?

What are my leadership strengths and weaknesses?

How consistent is my view of my leadership with how others see me?

What do I need to do to improve my abilities to move the organization forward?

Where do I think the organization should be headed during the next 10 years?

How clear are others about our shared vision of the future?

How much do I understand about what is going on in the organization and the world in which it operates?

What are the challenges we face? How prepared are we to deal with them?

How prepared am I to handle the complex problems that now confront my organization?

What gives me the courage to continue in the face of uncertainty and adversity?

How will I handle disappointments, mistakes, and setbacks?

What keeps me from giving up?

Continued

BOX 1.5 Questions to Ask Yourself for Exemplary Leadership–cont'd

How solid are my relationships with my constituents?

How much do my constituents trust me and trust one another?

How can I keep myself motivated and encouraged?

How am I doing at sharing the credit and saying thank you?

What can I do to keep hope alive–in myself and others?

Am I the right one to be leading at this very moment? Why?

_____

Source: Grossman, S., & Valiga, S. (2009). *The new leadership challenge* (3rd ed.). Philadelphia, PA: F.A. Davis.

References

Antonakis, J. (2012). Transformational and charismatic leadership. In D. V. Day & J. Antonakis (Eds.), *The nature of leadership* (2nd ed., pp. 256–288). Thousand Oaks, CA: Sage.

Aronson, J., Walker, M., Arries, E., Maposa, S., Telford, P., & Berry, L. (2014). Qualities of exemplary nurse leaders: perspectives of frontline nurses. *Journal of Nursing Management, 22,* 127–136.

Avolio, B. (2011). *Full range leadership development* (2nd ed.). Thousand Oaks, CA: Sage.

Avolio, B. J., Walumbwa, F. O., & Weber, T. J. (2009). Leadership: Current theories, research and future directions. *Annual Review of Psychology, 60,* 421–449.

Bacha, E., & Walker, S. (2013). The relationship between transformational leadership and followers' perceptions of fairness. *Journal of Business Ethics, 116,* 667–680.

Bamford, M., Wong, C., & Laschinger, H. (2013). The influence of authentic leadership and areas of work life on work engagement of registered nurses. *Journal of Nursing Management, 21,* 529–540.

Bass, B. (1990). *Bass and Stogdill's handbook of leadership: Theory, research and management applications* (3rd ed.). New York, NY: Free Press.

Bass, J., Avolio, B., & Jung, D. (1999). Re-examining the components of transformational and transactional leadership using the Multifactor Leadership Questionnaire. *Journal of Occupational and Organizational Psychology, 72:* 441–462.

Belle, N. (2013). Leading to make a difference: A field experiment on the performance effects of transformational leadership, perceived social impact, and public service motivation. *Journal of Public Administration Research and Theory, 24,* 109–136.

Bing, J. W. (2004). Hofstede's consequences: The impact of his work on consulting and business practices. *Academy of Management Executive, 18*(1), 80–87.

Blake, R. R., & Mouton, J. S. (1985). *The managerial grid III.* Houston, TX: Gulf.

Borkowski, N. (2011). *Organizational behavior in health care.* Sudbury, MA: Jones & Bartlett.

Braun, S., Peus, C., Weisweiler, S., & Frey, D. (2012). Transformational leadership, job satisfaction and team performance: A multilevel mediation model of trust. *The Leadership Quarterly, 24,* 270–283.

Buell, J. M. (2008, November–December). Living the organization's mission, vision, and values. *Healthcare Executive,* 21–24.

Bulmer, J. (2013). Leadership aspirations of registered nurses: Who wants to follow us? *Journal of Nursing Administration, 45*(3), 130–134.

Casida, J., & Parker, J. (2011). Staff nurse perceptions of nurse manager leadership styles and outcomes. *Journal of Nursing Management, 19*, 478–486.

Caldwell, C., Dixon, R., Floyd, L., Chaudoin, J., Post, J., & Cheokas, G. (2011). Transformative leadership: Achieving unparalleled excellence. *Business Ethics*, 109: 175–187.

Chen, C., Chen, C., & Li, C. (2013). The influence of leader's spiritual values of servant leadership on employee motivational autonomy and eudaemonic well-being. *Journal of Religious Health, 53*, 418–438.

Clavelle, J., & Drenkard, K. (2012). Transformational leadership practices of chief nursing officers in Magnet organizations. *Journal of Nursing Administration, 42*(4), 195–201.

Cowden, T., Cummings, G., & McGrath, J. (2011). Leadership practices and staff nurses' intent to stay: A systematic review. *Journal of Nursing Management, 19*, 461–477.

Crowell, D. M. (2011). Leadership in complex nursing and health systems. In A. W. Davidson, M. A. Ray, & M. C. Turkel, (Eds.), *Nursing, caring, and complexity science.* New York, NY: Springer.

Curtis, E., & O'Connell, R. (2011). Essential leadership skills for motivating and developing staff. *Nursing Management, 18*(5), 32–34.

Davidson, A. W., Ray, M. A., & Turkel, M. C. (2011). *Nursing, caring, and complexity science.* New York, NY: Springer.

Dent, E. B. (2000). Complexity science: A worldview shift. *Emergence, 11*(4), 73–87.

Deutschendorf, H. (2014, June 16). 5 crucial emotional intelligence traits of highly effective leaders. *Fast Company.* Retrieved from http://www.fastcompany.com/3031708/the-future-of-work/5-crucial-emotional-intelligence-traits-of-highly-effective-leaders

Dorfman, P. W., Hanges, P. J., & Brodbeck, F. C. (2004). Leadership and cultural variation: The identification of culturally endorsed leadership profiles. In R. House, P. Hanges, M. Javidan, P. Dorfman, V. Guta, & Associates (Eds.), *Culture, leadership and organizations: The GLOBE study of 62 societies* (pp. 669–722). Thousand Oaks, CA: Sage.

Drenkard, K. (2013). Transformational leadership. *Journal of Nursing Administration, 43*(2), 57–58.

Ellis, P., & Abbott, J. (2013). The emotionally resilient renal manager: Understanding the language of emotion. *Journal of Renal Nursing, 5*(5), 256–257.

Erfureten, A., Cemalcilar, Z., & Aycan, Z. (2013). The relationship of downward mugging with leadership style and organizational attitudes. *Journal of Business Ethics, 116*, 205–216.

Failla, K. R., & Stichler, J. F. (2008). Manager and staff perceptions of the manager's leadership style. *Journal of Nursing Administration, 38*(11), 480–487.

Fayol, H. (1916). *General and industrial management.* London, England: Pitman.

Fiedler, F. E. (1967). *A theory of leadership effectiveness.* New York, NY: McGraw Hill.

French, J. R., & Raven, B. (1959). The bases of social power. In D. Cartwright (Ed.), *Studies in social power* (pp. 259–269). Ann Arbor, MI: Institute for Social Research.

Garber, J. S., Madigan, E. A., Click, E. R., & Fitzpatrick, J. J. (2009). Attitudes towards collaboration and servant leadership among nurses, physicians, and residents. *Journal of Interprofessional Care, 23*(4), 331–340.

Graeff, C. L. (1997). Evolution of situational leadership theory: A critical review. *Leadership Quarterly, 8*(2), 153–170.

Greenleaf, R. K. (1970). *The servant as leader.* Westfield, IN: The Greenleaf Center for Servant Leadership.

Grossman, S., & Valiga, T. (2009). *The new leadership challenge* (3rd ed.). Philadelphia, PA: F. A. Davis.

Grove, C. (2005). *Worldwide differences in business values and practices: Overview of GLOBE research findings.* Retrieved from http://www.grovewell.com/pub-GLOBE-dimensions.html

Hansbrough, T. K. (2012). The construction of a transformational leader: Follower attachment and leadership perceptions. *Journal of Applied Social Psychology, 42*(6), 1533–1549.

Holden, L. M. (2005). Complex adaptive systems: Concept analysis. *Journal of Advanced Nursing, 52*(6), 651–657.

House, R., Hanges, P., Javidan, M., Dorfman, P., Guta, V., & Associates. (Eds.). (2004). *Culture, leadership and organizations: The GLOBE study of 62 societies* (pp. 669–722). Thousand Oaks, CA: Sage.

Hunter, E., Neubert, M., Perry, S., Witt, L., Penney, L., & Weinberger, E. (2013). Servant leaders inspire servant followers: Antecedents and outcomes for employees and the organization. *The Leadership Quarterly, 24*, 316–331.

Jacobs, G., van Witteloostuijn, A., & Christe-Zeyse, J. (2013). A theoretical framework of organizational change. *Journal of Organizational Change Management, 26*(5), 772–792.

Johnson, S. (1998). *Who moved my cheese?* New York, NY: Putnam.

Judge, T. A., Bono, J. E., Illies, R., & Gerhardt, M. W. (2002). Personality and leadership: A qualitative and quantitative review. *Journal of Applied Psychology, 87*, 765–780.

Kark, R., Manor, R., & Shamir, B. (2012). Does valuing androgyny and femininity lead to a female advantage? The relationship between gender-role, transformational leadership and identification. *The Leadership Quarterly, 23*, 620–640.

Kaslow, N., Falender, C., & Grus, C. (2012). Valuing and practicing competency-based supervision: A transformational leadership perspective. *Training and Education in Professional Psychology, 6*(1), 47–54.

Katz, R. L. (195). Skills of an effective administrator. *Harvard Business Review, 33*(1), 33–42.

Kerfoot, K. (2006). Authentic leadership. *Nursing Economics, 24*(2), 116–117.

Kotter, J. P. (1990). *A force for change: How leadership differs from management.* New York, NY: Free Press.

Kotter, J. P. (1996). *Leading Change.* Boston, MA: Harvard Business School Press.

Kouzes, J., & Posner, B. (2012). *The leadership challenge* (5th ed.). San Francisco, CA: Jossey-Bass.

Kovjanic, S., Schuh, S., & Jonas, K. (2013). Transformational leadership and performance: An experimental investigation of the mediating effects of basic needs satisfaction and work engagement. *Journal of Occupational and Organizational Psychology 86*, 543–555

Laschinger, H., & Smith, L. (2013). The influence of authentic leadership and empowerment on new-graduate nurses' perceptions of interprofessional collaboration. *Journal of Nursing Administration, 43*(1), 24–29.

Laschinger, H., Wong, C., & Grau, A. (2012). The influence of authentic leadership on newly graduated nurses' experiences of workplace bullying, burnout, and retention outcomes: A cross-sectional study. *International Journal of Nursing Studies, 49*, 1266–1276.

Leroy, H., Palanski, M., & Simons, T. (2012). Authentic leadership and behavioral integrity as drivers of follower commitment and performance. *Journal of Business Ethics, 107*, 255–264.

Lewin, K. (1947). Frontiers in group dynamics. *Human Relations, 1*(1), 5–41.

Liden, R. C., Panaccio, A., Meuser, J. D., Hu, J., & Wayne, S. J. (2013). Servant leadership: Antecedents, processes, and outcomes. In *The Oxford handbook of leadership and organizations.* Oxford, England: Oxford University Press.

Liden, R. C., Wayne, S., Zhao, H., & Henderson, D. (2008). Servant leadership: Development of a multidimensional measure and multi-level assessment. *The Leadership Quarterly, 19*, 161–177.

Lippitt, G. L. (1973). *Visualizing change: Model building and the change process.* La Jolla, CA: University Associates.

Malloy, T., & Penprase, B. (2010). Nursing leadership style and psychosocial work environment. *Journal of Nursing Management, 18*, 715–725.

Markham, S. E. (2012). The evolution of organizations and leadership from the ancient world to modernity: A multilevel approach to organizational science and leadership (OSL). *The Leadership Quarterly, 23*, 1134–1151.

McFadden, K., Henagan, S., & Gowen, C. (2009). The patient safety chain: Transformational leadership's effect on patient safety culture, initiatives, and outcomes. *Journal of Operations Management, 27*, 390–404.

McMullen, C., Schneider, J., Firemark, A., Davis, J., & Spofford, M. (2013). Cultivating engaged leadership through learning collaborative: Lessons from primary care renewal in Oregon safety net clinics. *Annals of Family Medicine, 11*(Suppl. 1), 534–541.

McSherry, R., Pearce, P., Grimwood, K., & McSherry, W. (2012). The pivotal role of nurse managers, leaders, and educators in enabling excellence in nursing care. *Journal of Nursing Management, 20*, 7–19.

Mitra, R. (2013). From transformational leadership to leadership transformations: A critical dialogic perspective. *Communication Theory, 23*: 395–416.

Mueller, C. (2011, September–October). Servant leadership: The way forward? *Health Progress,* 21–24.

Mumford, M. D., Zaccaro, S. J., Connelly, M. S., & Marks, M. A. (2000). Leadership skills: Conclusions and future directions. *Leadership Quarterly, 11*(1), 155–170.

Murphy, L. (2012). Authentic leadership: Becoming and remaining an authentic nurse leader. *Journal of Nursing Administration, 42*(11), 507–512.

Neilsen, K., & Daniels, K. (2012). Does shared and differentiated transformational leadership predict followers' working conditions and well-being? *The Leadership Quarterly, 23*, 383–397.

Nicholson, N. (2013). *The "I" of leadership: Strategies for seeing, being, and doing.* San Francisco, CA: John Wiley & Sons.

Northouse, P. (2015). *Leadership: Theory and practice* (7th ed.). Thousand Oaks, CA: Sage.

Oc, B., & Bashshur, M. (2013). Followership, leadership, and social influence. *The Leadership Quarterly, 24*, 919–934.

O'Neill, J. A. (2013). Advancing the nursing profession begins with leadership. *Journal of Nursing Administration, 43*(4), 179–181.

Perkins, K. (2013). Investation: An original leadership concept. *Nursing Management, 4*, 35–38.

Plsek, P., & Greenhalgh, T. (2001). The challenge of complexity in health care. *British Medical Journal, 323*, 625–628.

Rankin, B. (2013). Emotional intelligence: Enhancing values-based practice and compassionate care in nursing. *Journal of Advanced Nursing, 69*(12), 2717–2725.

Rego, A., Vitoria, A., Magalhaes, A., Ribeiro, N., & Cunha, M. (2013). Are authentic leaders associated with more virtuous, committed and potent teams? *The Leadership Quarterly, 24*, 61–79.

Salanova, M., Lorente, L., Chambel, M., & Martinez, I. (2011). Linking transformational leadership to nurses' extra-role performance: the mediating role of self-efficacy and work engagement. *Journal of Advanced Nursing, 67*(10), 2256–2266.

Sanger, M., & Giddings, M. (2012). Teaching Note: A simple approach to complexity theory. *Journal of Social Work Education, 48*(2), 269–367.

Shankman, M. L., & Allen, S. J. (2008). *Emotionally intelligent leadership: A guide for college students.* San Francisco, CA: Jossey-Bass.

Shirey, M. (2009). Authentic leadership, organizational culture, and healthy work environments. *Critical Care Nursing Quarterly, 52*(3), 189–198.

Shirey, M. (2013). Lewin's theory of planned change as a strategic resource. *Journal of Nursing Administration, 43*(2), 69–72.Smith, M. (2011). Philosophical and theoretical perspectives related to complexity science in nursing. In A. W. Davidson, M. A. Ray, & M. C. Turkel (Eds.), *Nursing, caring, and complexity science.* New York, NY: Springer.

Sosik, J., & Cameron, J. (2010). Character and authentic transformational leadership behavior: Expanding the ascetic self toward others. *Consulting Psychology Journal: Practice and Research, 62*(4), 251–269.

Stone, B. (2011). The return. *Bloomberg BusinessWeek, 4249*, p. 40.

Summerfield, M. (2014). Leadership: A simple definition. *American Journal Health Systems Pharmacy, 71*, 251–253.

Tomlinson, J. (2012). Exploration of transformational and distributed leadership. *Nursing Management, 19*(4), 30–34.

Tremblay, M. (2010). Fairness perceptions and trust as mediators on the relationship between leadership style, unit commitment, and turnover intentions of Canadian Forces Personnel. *Military Psychology, 22,* 510–523.

Tse, H., & Chiu, W. (2014). Transformational leadership and job performance: A social identity perspective. *Journal of Business Research, 67,* 2827–2835.

Van Dierendonck, D. (2011). Servant leadership: A review and synthesis. *Journal of Management,* 37(4), 1228–1261.

Vroom, V. H., & Yetton, D. W. (1973). *Leadership and decision-making.* Pittsburgh, PA: University of Pittsburgh Press.

Walumbwa, F. O., Avolio, B. J., Gardner, W. L., Wernsing, T. S., & Peterson, S. J. (2008). Authentic leadership: Development and validation of a theory-based measure. *Journal of Management,* 34(1), 89–126.

Walumbwa, F. O., & Hartnell, C. (2011). Understanding transformational leadership-employee performance links: The role of relational identification and self-efficacy. *Journal of Occupational and Organizational Psychology, 84,* 153–172.

Walumbwa, F. O., Wang, P., Wang, H., Schaubroeck, J., & Avolio, B. J. (2010). Psychological processes linking authentic leadership to follower behaviors. *The Leadership Quarterly, 21,* 901–914.

Wang, A., Chiang, J., Tsai, C., Lin, T., & Cheng, B. (2013). Gender makes the difference: The moderating role of leader gender on the relationship between leadership styles and subordinate performance. *Organizational Behavior and Human Decision Processes, 122,* 101–113.

Wang, P., & Rode, J. (2010). Transformational leadership and follower creativity: The moderating effects of identification with leader and organizational climate. *Human Relations, 64*(8), 1105–1128.

Waterman, H. (2011). Principles of servant leadership and how they can enhance practice. *Nursing Management, 27*(9), 24–26.

Wenberg, D. (2012). Complexity leadership: A healthcare imperative. *Nursing Forum, 47*(4), 268–276.

Wexford, C. (2002). Matching theory to practice. *Nursing Management 9*(4), 7–11.

Wheatley. M. (2006). *Leadership and the new science* (3rd ed.). San Francisco, CA: Berrett-Koehler.

Wheelen T. L., & Hunger, J. D. (1997). *Strategic management and business policy* (6th ed.). Upper Saddle River, NJ: Addison-Wesley.

Whittington, J. L., Coker, R. H., Goodwin, V. L., Ickes, W., & Murray, B. (2009). Transactional leadership revisited: Self-other agreement and its consequences. *Journal of Applied Social Psychology, 39* (8), 1860–1886.

Wilson, M. (2009). Complexity theory. *Whitireia Nursing Journal, 16,* 18–24.

Wiseman, L., & McKeown, G. (2010). *Multipliers: How the best leaders make everyone smarter.* New York, NY: HarperCollins.

Wong, C., & Giallonardo, L. (2013). Authentic leadership and nurse-assessed adverse patient outcomes. *Journal of Nursing Management, 21,* 740–752.

Wong, C. A., & Laschinger, H. K. (2013) Authentic leadership, performance, and job satisfaction: The mediating role of empowerment. *Journal of Advanced Nursing 69*(4), 947–959.

Yang, F., Wu, M., Chang, C., & Chien, Y. (2011). Elucidating the relationships among transformational leadership, job satisfaction, commitment foci, and commitment bases in the public sector. *Public Personnel Management, 40*(3), 265–278.

Zaccaro, S. J., Kemp, C., & Bader, P. (2004). Leader traits and attributes. In J. Antonakis, A. Cianciolo, & R. Sternberg (Eds.), *The nature of leadership* (pp. 101–124). Thousand Oaks, CA: Sage.

Zaleznik, A. (1977). Managers and leaders: Are they different? *Harvard Business Review, 55,* 67–78.

2

Workplace Leadership Opportunities

Over the past decade, the call for health-care transformation has been loud and clear. Nurse leaders have been challenged not just to make a few changes to repair one situation, but also to incorporate new ways of thinking, practicing, developing, and sustaining relationships within an entire system (Mason & Wesorick, 2011; Parsons & Cornett, 2011). The terms "quality," "safety," "satisfaction," "transparency," "communication," "outcomes," and "systems" are common in current health-care literature. This chapter focuses on the pressing workplace issues impacting these concepts including organizational ethics, workplace and workforce safety, governance (particularly shared governance), teamwork, and diversity (Box 2.1).

ORGANIZATIONAL ETHICS

The study of ethics has religious, cultural, and philosophical underpinnings. Although what constitutes ethics and ethical behavior has been studied and debated for centuries, the discussion of organizational ethics is a relatively new phenomenon. Nursing students explore the Nursing Code of Ethics (American Nurses Association, 2010) in order to provide a framework for an individual's practice of nursing; however, the discussion of organizational ethics is not strongly emphasized in most nursing programs.

"Organizational ethics examines ethical principles and moral or ethical problems that arise in a business environment. It applies to all aspects of business conduct and is relevant to the conduct of individuals and entire organizations" ("Business Ethics," 2008). Leaders are constantly facing decisions that cause conflict (for example, weighing human rights against fiscal goals). Early research into organizational ethics identified the following nine tenets:

1. Sound ethics is important for business.
2. Profit should not be the only business motivator.
3. At middle- and lower-management levels, pressure to compromise personal values is strongly felt.
4. Competition can force individuals to ignore ethical considerations.

BOX 2.1 **Sustaining Workplace Relationships**

As you read this chapter, think about how you and your organization currently approach these workplace issues and what suggestions you, as a leader, might make for improvement.

---

5. A well-defined personal code of ethics is important to acting ethically in business.
6. Pressure from leadership can cause employees to engage in unethical behaviors.
7. Employees who strongly identify with the organization are more likely to abdicate personal responsibility for their actions.
8. Interpersonal communication and organizational ethics are related.
9. Persons who engage in small unethical behaviors often later expand into more serious unethical practices (Lewis, 1985; Schumacher & Wasieleski, 2013).

Key Components of Organizational Ethics

Three key components make up organizational ethics: values, the ethical climate, and trust.

Values

Organizational values address not only what ought to be but also what is good and desirable. They can be observed through spoken and written communication and physical actions. Ethical marketing issues include marketing redundant or dangerous products/services; transparency about environmental risks, product ingredients (genetically modified organisms), possible health risks, or financial risks; respect for consumer privacy and autonomy; advertising truthfulness; and fairness in pricing and distribution.

Examples of organizational ethics include sales practices; tax payments; external and internal audits; recruitment selection and appraisal of employees; and discrimination by age, gender, sexual orientation, race, religion, disability, weight, and perceived attractiveness. Issues related to ethical marketing often appear in the news regarding product ingredients, possible health risks, respect for consumer privacy and autonomy, truth in advertising, and price fairness ("Ethical Issues," 2014).

Recent research (Van Der Wal, 2011) on organizational values identified the following concepts that are important to leadership within organizations:

- Responsiveness: addressing stakeholder wishes and demands
- Transparency and accountability: acting openly and visibly, being able to justify actions to stakeholders
- Lawfulness: acting in accord with existing laws, rules, and codes of conduct
- Consistency, reliability, and incorruptibility: acting in a trustworthy and consistent manner
- Efficiency and effectiveness: focusing on the interrelatedness of moral, financial, and policy considerations

Values have been linked to organization sustainability. Organizational sustainability includes the economic, social, and environmental practices that the organization demonstrates. Leadership values, an integral part of sustainability, are therefore strongly linked to the practice of values supporting organizational sustainability (Table 2.1). These values include altruism, empathy, reciprocity, and self-effacement (Box 2.2).

Ethical Climate

Ethical work climates provide employees with the foundation for thinking about moral issues within the organization. Work climates are defined as the shared perceptions that employees hold about policies, procedures, and practices supported by the organization. The ethical climate translates to ethical behaviors in employees insofar as it is related to ethical decision making and behaviors. In the unethical organization, for example, this behavior includes theft, lying, falsifying information, and bribes (Arnaud & Schminke, 2012). Leadership plays a critical role in developing and supporting the ethical climate. Viinamaki (2011) and Credo, Armenakis,

TABLE 2.1 Leadership Practices and Organizational Sustainability

Leadership Practice	Value
Succession planning	Altruism
Development of critical competencies	Altruism
Communication of clear expectations and goal alignment	Empathy
Flexible work arrangements	Altruism
Developmental activities such as on-boarding and coaching	Altruism Empathy Reciprocity Self-effacement
Identification of skill gaps and performance deficiencies	Empathy Self-effacement
Quality of life and work-life balance	Empathy Self-effacement

BOX 2.2 **Values Supporting Organizational Sustainability**

Altruism: Altruistic behaviors affect others by helping with organizationally relevant problems. The opposite of self-interest, altruistic behaviors and practices often promote healthier work and home environments.

Empathy: The personal value of empathy reflects one's ability to recognize and respond to others' emotional behaviors. Empathy is demonstrated through compassion, tenderness, and sympathy. Empathy is an organizational function in which leaders put aside their own pursuits and interests to help employees.

Reciprocity: Reciprocity postulates that people should help and not harm those who have not helped them. This value promotes stability in the leader–employee relationship, encourages trust, and promotes formation of networks and activities within the organization.

Self-Effacement: Self-effacement is defined as humility, unpretentiousness, or a lack of arrogance. Leaders with a strong sense of self-effacement demonstrate a lack of arrogance and strong ties to the organization.

Field, and Young (2010) cite essential issues important to successful leadership in 21st-century organizations:

- Traditional power is often powerless in professional organizations: Organizations today must decentralize to create consensual decision making and cohesive authority on the basis of shared values, as well as receiving and providing feedback actively.
- Stakeholder participation needs to be intensive and extensive: Ensure that stakeholders are motivated and empowered and aware of the organizations' goals and values.
- New forms of control and feedback are essential: The leader needs to move from controller to enabler, making clear to participants how these roles will be operationalized.
- Values should be communicated clearly: Leaders should provide guidance when decisions are ambiguous and demonstrate a clear value-based image.

Trust

Nurses are well aware of the need for trust in the nurse–patient relationship. Trust is also an important condition within organizations. In organizations, the trustee is vulnerable, reliant, and dependent on the organization. In a leader, demonstrating acceptance, respect for others, knowledge, openness, beneficence, confidentiality, and a commitment to competence influence others' ability to trust (Box 2.3).

Leadership Responsibilities

Organizations with strong foundational ethics can be viewed as human communities. The human community emphasizes the uniqueness of both the individuals and the

BOX 2.3 **Inspiring Trust**

How do you demonstrate the behaviors of a leader to others? How might you improve yourself or your organization in demonstrating these behaviors?

Source: Goold, S. (2001). Trust and the ethics of health care institutions. *Hastings Center Report 31*(6), 26–33.

community as a whole. More than a constellation of interests, the human community consists of interpersonal and social exchanges and links. Within this human community, the leader can contribute to significant changes in the life of individuals and organizations by demonstrating moral leadership, developing a social–moral climate (SMC), asking the right questions, establishing an ethical decision-making (EDM) process, and providing organizational ethics training (Mele, 2011; Verdorfer, Weber, Unterrainer, & Seyr, 2013).

Moral Leadership

Four leadership styles (as discussed in Chapter 1) exemplify ideas associated with moral leadership (Bjarnason & LaSala, 2011; Hannah, Avolio, & Walumbwa, 2011):

- Transformational leadership: This leadership style involves motivating others through coaching, mentoring, and shared governance and effectively communicating organizational mission, vision, goals, and values.
- Authentic leadership: The authentic leader is viewed as real, trustworthy, sincere, and possessing integrity and self-discipline with a leadership style characterized by personal values and beliefs, forming a strong sense of self. Authentic leadership has demonstrated a positive relationship to followers' displays of moral courage and ethical behaviors.
- Servant leadership: The servant leader focuses on team success and a collective group approach to planning and decision making with a strong sense of improving society.
- Evidence-based leadership: Developing collaborative work environments to build team-focused goals characterizes evidence-based leadership.

Develop a Social–Moral Climate

Explored since the 1980s, SMC represents a subcategory of the organizational climate. It refers to the principles of communication, teamwork, and collective problem-solving and decision making. Leadership responsibilities for promoting a strong SMC include the following:

- Open confrontation of employees with conflicts
- Reliable and constant appreciation, care, and support by supervisors and colleagues
- Open communication and participative cooperation

- Trust-based assignment and allocation of responsibility corresponding to the respective employees' capabilities
- Organizational concern for the individual
- Establishment of an atmosphere of workplace fairness (De Schrijver, Delbeke, Maesschalck, & Pleysier, 2010; Verdorfer et al., 2013)

Ask the Right Questions

The nursing leader is an essential conduit between the organization and the individuals it serves. Ethical issues often arise that exist on a continuum between the clinical and the organizational. These ethical issues often have high-stakes consequences. Leader EDM requires recognition and proper representation of multiple pieces of information. Thiel et al. (2012) recommend that leaders use a sense-making model for EDM. This multifaceted process allows leaders to engage in multiple complex cognitive strategies. The EDM model consists of four steps: (1) emotional regulation, (2) self-reflection, (3) forecasting, and (4) information integration, as described in Table 2.2. The EDM process requires careful scanning, interpreting, and analyzing of complex ethical dilemmas. The process assists the leader to assess individual, environmental, and social pressures that might impact the accuracy and completeness of decision making.

Establish an Ethical Decision-Making Process

Ethical decisions are rarely easy to make. Developing an EDM process that allows review of ethical issues in a planned, systematic manner may help to clarify ethical conflict,

TABLE 2.2 Sense-Making Strategies

Strategy	Behavior
Emotional regulation	Behaviorally and/or cognitively appraising and reappraising the emotional reactions to the situation
Self-reflection	Using experiential or academic knowledge that has been personally acquired or learned vicariously
Forecasting	Reflecting on positive past experiences or other learning applications to enhance future ethical decision making
Information integration	Framing the issue from an organizational perspective

Adapted from: Thiel, C., Bagdasarov, Z., Harkrider, L., & Mumford, M. (2012). Leader ethical decision-making in organizations: Strategies for sensemaking. *Journal Business Ethics, 107*, 49–64.

structure reasoning, and support the leader's ethical practice. These eight steps represent just such a system:

Step 1: Clarify the ethical conflict.
Step 2: Identify all affected stakeholders and their values.
Step 3: Understand the circumstances surrounding the issue.
Step 4: Identify the ethical perspective relevant to the issue.
Step 5: Identify different options for action.
Step 6: Select among the options.
Step 7: Share and implement the decision.
Step 8: Review the decision to ensure it achieves the desired goal.

Provide Organizational Ethics Training

Ethics training is vital to decreasing disciplinary and legal ramifications. Even more important is the need for a proactive approach that will instill the organizational beliefs and values to help employees be better prepared to face ethical challenges. Bayley (2012) cautions against using a case-based reactionary approach instead of a more conceptual proactive framework. Lawrence and Maitlis (2012) supported this conceptual approach by recommending that organizations establish an ethic of care from the perspective that persons within organizations are relational and interdependent rather than independent and self-sufficient (Box 2.4).

WORKPLACE SAFETY

Leaders must focus on two vital components of workplace safety: patient safety and employee safety. A 2012 phenomenological study of health-care executives suggested that honesty, inclusiveness, clear accountability, empowering others, and acting as transformational leaders all contributed to developing a culture of safety. A meta-analysis of 57 studies concluded that supportive leadership was one of the components associated with improved performance outcomes (Bohan & Lang, 2012; Brand et al., 2012).

An aging workforce, increasing demands of aging clients requiring more complex care, and increased costs have come together to create the "perfect storm" economists cite when talking about the challenges to successful delivery of safe care (Leonard & Frankel, 2010). Krause (2005) identifies that organizations that lead in safety are also operationally efficient and cost effective. He points out that leaders in safe organizations define specific values that create safety, hold everyone accountable to behaviors that support these values, and continually work to improve the culture.

BOX 2.4 Becoming an Ethically Supportive Leader

Ethics is emerging as one of the most critical issues facing leaders and organizations. The complex health-care environment will continue to offer leadership challenges. How can you become an ethically supportive leader across the many levels of the organization?

According to the Agency for Healthcare Research and Quality (AHRQ, 2014), a culture of patient safety demonstrates the following features:

- Acknowledgment of the high-risk nature of an organization's activities and the determination to achieve consistently safe operations
- A blame-free environment in which individuals are able to report errors or near misses without fear of reprimand or punishment
- Encouragement of collaboration across ranks and disciplines to seek solutions to patient safety problems
- Organizational commitment of resources to address safety concerns

A 2010 meta-analysis (Sammer, Lykens, Singh, Mains, & Lackan, 2010) identified seven concepts (also referred to as "subcultures") within the definition of a patient safety culture: leadership, teamwork, communication, basis in evidence, learning, justice, and centering on the patient (Table 2.3).

Patient Safety

The first step in making safety leadership more effective is to assess the existing safety culture. Galloway (2010) suggests following these seven steps:

1. Review documentation, programs, and policies. What are the current and past programs, initiatives, previous incidents, and audits? How has safety been rewarded and recognized in the past?
2. Communicate prior to employee interaction. Notify all employees that a safety audit is being conducted to focus on current strengths while identifying opportunities to further improve.
3. Conduct a location walk. Visit major sites within the organization. Observe differences and similarities in group and individual behaviors that might contribute to a positive and negative safety culture.
4. Complete a leadership discussion. Make sure to include all key personnel in an early discussion regarding the goal of the assessment. Reinforce the idea that the assessment is not a fault-finding process, but rather an opportunity to identify approaches to excellence.
5. Utilize a customized safety perception survey. Many perception surveys are available; however, it is usually more beneficial to develop a perception survey based on the specific organization.
6. Conduct group and individual interviews. Both focus groups and one-on-one interviews may be useful in obtaining a deeper understanding of perceptions, workplace realities, past history, and the interconnectivity of people and departments related to safety.
7. Provide a report focusing on internally actionable items. Schedule an exit meeting with all key personnel on the last day of the assessment. Discuss preliminary findings and next steps.

With a thorough assessment in place, it is time to transform the organization using the following steps (Galloway, 2010; Leonard & Frankel, 2010; Llorens, 2010; Ring & Fairchild, 2013; Sammer et al., 2010):

- *Be a safety leader.* Acknowledge the high risks associated with the health-care environment. Align vision and mission and fiscal and human resources with

TABLE 2.3 Subculture/Concept Properties

Leadership	Teamwork	Communication	Evidence-Based	Learning	Justice	Patient-Centered
Accountability	Alignment	Assertion/speak up	Best practices	Awareness/ informed	Blame-free	Community/grass roots
Change management	Deference to expertise	Hand-offs	High reliability/ zero deficits	Celebrate success/ rewards	Disclosure	Compassion/ caring
Commitment	Flattened hierarchy	Linkages between executives and front line	Outcomes driven	Data driven	Non-punitive reporting	Empowered patients/ families
Executive rounds	Multidisciplinary/ multigenerational	Bottom-up approach	Science of safety	Education/ training/ including physicians	No at-risk behaviors	Exemplary patient experiences
Governance	Mutual respect	Clarity	Standardization: Protocols/ checklists	Learn from mistakes/ evaluation	Systems focused	Formal participation in care
Open relationships	Psychological safety	Resolution/ feedback	Guidelines	Monitor/ benchmark	Trust	Health promotion
Physician engagement	Readiness to adapt/flexibility	Safety briefings/ debriefings	Technology/ automation	Performance improvement		Informed patients/ families
Priority	Supportive	Structured techniques		Proactive		Patient stories
Resources		Transparency		Root-cause analysis		
Role model				Share lessons learned		
Support						
Vigilance						
Visibility						
Vision/ mission						

Adapted from: Lykens, K., Singh, K., Mains, D., & Lackan, N. (2010). What is patient safety culture? A review of the literature. *Journal of Nursing Scholarship, 42*(2), 156–165.

safety initiatives. Survey people regularly on how they are addressing critical issues, and build ongoing dialogue around a culture of accountability.

• *Establish a just culture.* The success of a patient safety culture rests strongly on a just culture that balances accountability between individuals and systems. Recognizing the principles of accepting human fallibility, managing risk, learning from errors, evaluating the system responsibly, and counseling or punishing, the just culture encompasses the other key components of transformational leadership, teamwork, evidence-based practice, and clear communication.

• *Encourage teamwork.* Identify individuals who are willing to become champions of safety, support them, and foster their growth as informal leaders of safety. Senior leaders, front-line clinicians, and physicians also need to model effective safety leadership behaviors. Promote a spirit of collegiality, cooperation, and collaboration.

• *Encourage learning.* A transformational leader cannot fully engage without becoming a steward of organizational energy. Invigorate safety meetings into involved activities that support an environment of continuous learning and improvement. Invest in training and establish discussions with candor and accountability.

• *Customize your safety leadership.* There is no lack of guidelines, policies, checklists, and experts in the area of health-care safety; however, each organization needs individualized ideas. Use of structured communication tools customized to the organization such as situation, background, assessment, recommendation (SBAR) debriefings, use of critical language, and the creation of an environment of psychological safety can be effective leadership tools in promoting safety.

• *Build community.* Safety needs to have a personal touch. It needs to be infused throughout the organization in a way that participants care and support one another and the culture. Another part of building a community is providing reliable processes of care that will offer predictability and a stable platform for measurement and improvement.

• *Invite communication.* Open communication about perceptions of leadership, teamwork, conflict resolution, how nursing input is received, and errors discussed in an atmosphere of safety can lead to changes in safety culture. Invite communication by rewarding and publically highlighting employees who speak up and support change, while simultaneously holding senior management accountable for responding to and welcoming crucial conversations.

• *Emphasize patient- and family-centered care.* An important aspect of patient safety is supporting the concept of family-centered care. Most caregivers perceive the caregiving process from a technical standpoint—"Did I do everything right?"—rather than viewing patients' experience from their perspective. Leading the initiatives to prepare other team members to better prepare patients to understand and participate in their own care will support the patient safety process.

The airline industry, the military, and other high-risk groups such as firefighters have been diligently focusing on crew resource management as part of a safety culture (Barter, 2010). Communication, with the need for standardized protocols, checklists, SBAR, and briefings, is just one integral part of safety training. Others, such as workload management, situational awareness (SA), and error management, also need to become part of a health-care organization's safety culture.

Workload Management

Workload management becomes critical when nurses are confronted with task over-load and are unable to perceive system problems. Issues related to high workload levels, interruptions, and fatigue may contribute to errors. Leaders trained in staffing protocols, reorganization of work units, whole-picture thinking, conflict resolution, and complexity management can support the nurse's participation in the safety culture. Successful workload management includes weekly management team meetings during which leaders identify immediate problems, address unit and staff concerns, and plan for long-term goal setting. Successful workload management also involves leaders and managers who are highly visible and available for the staff at all times. Box 2.5 offers suggestions for promoting workload management.

BOX 2.5 Promoting Workload Management

Empowering the Staff: Provide unit-based committees; staff works together to embrace self-governance.

Rounding for Outcomes: Structured hourly rounding, or hourly visits to patients by the registered nurse and other health-team members, has been shown to improve patient satis-faction scores (Fabry, 2015). Using this approach, staff leaders who "round" with staff by walking around and soliciting staff feedback on improving the unit can ask three simple questions: What is working in the unit? What is not working in the unit? Who would you like to acknowledge?

Getting to Know You: Staff receive e-mails when their issues have been involved; staff are acknowledged during rounding for outcomes when their suggestions have been implemented.

Accountability: Staff and managers feel comfortable holding one another accountable. Accessi-bility to someone who has authority to "make things happen" is available at all times. Feedback and ongoing staff development are encouraged.

Professional Development: Leaders promote an atmosphere in which mentoring for advance-ment and professional growth is encouraged and recognized.

Fostering Work-Life Balance: Self-scheduling and managing one's workload are encouraged. Last-minute requests are honored and addressed.

Individual Worth of Each Person: Encourage diversity, respect differences, and foster an open-door policy promoting individual contributions to the team.

Celebrations: Holiday celebrations are always welcome, but creating unique and special cele-brations also shows ongoing appreciation.

Active Participation in Social Activities: Plan social activities for team building or special activ-ities through a social-planning committee.

Adapted from: Blake, N. (2012). A model of authentic leadership to promote a healthy workplace. *AACN Advanced Critical Care, 23*(4), 358–361.

Situational Awareness

SA is a well-understood concept used to maintain operational safety in many organizations. Nurses play a critical role in providing vigilance in health care, which is directly related to managing and improving patient outcomes. Thus, leadership within these contexts must involve interactions that facilitate the appraisal of hazards, risks, potential benefits, resources, and solutions using information that is often insufficient and equivocal. A leader's ability to perceive reality can be affected by stress, fatigue, distractions, ambiguity, complacency, or fixating on minutiae (Fore & Sculli, 2013). Leaders need to be able to continually assess the environment and challenge assumptions. Baran and Scott (2010), using their research on near-miss errors with firefighters, identified numerous leadership actions and processes related to SA (Box 2.6).

Error Management

A patient safety culture is only as strong as the procedures for identifying, tracking, and categorizing errors (Box 2.7). Nurse leaders should ask the following questions regarding errors: Are they design versus person induced? Are they variable or constant? Are they reversible or irreversible? Are they slips, lapses, mistakes, or violations? Are they the result of skills, rules, or knowledge errors? Are they caused by external factors, organizational factors, human factors, or technical failures? Leaders within high-reliability organizations focus on system, organizational support, training, and transforming care at the bedside (Barter, 2010; Oien, Utne, & Herra, 2011).

WORKFORCE SAFETY

Healthy work environments and workforce safety are addressed by the federal government as well as many national agencies. A 2013 Joint Commission publication

---

BOX 2.6 Situational Awareness

Direction setting: Ensuring personnel follow safety procedures

Talk: Repeating information until meanings are shared

Knowledge: Using information from both prior experience and training to purposefully guide action

Role-Play: Practicing doing expected tasks

Agility: Rapidly adjusting behavior due to changing conditions

Role Modeling: Personally enacting examples of mindful behavior

Trust: Believing in the reliability of coworkers and depending upon them when necessary

---

Adapted from: Baran, B. E., & Cliff, W. S. (2010). Organizing ambiguity: A grounded theory of leadership and sensemaking within dangerous contexts. *Military Psychology, 22,* (Suppl. I), S42–S69.

BOX 2.7 Enacting Safety Initiatives

The nuclear power industry applies the concept of "red rules" to its safety initiatives. Red rules refer to protocols that must be followed without any deviation. All work can stop until the protocol is reinitiated, and any person can call a red rule (Karsten, 2011). What situations would you identify that might warrant a red rule? As a leader, how would you introduce the concepts of red rules to your organization?

Consider the attitudes, values, and behaviors that reflect the culture in your work environment. Do you perceive them as conducive to the delivery of safe, quality, patient-centered care? What suggestions would you make to improve them?

Improving Patient and Worker Safety, contends that high rates of injuries and illnesses among health-care workers serve as a warning that the entire organization must be transformed. The Occupational Safety and Health Administration (OSHA) reports that more than 2 million acts of physical violence, harassment, intimidation, or other threatening disruptive behavior occur annually in the workplace (OSHA, 2014). A 2014 quantitative analysis included a review of 136 articles providing data from 151,347 nurses. That analysis revealed that of the total reported acts on an international level, physical violence accounted for 36.4%, nonphysical violence 66.9%; 37.1% bullying 39.7% and 25% reported sexual harassment (Spector, Zhou, & Xin, 2014).

The importance of high-caliber interprofessional teams in the delivery of safe and quality health care is well documented in the literature (Institute of Medicine, 2004, 2011). Promotion of health and well-being at work includes preventive services, timely interventions, rehabilitation, activities that promote health and well-being, and teaching and training of leaders to encourage support of staff health and well-being. Negative workplace relationships and behaviors contribute to burnout, staff turnover, and poor patient outcomes (Becher & Visovsky, 2012). Unfortunately, nurses report one of the highest rates of workplace violence (WPV) among medical workers. Employees' perceptions of an organization's policies, procedures, and practices toward WPV are important contributors to the employees' health (Aytac & Dursun, 2012; Campbell et al., 2011). Most organizations have prevention training related to patient and visitor violence that nurses can use to de-escalate aggressive situations. When these strategies do not work, the leader's responsibility should include collaboration with other leaders, organizational development staff, law enforcement, and risk managers to develop coordinated and rapid responses available to support employees. This could include development of scenarios and practice preparing staff, reorganization of the physical layout, and debriefings after incidences (Hardin, 2012).

Along with WPV directed at employees from patients, lateral or horizontal violence is increasing. Table 2.4 describes basic themes of horizontal violence. Lateral violence includes both overt and covert behaviors imposed on an employee by another employee. Overt behaviors include sabotage, verbal and physical intimidation, and bullying. Covert behaviors such as failure to cooperate, failure to respect privacy, making distasteful facial expressions, undermining others, discouraging new staff, gossiping, and providing minimal guidance to new employees can be just as detrimental as overt behaviors. Research on horizontal violence has grown over the past two

TABLE 2.4 **Themes of Horizontal Violence**

Themes	Examples
Economy and workload	Nursing staff cutbacks and skill mix changes Standardized practices that are unevenly applied Unequal distribution of the workload
Lack of interpersonal skills	Marginalizing staff Continuous surveillance
Lack of management skills	Leading from a difference Lack of conflict management Acting as an agent of control Unfair appointment of others
Generational differences	Inability to address differences fairly
Hierarchical nature of nursing work	Making unfair assignments Lack of consistency in policies and procedures

Source: Croft, R., & Cash, P. (2012). Deconstructing contributing factors to bullying and lateral violence in nursing using a postcolonial feminist lens. *Contemporary Nurse 42*(2), 226–242.

decades. International occupational health research shows that lateral violence is an issue across many workplaces, decreasing job satisfaction and commitment and increasing costs (Ceravolo, Schwartz, Foltz-Ramos, & Castner, 2012).

Table 2.5 demonstrates that horizontal violence has many roots including individuals, groups, organizations, and even society at large. A 2012 qualitative study from the British Nurses Union identified five themes similar to previous decades of research: economy and workload, lack of interpersonal skills, lack of management skills, generational differences, and the hierarchical nature of nursing work (Croft & Cash, 2012; Griffin, 2011; Samnai & Singh, 2012).

Center (2011) has developed excellent assessment questions a leader should ask to create a culture of civility (Box 2.8).

Gurt, Schwennen, and Elke (2011) studied whether there is an association between leader consideration for the health of employees and their levels of stress and their well-being. Previous research demonstrates a significant relationship between leadership styles and practices and employee health through both leader initiation and support of organizational policies and systems as well as personal interactions and communication (Gurt, Schwennen, & Elke, 2011; Kuoppala, Lamminpaa, Liira, & Vainio, 2008; Laschinger, Wong, & Grau, 2012).

TABLE 2.5 **Roots of Horizontal Violence**

Roots	Consequences	
Perpetrator	*Personality and traits*: aggressive *Demographics*: male	
Group factors	Group norms Status inconsistency Situational factors: team autonomy	
Organizational factors	Leadership and management style Organizational culture Organizational policies Situational factors: reward systems	
Target	*Personality and traits* Neuroticism Introversion Agreeableness Conscientiousness Negative affect Low self-esteem	*Demographics* Female Ethnic minority
Consequences	*Individual* Psychological well-being Suicide Absenteeism Intent to leave Job satisfaction	*Group* Team effectiveness Team norms *Organizational* Organizational performance Organizational culture *Societal* Unemployment Legal costs Interpersonal relationships
Broad societal factors	National culture	

Adapted from: Samnai, A., & Singh, P. (2012). 20 years of workplace bullying research: A review of the antecedents and consequences of bullying in the workplace. *Aggression and Violent Behavior, 17*, 581–589.

BOX 2.8 **Culture of Civility**

How are incidents handled when they occur? Are they ignored, indirectly demonstrating accept-ability? Do finger-pointing, blaming, and disciplinary actions create fear and a culture of silence? Are the incidents viewed, instead, as growth and improvement opportunities? Do staff feel empowered to confront issues as a quality improvement initiative?

- How is the incident investigated? Is the issue viewed as a system breakdown or is there an immediate assumption of individual blame?

- How are incidents discussed and shared with others? Is there open dialogue or are incidents kept hidden?

- Is everyone held to the same standards and accountability for incivility? Is there immediate coaching when incidents occur?

- Is there a zero-tolerance policy toward incivility? Who is responsible for looking at system patterns of uncivil behavior?

- How has horizontal violence impacted such resources as sick time, staff turnover, poor job satisfaction, mental health, and organizational commitment?

- What is the current organizational commitment to addressing an issue?

Support of Organizational Policies

A 2008 study by Gurt et al. identified differences in leadership activities between general leadership and health-specific leadership. Health-specific leadership incorporated behaviors that assumed responsibility for employee health, set the agenda for health-promotion activities, and motivated and supported employees in health-promotion activities. In addition, health-specific leaders were role models and demonstrated positive attitudes toward employees' healthy behaviors with an attitude of respect, trust, and openness.

Personal Interactions

Personal leadership includes behaviors used to influence others through personal interactions and communication. Effective leadership styles are explored in other areas of this text; in this section, communication behaviors as a means to decrease horizontal violence are examined.

Communication falls into four categories: tone, tools, processes, and role.

Tone

As the saying goes, "It's not what you say but how you say it." Does a good leader sound overwhelmed and stressed in speaking to others? Is he or she inconsistent in tone of communication or does he or she try to avoid communication with others? Does the leader carve out time for employees? Does he or she set a good example in communication style?

Tools

What methods does the leader use to disseminate information? In e-mail, meetings, memos, and verbal instructions, a leader should continue to learn and practice effective communication skills.

Processes

A leader should ensure that effective communication is part of all employees' training, especially managers and preceptors. The leader should also promote organizational processes that promote staff empowerment and shared governance.

Role

A nurse leader has a crucial impact on workplace health for both patients and employees. Making a thorough assessment of current practices for both workplace and workforce safety, developing effective organizational strategies for improvement, and above all critically evaluating his or her own leadership and communication style will go a long way in making employees and patients feel safe (Box 2.9). Table 2.6 offers suggestions for promoting effective communication and decreasing horizontal violence that have worked for other leaders (Hartung & Miller, 2013).

GOVERNANCE

Does type of governance influence the organizational culture, satisfaction, and retention rate of registered nurses? Does type of governance influence patient satisfaction with registered nurse care? As early as 2001, the answer from both patients and registered nurses was a resounding yes (Stumpf, 2001). More than decade ago, research on registered nurse satisfaction cited pay, autonomy, task requirements, organizational policies, and professional practice climate as important. At the same time, authoritarian leadership and poor access to information were linked to feelings of disempowerment (Kuokkanen & Katajisto, 2003; Martin, Gustin, Uddin, & Risner, 2004). Research continues to support nurses' desire to be autonomous and have control over their practice environment (Twigg & McCullough, 2014).

Shared Governance

Creating a successful professional environment is extremely challenging in today's environment of increased competition, declining reimbursement, escalating patient needs, and evolving technology. The foundation for a strong shared governance structure must start with the leader demonstrating a solid foundation of nursing professionalism,

---

BOX 2.9 Nurse Leader Communication Style

How do you handle the feelings of "being pulled in different directions" and being "spread too thin"?

TABLE 2.6 **Effective Communication Strategies to Decrease Horizontal Violence**

Category	Recommendations
Tone of communication	• Develop an approachable, visionary, open leadership style • Ensure accessibility and be approachable • Encourage honest, open, and frank dialogue • Develop listening skills that encourage problem-solving • Critically evaluate your own communication tone
Tools of communication	• Evaluate methods of communication throughout the organization • Work with organizational development to support and encourage formal and continuing communication education • Model effective communication behaviors • Critically evaluate your own communication methods • Encourage team building and debriefings
Processes for healthy communication	• Plan regular and consistent meetings with staff • Seek other perspectives and value input • Evaluate methods to increase efficiency of information throughout the organization • Take responsibility for effective communication
Role	• Ensure your commitment to becoming a transformational, authentic leader

Adapted from: Hartung, S., & Miller, M. (2013). Communication and the healthy work environment. *Journal of Nursing Administration, 43*(5), 266–273.

philosophical underpinnings, and a vision for the future (Start, Wright, Murphy, McIntosh, & Catrambone 2013):

- Nursing professionalism: Shared governance embraces a philosophy of nursing excellence and accountability for providing safe, high-quality care.
- Philosophical underpinnings: Embracing the philosophy of total staff involvement from the beginning in planning a shared governance model is important to success. Make sure that everyone involved understands the importance of shared governance to the satisfaction of nurses and patients.
- Nursing vision: Shared governance leaders must begin planning with a vision that nursing should be a full professional partner with medicine and

health-care administration. Bylaws that include mission statement, eligibility for membership, officers and executive board, meetings, election process, committees and subcommittees, and amendment procedures for changing the bylaws are imperative to a strong shared governance structure.

Magnet Recognition

Current nursing literature provides numerous examples of successful shared governance models. The most widely recognized is the American Nurses Credentialing Center Magnet Recognition Program. Since the program's inception in 1992, more than 400 facilities have attained Magnet designation. Nurses in Magnet facilities often rate their opportunities to influence workplace organization and participation in shared governance higher than do nurses in non-Magnet facilities. Based on the 14 Forces of Magnetism, facilities credentialed with the Magnet designation are recognized for their excellence in nursing practice. Magnet facilities must demonstrate the following attributes and their application to quality patient outcomes (American Nurses Credentialing Center, 2014; Hess, DesRoches, Donelan, Norman, & Buerhaus, 2001; Upenieks & Sitterding, 2008):

1. Quality of nursing leadership
2. Organizational structure
3. Management style
4. Consultation and resources
5. Autonomy
6. Community and health-care organization
7. Personnel policies and programs
8. Professional models of care
9. Nurses as teachers
10. Image of nursing
11. Quality of care
12. Interdisciplinary relationships
13. Quality improvement
14. Professional development

Creating Positive Practice Environments

Porter-O'Grady, in his *Shared Governance Implementation Manual*, cautions us that "shared governance really does not take form until it is present in the places where the staff does its work" (p. 71). Strategies to embark on any shared governance journey include encouraging nurse participation in hospital affairs, promoting meaningful foundations for quality care, adopting a leadership style that supports and encourages staff, encouraging collaborative interdisciplinary relationships, and effectively managing resources (Twigg & McCullough, 2013). Table 2.7 offers activities related to each strategy.

The association between nurse involvement in governance and work satisfaction has been discussed. Although not limited to a formal structure, research on nurse involvement in decision making, quality improvement, organizational commitment, and improved patient outcomes is documented in the literature (Erickson, Ditomassi, & Jones, 2008; Houser, Erkenbrack, Handberry, Ricker, & Stroup, 2012; Moore & Wells, 2010; Nolan, Wary, King, Laam, & Hallick, 2011). A 2010 systematic review of leadership

TABLE 2.7 Activities That Promote Positive Practice Environments

Strategy	Activity
Encourage nurse participation in hospital affairs	• Provide access to information, support, opportunities, and resources • Promote shared governance structure with time to participate • Recognize achievements in publications and other activities • Provide a flat, flexible, and decentralized organizational structure • Be accessible • Provide explanations and understanding of organizational decision making
Promote meaningful foundations for quality care	• Promote nurses as independent practitioners • Encourage flexibility and decision making about patient care with trust and respect • Develop clinical ladder programs, specialty certification, and other activities that promote scholarship and professional role development; support with salary increases • Develop leadership skills in staff
Provide a leadership style that supports and encourages staff	• Be visible, accessible, responsive, and accountable • Role model professional development • Be innovative, confident, knowledgeable, and communicative
Encourage collaborative interdisciplinary relationships	• Promote interdisciplinary respect and competence • Develop processes for conflict resolution • Define roles and responsibilities based on current best practices
Effectively manage resources	• Manage work demands that promote safe, effective care and work-life balance

Adapted from: Twigg, D., & McCullough, K. (2014). Nurse retention: A review of strategies to create and enhance positive practice environments in clinical settings. *International Journal of Nursing Studies, 51,* 85–92.

styles and staff satisfaction with work environments resulted in 53 studies (Cummings et al., 2010). Outcomes were grouped into five categories: staff satisfaction with work, role, and pay; staff relationships with work; staff health and well-being; work environment factors; and productivity and effectiveness. The results clearly supported that leadership styles focusing on people and relationships rather than tasks were associated with better outcomes in all categories (Box 2.10).

BOX 2.10 Leadership Models

Review the leadership models discussed in Chapter 1. How will you develop effective leadership behaviors in yourself and others? What leadership model do you feel will work most effectively for you?

Challenges to Shared Governance

Moving to a shared model of governance is not without challenges. Change to a shared governance model may require shifts in preconceptions resulting in staff being unable to make any meaningful decisions. Staff would not be released from clinical responsibilities to participate in meetings, and the full development of a shared governance model would be arduous and far too time consuming to be of value (Ballard, 2010; Dunbar et al., 2007). To promote success of a shared governance model, the leader must overcome lack of support, time, and money; lack of planned communication processes; decisions being overruled or ridiculed by other leaders; failure to follow through on agreements or replace autocratic processes; and lack of staff participation. However, a successful shared governance model will reflect the removal of barriers while facilitating unit accountability and decision making, council involvement in most projects, excellent council communication to staff regarding decisions and successes, and manager delegation of accountability and authority for unit decisions (Box 2.11) (Ballard, 2010).

Table 2.8 identifies human and structural factors that are important in the success of shared governance implementation.

TEAMWORK

One of the major challenges facing the nurse leader is preparing staff to work in effective teams. Research has demonstrated the complexity of team relationships and the many different situations that may arise in health-care delivery—70% to 80% of health-care errors have been attributed to ineffective teamwork. Conversely, effective teams have been associated with better patient outcomes, reduced risk of duplication and fragmentation of services, reduced costs, and improvements in workplace satisfaction (Institute of Medicine, 2004; Mitchell, Parker, & Giles, 2011; Xyrichis & Ream, 2008).

Team learning has been viewed as the collective process of taking action, reflecting on feedback, and making changes. Team learning has been shown to have a positive

BOX 2.11 Successful Shared Governance

Based on the factors listed in Table 2.8, what strategies can you identify that will work in your organization to promote staff empowerment through shared governance?

TABLE 2.8 **Factors for Shared Governance Success**

Human Factors	Structural Factors
Leadership vision	Ongoing education and training
Management and staff understanding	Effective decision-making structure
Transition plan	Clear identification of issues
Realistic goals and time frame	Staff support and time for meetings
Coaching and mentoring of council chairs and members	Technology and clerical support to facilitate dissemination of information
Support and recognition of decisions by leadership	Support for data analysis and evaluation of outcomes

Adapted from: Ballard, N. (2010). Factors associated with success and breakdown of shared governance. *Journal of Nursing Administration, 40*(10), 411–416.

influence on team performance. Team beliefs about self and other team members may impact team learning. Team beliefs include psychological safety, perceived team task interdependence, and group potency (Ortega, Sanchez-Manzanares, Gil, & Rico, 2012), as outlined in the following:

- Psychological safety is the belief that the team is a safe place to take interpersonal risks such as ask questions, express ideas, and voice concerns.
- Team task interdependence is the perceived extent to which team members depend on each other to achieve objectives and demonstrate cooperation, mutual help, and role flexibility.
- Group potency is the shared belief that the team can perform effectively in all areas of the work in which they are involved rather than just have the capacity to meet the task.

Both interprofessional and nurse teamwork have positive consequences for individuals, patients, and organizations. Assisting in supporting the development and maintenance of effective teams is imperative for nursing leaders.

Interprofessional Teamwork

As early as 1998, strategies proposed for the creation of interprofessional practice as a means of decreasing errors and increasing quality appeared in the literature. Current literature supports a widespread interest in interprofessional practice; however, implementation and long-term commitment have been disappointing and attributed to the understanding of leadership issues within the context of interprofessional teams. Research suggests that interprofessional teams may experience friction, hostility, and barriers to knowledge sharing (Mitchell et al., 2011; Suter et al., 2013).

A 2008 concept analysis completed by Xyrichis and Ream provides the following definition of interprofessional teamwork:

> A dynamic process involving two or more health professionals with complementary backgrounds and skills, sharing common health goals and exercising concerted physical and mental effort in assessing, planning, or evaluating patient care. This is accomplished through interdependent collaboration, open communication, and shared decision-making. This in turn generates value-added patient, organizational, and staff outcomes. (p. 238)

Table 2.9 identifies individual, group, and organizational factors impacting interprofessional teams (Willumsen, Ahgren, & Odegard, 2012).

Of utmost importance for leaders in promoting interprofessional teamwork is the need to build psychologically safe environments where all employees feel free to share their knowledge, solve problems, and reflect together. Strategies to improve interprofessional teamwork include organizational development team-training initiatives, team meetings to review treatment plans and receive team feedback, team leadership coaching, and assertiveness training and communication support. One of the most effective training programs for interprofessional teamwork is the joint AHRQ and Department of Defense TeamSTEPPS program (AHRQ, 2014). With more than 20 years of evidence to support the program approach, it provides materials and a full curriculum to integrate teamwork principles into health-care organizations. Training includes skills in leadership, communication, situation monitoring, and mutual support and

TABLE 2.9 Factors Influencing Interprofessional Teams

Individual Factors	Group Factors	Organizational Factors
Work motivation	Leadership	Culture
Role expectations	Coping	Mission
Personality	Communication	Environment
Professional power	Social support	

has been demonstrated to improve teamwork performance, knowledge, and attitudes. Information on the program and contact information is found at teamstepps. ahrq.gov/.

Nursing Teamwork

Teamwork is essential for nursing teams. Nursing teams must not only produce nursing care, but also respond to the many innovations that occur on a daily basis such as clinical guidelines, protocols, and changes in delivery systems. Teams must not only obtain knowledge of these innovations, but must also retrieve and implement the innovations. Rather undergoing than a linear process, nursing teams receive different types of information continually in a crossover fashion, requiring the need for the creation of different learning tasks at different points in time. For instance, nurses might need to understand how to operate a new piece of equipment, while at the same time need to be able to discern when to use this piece of equipment rather than a similar piece of equipment.

A 2012 study from Timmermans, Van Linge, Van Petegem, Van rompacy, and Denekens described a sample of 469 nurses representing 30 nursing teams. The study supported team-learning activities as an important component of addressing innovations that improved patient outcomes, including use of the TeamSTEPPS program (Castner, Foltz-Ramos, Schwartz, & Ceravolo, 2012). The TeamSTEPPS Master Trainer Course is an outstanding opportunity for leaders to prepare to implement a strong team presence in their institution.

Leadership is important in modeling and setting expectations for team interaction and assigning, coordinating, and evaluating team member performance workers. Sorra and Dyer's (2010) study of morethan 50,000 health-care workers found moderate to strong correlation between leadership support and patient safety outcomes. Their study revealed that leadership variables demonstrated greater correlation with patient safety than did communication, handoffs, feedback, staffing, or teamwork.

DIVERSITY

Traditionally, "diversity" has been described as differences in ethnicity and gender. An expanded definition of the concept of diversity may include any attribute that people differ on such as gender, race, ethnicity, functional background, age, sexual orientation, religion, or marital status (Dolan, 2012).

Diversity is a difficult concept to measure. Concepts aligned with diversity include tolerance, cultural competence, and cultural sensitivity. Table 2.10 explores the key similarities among these concepts that align them with diversity. Analyses of these three concepts reveal improved understanding, broadened perspectives, and increased understanding of others leading to improved patient outcomes and workplace satisfaction (Dudas, 2013; Foronda, 2008; Moore & Walker, 2012; Peery et al.,2013).

Workforce Diversity

Workforce diversity has become increasingly important during the past decade. Top management diversity research has attempted to support the premise that high levels

TABLE 2.10 **Diversity Concepts**

Cultural Sensitivity	Tolerance	Cultural Competence
Knowledge	Respect	Awareness
Understanding	Acceptance	Attitude
Respect	Empathy	Behaviors
Consideration	Willingness to allow listen	

of diversity among top management contributes to improve performance. However, a 2013 systematic review on top management team diversity (Homberg & Bui, 2013) reveals that top management diversity alone does not support improved performance, but that organizational policies that work toward equal opportunity and the values of multiculturalism are important to workforce diversity. This research is supported by other organizational research stating that diversity can lead to desirable work outcomes, but only if other human resources initiatives exist that support effective diversity management. Initiatives often include meeting human resources objectives such as attracting and retaining a wider talent pool, reducing labor costs, improving employee satisfaction, and implementing diversity training and mentorships. Research does support that how organizations and employees respond to diversity is determined both by individual and organizational values. Actions of leaders in modeling positive diversity values and practices and procedures that emphasize the value of diversity may contribute to a more positive diversity culture (Guillaume, Dawson, Woods, Sacramento, & West, 2013).

Although we often focus on surface-level diversity, psychological diversity related to values, personality, and attitudes may affect team effectiveness even more greatly. A 2012 study by Woehr, Arciniega, and Poling on the effects of value diversity on team effectiveness revealed 10 value constructs having the potential to impact the ability of a team to work together (Table 2.11).

Diversity is driven by and the responsibility of leadership. Diversity in the workplace is complex and multifaceted. It encompasses both surface diversity, such as age, race and ethnicity, and value diversity, as identified in Table 2.11. Diversity training has been shown to have a positive impact on reducing ethnic discrimination and increasing job satisfaction; however, effective diversity leadership requires focus, communication, passion, and an organizational commitment to the value and vision of a diversity program Pieterse, Knippenberg, & Dierendonck, 2013).

A leader's first step in implementing a diversity program is to determine how the organization defines diversity, what the goals of the diversity initiative should be, and

TABLE 2.11 **Value Constructs**

Value Construct	Example
Power	Likes to be in charge and tell others what to do
Achievement	Likes to stand out and impress others; wants to be seen as successful
Hedonism	Wants to enjoy life and have a good time above all else
Stimulation	Likes to take risks; adventuresome
Self-direction	Curious; wants to understand and learn
Universalism	Justice is important for everyone; everyone should be treated equally
Benevolence	Important to care for people one knows and likes
Tradition	Important to follow family traditions and customs
Conformity	Do what you are told; always follow rules
Security	Safety of country is of upmost importance

Adapted from: Woehr, D., Arciniega, L., & Poling, T. (2012). Exploring the effects of value diversity on team effectiveness. *Journal Business Psychology, 28,* 107–121.

whether such a program is a strategic priority for the organization. The next step is to understand the diversity makeup of the employees and the community: make diversity a part of employment, succession planning, and mentoring; communicate the value of cultural differences among employees and patients; and implement diversity education programs that include strategies to prevent unacceptable or unprofessional behaviors (Bell, 2012; Clapp, 2010).

Eliminating exclusion, prejudices, and misunderstandings based on diversity is not a simple fix. Changing attitudes, habits, and values cannot be accomplished with policy alone. Leaders must actively demonstrate the importance of diversity and their commitment to coworkers and patients on a daily basis.

CONCLUSION

Research supports the premise that work is an effective way to improve the well-being of individuals, their families, and their communities. Work has the opportunity to contribute to both physical and mental health (Black, 2012). This chapter has explored leadership challenges in the workplace that have demonstrated their impact on workforce satisfaction and ultimately patient outcomes. The ability of the leader to develop organizational ethics and emphasize workplace and workforce safety is necessary in today's complex health-care environment. Moreover, a visible, empowering leadership that encourages teamwork and embraces diversity within a shared governance structure is closely related to nurses' level of professional commitment (Lu, Barriball, Zhang, & White, 2012).

References

Agency for Healthcare Research and Quality. (2014). *Patient safety network*. Retrieved from http://psnet.ahrq.gov/primer.aspx?primerID=5

Agency for Healthcare Research and Quality. (2015). TeamSTEPPS. Retrieved from http://teamstepps.ahrq.gov/aboutnationalIP.htm

American Nurses Association. (2010). *Guide to the code of ethics for nurses: Interpretation and application*. Retrieved from http://www.nursesbooks.org/Main-Menu/Ethics/Guide-to-the-Code-of-Ethics-for-Nurses.aspx

American Nurses Credentialing Center. (2014). *14 forces of magnetism*. Retrieved from http://nursecredentialing.org/Magnet/ProgramOverview/HistoryoftheMagnetProgram/ForcesofMagnetism

Arnaud, A., & Schminke, M. (2012). The ethical climate and context of organizations: A comprehensive model. *Organization Science, 23*(6), 1767–1780.

Aytac, S., & Dursun, S. (2012). The effect on employees of violence climate in the workplace, *Work, 41*, 3026–3031.

Ballard, N. (2010). Factors associated with success and breakdown of shared governance. *Journal of Nursing Administration, 40*(10), 411–416.

Baran, B. E., & Scott, C. W. (2010). Organizing ambiguity: A grounded theory of leadership and sensemaking within dangerous contexts. *Military Psychology, 22*(Suppl. 1), S42–S69.

Barter, M. (2010, April). Organizational support for safety programs: Lessons from the military and airline industry. *Nurse Leader, 8*(2), 35–39.

Bayley, B. (2012). Organizational ethics training: A proactive perspective. *Journal for Quality and Participation, 7*, 15–21.

Bean, S. (2011). Navigating the murky intersection between clinical and organizational ethics: A hybrid case taxonomy. *Bioethics, 25*(6), 320–325.

Becker, J., & Visovsky, C. (2012). Horizontal violence in nursing. *MEDSURG Nursing, 21*(4), 210–232.

Bjarnason, D., & LaSala, C. (2011). Moral leadership in nursing. *Radiology Nursing, 30*(1), 18–24.

Black, C. (2012). Why healthcare organizations must look after their staff. *Nursing Management, 19*(6),

Blake, N. (2012). A model of authentic leadership to promote a healthy workplace. *AACN Advanced Critical Care, 23*(4), 358–361.

Bohan, P., & Laing, M. (2012). Can leadership behavior affect quality and safety? *British Journal of Healthcare Management, 18*(4), 184–190.

Brand, C., Barker, A., Morello, R., Vitale, M., Evans, S., Scott, I., . . . Cameron, P. (2012). A review of hospital characteristics associated with improved performance. *International Journal for Quality in Health Care, 24*(5), 483–394.

Business ethics. (2008). *Stanford encyclopedia of philosophy*. Retrieved from http://plato.stanford.edu/entries/ethics-business/

Campbell, J., Messing, J., Kub, J., Agnew, J., Fitzgerald, S., Fowler, B., . . . Bolyard, R. (2011). Workplace violence: Prevalence and risk factors in the safe at work study, *Journal of Occupational and Environmental Medicine, 53*(1), 82089.

Castner, J., Foltz-Ramos, K., Schwartz, D., & Ceravolo, D. (2012). A leadership challenge: Staff nurse perceptions after an organizational TeamSTEPPS initiative. *Journal of Nursing Administration, 42*(10), 467–472.

Center, D. (2011). Mandates for patient safety: Are they enough to create a culture of civility in healthcare? *Journal of Continuing Education in Nursing, 42*(1), 17–18.

Ceravolo, D., Schwartz, D., Foltz-Ramos, K., & Castner, J. (2012). Strengthening communication to overcome lateral violence. *Journal of Nursing Management, 20*, 590–606.

Clapp, J. R. (2010). Diversity leadership: The Rush University Medical Center experience. *Hospital Topics, 88*(2), 61–66.

Credo, K., Armenakis, A., Field, H., & Young, R. (2010). Organizational ethics, leader-member exchange, and organizational support: Relationship with workplace safety. *Journal of Leadership & Organizational Studies, 17*(4), 325–334.

Croft, R., & Cash, P. (2012). Deconstructing contributing factors to bullying and lateral violence in nursing using a postcolonial feminist lens. *Contemporary Nurse, 42*(2), 226–242.

Cummings, G., MacGregor, T., Davey, M., Lee, H., Wong, C., Lo, E., . . . Stafford, E. (2010). Leadership styles and outcome patterns for the nursing workforce and work environment: A systematic review. *International Journal of Nursing Studies, 47*, 363–385.

De Schrijver, A., Delbeke, K., Maesschalck, J., & Pleysier, S. (2010). Fairness perceptions and organizational misbehavior: An empirical study. *American Review of Public Administration, 40*(6), 691–703.

Dolan, T. (2012). Inclusion for all. *Healthcare Executive*, July/August, 6.

Dudas, K. (2013). Cultural competence: An evolutionary concept analysis. *Nursing Education Perspectives, 33*(5), 317–322.

Dunbar, B., Park, B., Berger-Wesley, M., Cameron, T., Lorenz, B., Mayes, D., & Ashby, R. (2007). Shared governance: Making the transition in practice and perception. *Journal of Nursing Administration, 37*(4), 177–183.

Ethical issues at an organizational level. (2014, June 27). Boundless Business. Retrieved from https://www.boundless.com/business/textbooks/boundless-business-textbook/business-ethics-and-social-responsibility-3/business-ethics-33/ethical-issues-at-an-organizational-level-174-7767/

Erickson, J., Ditomassi, M., & Jones, D. Interdisciplinary institute for patient care: Advancing clinical excellence. *Journal of Nursing Administration, 38*(6), 308–314.

Fabry, D. (2015). Hourly rounding: Perspectives and perceptions of the frontlinenursing staff *Journal of Nursing Management, 23*, 200–210.

Florea, L., Cheung, Y., & Herndon, N. (2013). For all good reasons: Role of values in organizational sustainability. *Journal Business Ethics, 114*, 393–408.

Fore, A., & Sculli, A. (2013) A concept analysis of situational awareness in nursing. *Journal of Advanced Nursing, 69*(12), 2613–2621. doi:10.1111/jan.12130

Foronda, C. (2008). A concept analysis of cultural sensitivity. *Journal of Transcultural Nursing, 19*(3), 207–212.

Galloway, S. (2010). Assessing your safety culture in seven simple steps. *EHS Today*. Retrieved from http://www.ehstoday.com

Goold, S. (2001). Trust and the ethics of health care institutions. *Hastings Center Report 31*(6), 26–33.

Griffin, C. (2011). Healthy work environments. *MedSurg Matters!, 20*(5), 4–5.

Guillaume, Y., Dawson, J., Woods, S., Sacramento, C., & West, M. (2013). Getting diversity at work to work: What we know and what we still don't know. *Journal of Occupational and Organizational Psychology, 86*, 123–141

Gurt, J., Schwennen, C., & Elke, G. (2011). Health-specific leadership: Is there an association between leader consideration for the health of employees and their strain and well-being? *Work & Stress, 25*(2),108–127.

Hannah, S., Avolio, B., & Walumbwa, F. (2011). Relationships between authentic leadership, moral courage, and ethical and pro-social behaviors. *Business Ethics Quarterly, 21*(4), 555–578.

Hardin, D. (2012). Strategies for nurse leaders to address aggressive and violent events. *Journal of Nursing Administration, 42*(1), 5–7.

Hartung, S., & Miller, M. (2013). Communication and the healthy work environment. *Journal of Nursing Administration, 43*(5), 266–273.

Hess, R., DesRoches, C., Donelan, K., Norman, L., & Buerhaus, P. (2011). Perceptions of nurses in Magnet hospitals, non-Magnet hospitals, and hospitals pursuing Magnet status. *Journal of Nursing Administration, 41*(7/8), 315–323.

Homberg, F., & Bui, H. (2013). Top management & team diversity: A systematic review. *Group and Organization Management, 38*(4), 455–479.

Houser, J., Erkenbrack, L., Handberry, L., Ricker, F., & Stroup, L. (2012). Involving nurses in decisions: Improving both nurse and patient outcomes. *Journal of Nursing Administration, 42*(7/8), 375–382.

Institute of Medicine. (2004). *Keeping patients safe: Transforming the work environment of nurses.* Washington, DC: National Academies Press.

Institute of Medicine. (2011). *Crossing the quality chasm: The IOM Health Care Quality Initiative.* Washington, DC: National Academies Press.

The Joint Commission. Improving patient and worker safety: Opportunities for synergy, collaboration and innovation. Retrieved from http://www.jointcommission.org/

Karsten, M. (2011, August). Patient safety: Commitment versus compliance. *Nurse Leader,* 47–56.

Krause, T. (2005). *Leading with safety.* Hoboken, NJ: Wiley-Interscience.

Kuokkanen, L., & Katajisto, J. (2003). Promoting or impeding empowerment? *Journal of Nursing Administration, 33*(4), 209–215.

Kuoppala, J., Lamminpaa, A., Liira, J., & Vainio, H. (2008). Leadership, job well-being, and health effects: A systematic review and meta-analysis. *Journal of Occupational and Environmental Medicine, 50*(8), 904–915.

Laschinger, H., Wong, C., & Grau, A. (2012). The influence of authentic leadership on newly graduated nurses' experience of workplace bullying, burnout, and retention outcomes: A cross-sectional study. *International Journal of Nursing Studies, 49,* 1266–1676.

Lawrence, T., & Maitlis, S. (2012). Care and possibility: Enacting an ethic of care through narrative practice. *Academy of Management Review, 27*(4), 641–663.

Leonard, M., & Frankel, A. (2010). The path to safe and reliable healthcare. *Patient Education and Counseling, 80,* 288–292.

Lewis, P. (1095). Defining "business ethics": Like nailing Jello to a wall. *Journal of Business Ethics, 4,* 377–383.

Llorens, J. (2010, November). A culture of silence threatens to impede a safer workplace. *Intelligence Communication, 22.*

Lu, H., Barriball, L., Zhang, X., & White, A. (2012). Job satisfaction among hospital nurses revisted: A systematic review. *International Journal of Nursing Studies, 49,* 1017–1038.

Lykens, K., Singh, K., Mains, D., & Lackan, N. (2010). What is patient safety culture? A review of the literature. *Journal of Nursing Scholarship, 42*(2), 156–165.

Martin, P., Gustin, T., Uddin, D., & Risner, P. (2004). Organizational dimensions of hospital nursing practice. *Journal of Nursing Administration, 34*(12), 554–561.

Mason, J., & Wesorick, B. (2011, April). Successful transformation of a nursing culture. *Nurse Leader,* 31–36.

Mele, D. (2011). The firm as a "community of persons": A pillar of humanistic business ethos. *Journal of Business Ethics, 106,* 89–101.

Mitchell, R., Parker, V., & Giles, M. (2011). When do interprofessional teams succeed? Investigating the moderating roles of team and professional identity in interprofessional effectiveness. *Human Relations, 64*(10), 1321–1343.

Moore, H., & Walker, C. (2012). Tolerance: A concept analysis. *Journal of Theory Construction & Testing, 15*(2), 48–52.

Moore, S., & Wells, N. (2010). Staff nurses lead the way for improvement to shared governance. *Journal of Nursing Administration, 40*(11), 477–481.

Nolan, R., Wary, A., King, M., Laam, L., & Hallick, S. (2011). Geisinger's proven care methodology: Driving performance improvement within a shared governance structure. *Journal of Nursing Administration, 41*(5), 226–230.

Occupational Safety and Health Administration. (2014). Workplace violence. Retrieved from https://www.osha.gov/S LTC/workplaceviolence/

Oien, K., Utne, I., & Herrera, I. (2011). Building safety indicators: Part 1—theoretical foundation. *Safety Science, 49*, 148–161.

Ortega, A., Sanchez-Manzanares, M., Gil, F., & Rico, R. (2012). Enhancing team learning in nursing teams through beliefs about interpersonal context. *Journal of Advanced, Nursing, 69*(1), 102–111.

Parsons, M., & Cornett, P. (2011, August). Leading change for sustainability. *Nurse Leader*, 36–43.

Peery, A., Julian, P., Avery, J., & Susan, L. (2013). Diversity must start somewhere: The experience of one college of nursing. *Journal of Cultural Diversity, 20*(3), 120–124,

Pieterse, A., Knippenberg, D., & Dierendonck, D. (2013). Cultural diversity and team performance: The role of team member goal orientation. *Academy of Management Journal, 56*(3), 782–804.

Porter-O'Grady, T. (2004). *Shared governance implementation manual.* St. Louis, MO: Mosby-Year Book.

Ring, L., & Fairchild, R. (2013). Leadership and patient safety: A review of the literature. *Journal of Nursing Regulation, 4*(1), 52–56.

Samnai, A., & Singh, P. (2012). 20 years of workplace bullying research: A review of the antecedents and consequences of bullying in the workplace. *Aggression and Violent Behavior, 17*, 581–589.

Sammer, C., Lykens, K., Singh, K., Mains, D., & Lackan, N. (2010). What is patient safety culture? A review of the literature. *Journal of Nursing Scholarship, 42*(2),156–165.

Schumacher, E., & Wasieleski, D. (2013). Institutionalizing ethical innovation in organizations: An integrated causal model of moral innovation decision processes. *Journal of Business Ethics, 113*, 15–37.

Sorra, J. S., & Dyer, N. (2010). Multilevel psychometric properties of the AHRQ hospital survey on patient safety culture. *BMC Health Services Research, 10*, 199–210.

Spector, P., Zhou, Z., & Xin, C (2014). Nurse exposure to physical and nonphysical violence, bullying, and sexual harassment: A quantitative review. *International Journal of Nursing Studies, 51*(1), 72–84.

Start, R., Wright, B., Murphy, M., McIntosh, E., & Catrambone, C. (2013). Building a strong shared governance foundation. *American Nurse Today, 8*(11), 14–15.

Stumpf, L. (2001). A comparison of governance types and patient satisfaction outcomes. *Journal of Nursing Administration, 31*(4), 196–202.

Suter, E., Goldman, J., Martimianakis, T., Chatalalsingh, C., DeMatteo, D., & Reeves, S. (2013). The use of systems and organizational theories in the interprofessional field: Findings from a scoping review. *Journal of Interprofessional Care, 27*, 57–64.

Thiel, C., Bagdasarov, Z., Harkrider, L., & Mumford, M. (2012). Leader ethical decision-making in organizations: Strategies for sensemaking. *Journal Business Ethics, 107*, 49–64.

Timmermans, O., Van Linge, R., Van Petegem, P., Van Rompacy, B., & Denekens, J. (2012). A contingency perspective on team learning and innovations in nursing. *Journal of Advanced Nursing, 69*(2), 363–373.

Twigg, D., & McCullough, K. (2014). Nurse retention: A review of strategies to create and enhance positive practice environments in clinical settings. *International Journal of Nursing Studies, 51*, 85–92.

Upenieks, V., & Sitterding, M. (2008). Achieving Magnet redesignation: A framework for cultural change. *Journal of Nursing Administration, 38*(10), 419–428.

Van Der Wal, Z. (2011). The content and context of organizational ethics. *Public Administration, 89*(2), 644–660.

Verdorfer, A., Weber, W., Unterrainer, C., & Seyr, S. (2013). The relationship between organizational democracy and socio-moral climate: Exploring effects of the ethical context in organizations. *Economic and Industrial Democracy, 34*(3), 423–449.

Viinamaki, O. (2012). Embedding value-based organization: An identification of critical success factors and challenges. *International Journal of Management Science and Information Technology, 1*(3), 37–67.

Wheeler, A., Halbesleben, J., & Shanine, K. (2010). Eating their cake and everyone else's cake too: Resources as the main ingredient to workplace bullying. *Business Horizons, 53*, 553–560.

Willumsen, E., Ahgren, B., & Odegard, A. (2012). A conceptual framework for assessing interorganizational integration and interprofessional collaboration. *Journal of Interprofessional Care, 26*, 198–204.

Woehr, D., Arciniega, L., & Poling, T. (2012). Exploring the effects of value diversity on team effectiveness. *Journal Business Psychology, 28*, 107–121.

Xyrichis, A., & Ream, E. (2008). Teamwork: A concept analysis. *Journal of Advanced Nursing, 61*(2), 232–241

3

Leading in Policy and Regulation

The world of nursing has dramatically changed over the past 50 years, including nurses' scope of practice, health-care settings, and health-care policies. One aspect of nursing that has remained constant, however, is the nurse's role as patient advocate. As the health-care system evolves, the nurse remains at the center of all actions related to the delivery of health care. Understanding the political facets of their role in health care will be paramount for nurses as we determine the future of the U.S. health-care system.

During this turbulent time in health care, nurses will be asked to sit at the decision-making table, and they must be able to articulate their unique perspective. Leaders should ask themselves, "As I review my role of registered nurse, do I see myself fulfilling all aspects of that role?" Although the majority of this chapter explores the role of the leader as it pertains to policy and regulation, it is imperative that all nurses understand the importance of advocacy for patients, the health-care system, health education, and epidemiological data trends in society.

The American Nurses Association (ANA) defines the registered nurse's (RN) role as follows. The RN is the only health-care professional who is specifically educated to:

- assess the patient to determine health status and risks, unhealthy lifestyles, minor health problems, and health education needs for patients and their families
- provide support and reassurance while caring for present and potential health problems
- advocate for primary and preventative care services (2013c, p. 4)

As advanced practice nurses (APNs) with master's degrees or higher, we must be prepared to be the voice for patient advocacy, nursing, and health care. The nursing profession is recognized for its noble mission of caring for all in a competent and ethical manner. The political arena is where we can advocate for improved outcomes and patient-care environments.

The nursing profession's undergraduate curriculum has shown only limited emphasis on the importance of the nurse's role in policy and advocacy. However, in graduate nursing education, nurses are given ever-bigger doses of policy and some of its fundamental processes. In fact, in its essentials for the bachelor of science in nursing (BSN), master of science in nursing (MSN), and doctor of nursing practice (DNP) degrees, the American Association of Colleges of Nursing (AACN) states that policy and advocacy are *fundamental* components of the curriculum. As nurses continue their education and obtain higher degrees, the importance of advocacy for the profession and discipline of the nursing profession likewise grows. As a contribution to the importance of sharing information on policy and politics with advanced degree nurses, this chapter prepares graduate students as a voice for nursing to ultimately drive the political process. See Reflection Box 3.1.

CRITICAL ANALYSIS OF POLICY AND REGULATION

As nurse leaders from practice or academia, we must feel comfortable participating in political processes. Whether responding to a proposed bill, developing a position statement, testifying at a legislative committee, or lobbying for a professional organization, being prepared to discuss and address the issues will provide the profession a path to political change.

Advocacy

"Advocacy" can be defined as a wide range of activities undertaken in support of individuals, families, systems, communities, and issues. As nurses, we advocate for patient and employee safety, best practices in health care, and improved health-care outcomes.

Although some nurses are actively engaged in the advocacy role, others have experienced barriers to becoming a voice to a cause or political position. Indeed, nursing as a licensed and regulated profession may be subject to many more barriers than are other, less regulated professions. Nurses may also walk a tightrope when balancing advocacy for patients with loyalty to their place of practice. In the academic arena, colleges of nursing educate all degree levels about nurses' roles in advocacy (although, as mentioned, the extent deepens at higher-level degrees). This advocacy can be related to patients (patient safety), nurse peers (healthy work environments), and professional organizations. The AACN provides essentials or standards through the Commission on Collegiate Nursing Education, the accreditation arm of its organization. Policy and advocacy are integrated in all of its accreditation standards.

REFLECTIONS 3.1 **Patient Advocacy**

As an APN, do you see yourself and your peers as a voice for patient advocacy? Make a list of political actions that you either personally vocalized or voiced through a professional organization.

Policy

"Policy" is a course of action taken by an individual or group dealing with a problem (Anderson, 2006). Policies are created in all legislative bodies, from small town councils and committees to the federal government. Definitions of policy differ based on context, such as public, private, and social realms. Examples of public policy initiatives, such as the Patient Protection and Affordable Care Act (PPACA), are discussed in the following sections.

Two other types of policies can be enacted when private concerns fail to achieve public objectives. *Allocative policy* is designed to provide benefits to a specific group, an example of which is the Medicare Act of 1965. *Regulatory policy* is used to influence behaviors of individuals or groups. The 1996 Health Insurance Portability and Accountability Act (HIPAA) focused on patient confidentiality and improvement of continuity and portability of health insurance coverage (Porter-O'Grady & Malloch, 2013)

Finally, *political analysis* measures the outcome of a policy related to political, social, economic, legal, or ethical aspects of proposed or instituted policies (Mason, Leavitt, & Chaffee, 2011). With their unique understanding of the importance of relationship building and detailed assessment, nurses have an advantage when engaging in political analysis. Both skills are imperative to the success of their political agenda. Knowing the health-care system, their analysis of how this potential policy will affect delivery of care and possible unforeseen consequences is a skill that most policy makers do not possess. Belonging to their professional political action groups provides them a voice and a way to reach legislators for potential modification of a bill before it is passed.

Patient Protection and Affordable Care Act

Enacted in March 2010, the PPACA is designed to improve the health-care system by improving and coordinating care, implementing technology and quality monitoring, and ensuring use of health-care teams' full scope of practice parameters (Box 3.1). It guarantees access to seamless quality affordable health care for all Americans, provides clinical practice incentives, and modifies the payment system to value and reward improved outcomes (Kocher, Emanual, & DeParle, 2010).

Accountable care organizations (ACOs) are voluntary networks of health-care providers that can slow the amount of spending while improving the quality of services. ACOs are key components of the PPACA. These financial reward systems are based on a local group of health-care professionals who agree to coordinate the quality of care delivered to a defined population. These providers should include at least the primary care physician, specialists, and hospital of choice. By delivering coordinated care, the ACO achieves its quality targets and receives a financial bonus from third-party payers but, conversely, can be fined for failing to meet their objectives (Mason et al., 2011).

American Recovery and Reinvestment Act

The American Recovery and Reinvestment Act of 2009 removes barriers to delivery of high-quality health care, such as unnecessary administrative oversight and limited access to primary care clinicians, and provides access to usable clinical data for outcome management and ultimate improvement. Such data include shared clinical outcomes, drug reconciliations, and alerts.

BOX 3.1 **PPACA and the Future of Health Care**

On March 23, 2010, the Patient Protection and Affordable Care Act (PPACA) was signed into law. The PPACA and the reconciliation bill that provided additional information are together considered the most significant social legislation since the 1965 passing of the Medicare bill. The PPACA starts the process of providing universal health care for up to 32 million adults by 2019. As of 2016, the PPACA has resulted in health-care insurance coverage for an estimated 20.0 million American adults who benefit broadly across racial and ethnic groups, an increase of 2.4 million since 2015 (U.S. Department of Health and Human Services, 2016). This policy initiative reduced the uninsured rate for nonelderly adults (aged 18–64 years) by 43% and has had a direct positive impact on health maintenance in the United States. The bill excludes insurance companies from denying coverage for costly illness or preexisting conditions and cannot apply lifetime caps on coverage. The landmark legislation will also have an effect on the U.S. health-care delivery system. To improve the U.S. health-care system outcomes, we must remodel the system to include a focus on health promotion, wellness, disease prevention, and management of chronic care (Katz, 2009).

Health Insurance Portability and Accountability Act

HIPAA provided guidance to the use, technology, and storage of health information as well as patients' rights to confidentiality. The law also made improvements related to the portability of health insurance coverage. Issues that are addressed in the law include the use and release of photographs and authorization of release of information that includes phone or in-person communication.

The Future of Nursing: Leading Change, Advancing Health

The 2010 report *The Future of Nursing: Leading Change, Advancing Health* was the result of a 2-year initiative by the Robert Wood Johnson Foundation and the Institute of Medicine (IOM) to evaluate and transform the nursing profession to accommodate the future of nursing. The following four recommendations resulted from their initiative:

1. Nurses should practice to the full extent of their education.
2. Nurses should achieve higher levels of education and training through an improved educational system that promotes seamless academic progression.
3. Nurses should be full partners with physicians and other health-care professionals in redesigning heath care in the United States.
4. Effective workforce planning and policy making require better data collection and information infrastructure (IOM, 2013).

Policy Process

The four components of the policy process provide the APN with a structure for getting the attention of the legislature and/or other branches of the federal government and encompass agenda setting, government response, policy and program implementation, and policy and program evaluation.

Step 1: Agenda Setting

This initial step includes the problem definition and problem statement and involves identifying and framing the problem from different sources. APNs must become comfortable speaking with legislators on health-care topics within a limited time frame (usually no more than 5 minutes) to present their talking points.

In preparing to speak to legislators on the topic of funding for type 2 diabetes, for example, the advocate should research the current literature and state of the problem as it relates to the health-care system in the United States. What is the cost to society? The presentation should include bulleted talking points to help the nurse advocate stay on topic and to be concise (less than 5 minutes). So that the legislators can review the presentation later, the nurse advocate should provide a handout that outlines his or her main talking points and also includes his or her contact information.

Step 2: Government Response

The response usually comes in the form of laws, regulations, and programs that are designed to address public health concerns. The legislative branch of the federal government (the Senate and the House of Representatives) uses a committee format to hear proposed bills. The process is not clear cut, and many interested parties try to influence the progression of the bill. The committee structure is very powerful, and the lobbying efforts of interest groups become apparent when the bill is passing through committee and undergoes the various changes that each group requests. Government programs are usually a legislative joint effort based on a design that includes budgetary concerns, agency selection, criteria for eligibility, and political feasibility, of which the passing of PPACA is a prime example.

President Barack Obama was not the first president to try to pass a health-care reform bill—Democratic presidents such as Harry Truman, Lyndon Johnson, Jimmy Carter, and Bill Clinton had all tried to garner bipartisan support for health-care reform with no success. However, when the effects of the economy and rising health-care costs (such as those associated with type 2 diabetes and its many comorbidities) combined with powerful stakeholder backing from employers, corporations, and insurance companies, the bill was finally able to pass.

Step 3: Policy and Program Implementation

It is important to remember that the implementation process of policies or programs is not linear. In this phase, it is paramount for content experts to voice their opinions on the particulars prior to and during planning. Legislative representatives will look to experts to weigh in on the feasibility and technology concerns and, most important, to provide feedback about meeting the needs of the population earmarked for this service. For program funding for patients with type 2 diabetes mellitus, the legislature might call upon endocrinologists, certified diabetes educators, registered dietitians, exercise specialists, and their professional organizations for their expert input. Nurses, moreover, are the experts in the area of access to care among underserved and uninsured populations and must articulate their experiences and ideas to the legislature.

Step 4: Policy and Program Evaluation

This important stage addresses whether the policy or program accomplished what it was intended to do—that is, did it meet the public need by creating resources to address an ever-present societal issue? Evaluation is based on data collection, which should start prior to program implementation. Comparing these data with after-implementation data provides sound evaluation principles. "Evaluation is conducted 'to benefit the human condition to improve profit, to amass influence and power, or to achieve other goals'" (Rossi & Freeman, 1995, p. 6).

Policy evaluation is important because it proves through data that the policy was or was not effective in delivering the service. This becomes critical when the opportunity for continued funding may be at risk. If funding for a type 2 diabetes education program is contingent on patients lowering their hemoglobin A_{1c} blood levels within 6 months of participation, data representing that improvement must be available.

POLITICS

"Politics" is a term that is sometimes used interchangeably with policy; however, their two definitions are actually quite distinct. *Politics* is an action and process that drive the legislative agenda. Through political action, the influence of positions for and against is developed with the emphasis on a political outcome. It is the political voice that takes a stand on an issue and articulates why the issue is important to society, culture, human rights, and health care. For nurses with advanced practice and graduate education, this verbalization is referred to as "professional advocacy." Professional advocacy is a fundamental component of a profession or discipline. The ability to unemotionally address facts related to a proposed bill provides the legislature and the public with valid issues to think about before committing to the political action.

Nurses have historically responded to political actions, and our national nursing organizations are committed to providing the voice of nursing on multiple political issues. Lobbying, testifying to the legislature, grassroots education, and using evidence-based research data to support their political stand have been successful. Advancing nurses' political leadership includes developing skills such as networking, strategic planning, and agenda setting, all of which assist with their ability to respond to legislative and regulatory priorities, develop successful political strategies, and educate colleagues. The ANA created the American Nurses Advocacy Institute as a prestigious mentoring program for the purpose of developing nurses as political leaders. The submission requirements for this yearlong program include endorsement by a state nursing organization and full-time membership in the ANA and the state nurse association or student nurse association. Alumni of this prestigious institute are prepared to recommend political action strategies and educate members through the use of multiple sources such as publications, continuing education offerings, and conference presentations. The ANA advocacy resources include the Government Affairs Program Assessment Tool, Political Environment Scan, information on political action committees (PACs) and tracking and interpreting bills, tips on messaging to advance a legislative or regulatory agenda, and a Coalition Building Guide (ANA, 2013b) and can be found at www.nursingworld.org/AdvocacyResourcesTools.

Political Power and Strategies

Influencing the political process can be a daunting task but may be made easier by knowing strategies to assist in influencing and accomplishing the political agenda.

Power is the same as influence in the context of political action. Knowing "who has power, what kind of power, and the extent of power in relation to others" is the essence of influence (Lewenson & Truglio-Londrigan, 2015, p. 212). Influencing the political agenda starts with understanding the complete issue and how it will affect special interest groups. Another strategy is clarifying the position and backing it up with data to show that the nurse is prepared to deliberate the facts of the potential bill. Being concise and clear helps to build consensus for the position—remember that a majority of votes is needed for a successful outcome.

Forms of Political Actions

Political strategies call for long-range planning that is supported by an organization or group of individuals. Using the power in numbers (which means votes) and planning a political initiative call for persistence in getting your message to the power brokers in the legislature. Conveying a consistent message that bombards key stakeholders through multiple sources helps to ensure that your initiative is front and center in their minds. Coalitions, lobbyists, and PACs can assist with getting your message out through various publications, letter campaigns, legislative visits, and networking. A professional nursing organization's political action groups are great resources to propose bills and to advocate your professional organization's stand on the political issues. Talking points are usually available to members to help them articulate the political agenda.

Policy Draft

The policy draft presents an opportunity to weigh in on how the policy will affect society, the individual, and/or the profession. Whether it is a proposed rule or changes in regulation, it is the nurse's professional and societal responsibility to answer the call and provide a voice for the voiceless. The policy draft is a document that explains the proposed bill or rule in detail. This document is named based on the origin of the bill (either House or Senate) with an attached number that allows its progress to be monitored.

Policy Brief

The policy brief (known colloquially as a "one pager"), by contrast, is an excellent tool for communicating core information about an issue related to health care or nursing practice in a clear, concise, overview format. A typical policy brief includes a summary of the issue, background information, and policy alternatives with advantages and disadvantages listed. Frequently, these documents are shared with public entities to influence support for policy action or to make policy makers and/or the public aware of a particular viewpoint related to a proposed law or an existing one. The nurse who is adept at writing a good policy brief plays a powerful role in policy decision making.

This written call to action succinctly outlines the rationale for a political action and is shared with specific organizations and professional groups that have a vested interest in the existing legislative policy. It should be grounded in evidence (for example, peer-reviewed journal references) with proposals for practical application and, if appropriate, nursing implications.

Policy briefs should include the following elements:

- **Key Stakeholders**—This section should be written from the vantage point of those most affected by the proposed bill. Include the bill sponsor and explain the sponsor's motivation for supporting it.
- **Financial Information**—This section should provide supporting financial data that represent the most current information on the subject.
- **Feasibility Factors**—This section is an evaluation of the economic, political, social, and technical justifications of the bill. It should also address the current possibility of the passage of the bill based on current affairs.
- **Nursing Implications**—This section addresses how the bill could affect nursing as a discipline and profession. Patient safety, healthy work environments, and quality measurements should be included.
- **Proposed Recommendations**—This section emphatically states the writer's position on the bill (either for or against) based on feasibility considerations.
- **Evaluation**—How will this bill be monitored going forward and evaluated for stated measured outcomes?
- **Conclusion**—What is the "takeaway" message?

Policy Analysis

Policy analysis usually follows a policy draft by providing an in-depth evaluation of the bill. Policy analysis and recommendations should address how the bill may possibly affect society, communities, organizations, and the individual in order to make the case for or against the policy change. Rarely is there one right or wrong way to proceed, and many times there are trade-offs whereby both sides of the debate get some enhancements. Making a policy analysis provides valuable experience for graduate students as they explore their role and responsibilities as advocates for patients and the profession. Being a voice for nursing is a sub-role of the APN through professional organizations, community activism, running for office, and networking with policy makers who may not have a nurse's knowledge about the possible side effects of passing the proposed bill.

Policy analyses should include the following:

- **Introduction**—This section identifies the organization being represented and clearly identifies the bill being analyzed.
- **Process Definition**—This section clearly states the meanings of any terms that may be misunderstood or unfamiliar, while providing examples of real-life applications. Statistics should be included to show the need for the bill and how it will affect society.
- **Process Analysis**—This section should address both sides of the argument including frequency of the problem, why people are concerned with the issue/bill, and the current impact on the public and the nursing profession.
- **Key Policy Events**—This section provides the history, addressing legislation that preceded this bill.

White Paper

A white paper is usually based on an organization's stand on an issue, how it may affect its members, and its possible short- and long-term effects on society. It concisely outlines the points of consideration that the organization wants to articulate to its audience of interest.

Legislative Visit

These visits usually last less than 5 minutes, so having talking points to keep the message consistent and the presenter on task is vital. The talking points should be left with the legislative representative in the form of a handout. Moreover, even with a scheduled appointment, the representative or senator might not be available, and the presentation is made instead to the legislative aide. A clear, concise handout that the aide can rely on when later conveying the salient points to the lawmaker is a valuable tool.

Letter-Writing Campaign

Letters should expose the legislator to the organization's or individual's views on a particular rule or law.

Networking

One of the most important components associated with political action, networking with legislators and their aides starts before an action is ever requested. Building a relationship with a legislator provides the opportunity for partnership. The partnership is based on mutual needs and provides each party the benefit of the other's expertise in and knowledge of a particular subject. These relationships should be continually cultivated.

Model of Political Action

In recent years, the Framework for Action, which was a model of political action for nurses and uses spheres of influence to graphically depict where nurses can influence policy, has been redesigned to include the workplace and workforce (Mason et al., 2011). The redesigned model demonstrates that nurses work in four spheres of influence that shape health and social policy: (1) the community, (2) the workforce and workplace, (3) the government, and (4) associations and interest groups. The Framework for Action now also includes the categories Health, Health and Social Policy, and Social Determinants of Health.

The Community

Nursing has a rich history of advocating for improvement in the health and well-being of the community it serves. Nurses as leaders in their community have traditionally been activists for societal health rights. Nursing leaders such as Lillian Wald, Dorothea Dix, and Florence Nightingale provided a voice for the societally voiceless by passionately believing in the ethical care of others. "Community" has multiple definitions and can be applied to local, state, regional, and national locations. The nurse's role in the community should include assisting with identification of the problem, using data, implementing strategies for change, and possessing the dedication to see the process to completion. Nurses need to be active in their communities because they offer so much insight and should feel competent to take on a leadership role in areas such as community boards, civic groups, faith-based organizations, and educational associations.

The Workforce and Workplace

Starting with the individual's ability to cast a vote in an election, making the nurse's voice heard through the political process is imperative. Political influence can be based on numbers, which is equivalent to votes. As nurses are positioned to be valuable members of the health-care team and voices for reform, they are seen as change agents and leaders. When nurses abdicate their decision-making power to others, they miss opportunities as well as possibly seeming to be ineffective as leaders. In a 2010 Gallup poll, an issue was identified as a reason that nurses have fallen short in influencing health-care reform: Nursing organizations on a national and state level are working together on issues of workplace safety, quality health care, and interprofessional communication. These joint efforts have the potential to reduce and to minimize health-care errors.

The Government

Government plays an important role in the designing and development of health policy. U.S. health care is considered to be a private sector enterprise, but government controls and regulates payment of such services. Government also influences nursing and nursing practice as a licensed profession. Individual states determine the scope of practice for nursing, with notable exceptions in the federal, veterans', and Indian health and public health services. "Federal and state governments determine who is eligible for care under specific benefits programs and who can be reimbursed for providing care" (Mason et al., 2011, p. 9). By controlling access to care and reimbursement, the government has great power to shape health-care policy. On a national level, the House of Representatives and the Senate have two overarching health committees. The House's Energy and Commerce Committee addresses public health concerns including Medicare and Medicaid, the Department of Health and Human Services, National Institutes of Health, Centers for Disease Control and Prevention, and a subcommittee on Indian Health Services (energycommerce.house.gov/subcommittee/health). The Senate Committee on Health, Education, Labor and Pensions oversees some of the same departments that the House of Representatives oversees but also includes the Agency on Healthcare Research and Quality, the Food and Drug Administration, and the Administration on Aging (www.help.senate.gov). The House Nursing Caucus is an informal group of legislators committed to assisting nursing. They have lobbied for federal funding to address nursing education and for loan-forgiveness programs for nursing faculty. Many similar committee structures exist on the state level and together influence societal health issues.

Associations and Interest Groups

Nursing associations play a significant role in influencing the health-care political agenda. Through their PACs, they provide support for policy change that potentially could affect the future of nursing. Through lobbying efforts, networking, and joining forces on common practice issues, nursing organizations can increase their influence. An example of working together as a coalition is the ANA as a member of Safer Chemicals, Healthy Families. United on common issues concerning toxic chemicals in the workplace and at home, these two groups have worked together to reduce exposure to toxic chemical products such as the persistent bioaccumulative toxicants and formaldehyde we once used daily. Another group that nursing organizations have been active in is the Coalition for Patients' Rights (www.patientsrightscoalition.org/). The coalition represents 35 health-care professional and nursing organizations that are working together to fight the American Medical Association's attempt to limit patient access to nonphysician providers (Coalition for Patients' Rights, 2015). Special interest groups are also influential and could provide a significant political opportunity for a nurse. The nurse educated in leadership and political process may help these groups with potential funding sources through grants and scholarships.

Health

Health is another element of this model insofar as patient optimal health is the ultimate goal for the nursing profession. Through policy development, the profession of nursing can advance the public safety of individuals, families, and populations by promoting access to care and positive health outcomes.

Health and Social Policy
As a new addition to the Framework for Action, health and social policy are represented in the first section of the model, especially because health-care systems and processes are changing so rapidly. Income, education, access to care, and housing as social factors influence society's health status. These factors are paramount to the social health-care agenda.

Social Determinants of Health
The addition of social determinants as they relate to health provides a lens for nurses to see the important role that they play in improving health care. Economic conditions and social factors can affect societal health. The poor and disadvantaged members of society often experience health care differently from the way that more affluent populations do. Based on issues of access to care and uninsured or underinsured status, those at the lower end of the socioeconomic scale have limited or no preventive care, shorter life spans, and minimal political voice. Addressing health-care disparity is a nursing profession responsibility that historically has been a part of our discipline.

REFLECTIONS 3.2 **Policy Process**

Using the policy process steps or the model of political action, provide a dialogue on a current policy issue that is facing health care, nursing, and/or patient access to care. Using the policy process steps, analyze your policy or program issue and suggest improvement strategies for the future.

LEADING THE REGULATORY CHARGE OF HEALTH CARE

It is interesting to consider how and why regulatory oversight is needed in health care. The reality is that the health-care field is not level and appropriate policy processes are essential for the safety and well-being of society. In this section, we discuss a wide range of regulatory concepts that are important to nurses as they continue to evolve in their educational and practice knowledge. Issues such as licensure, examination, endorsement, and certification as well as other important regulatory concepts are discussed.

Nurse Practice Act

The nurse practice act (NPA) of any state is a set of laws that address the actions of the nursing profession and provides governance of a board of nursing for the protection of the public. NPAs in the United States differ from state to state or state to territories, and the nurse is held accountable for knowledge of the act. NPAs are usually written in the form of acceptable scope of practice language and outline minimal requirements for practice. The board of nursing in its judicial capacity interprets and acts based on the authority set forth in the NPA, by the governor, and/or state legislature. The act establishes scope of practice professional standards, educational standards, and licensure, all resulting in the outcome of autonomous practice.

Disciplinary guidelines are also addressed in the NPA and outline the definitions and actions associated with continuing education, supervision, suspension, revocation, and other corrective actions. Disciplinary cases often appear in one of the following categories:

- Practice related: breakdowns or errors during nursing
- Drug related: mishandling, misappropriation, or misuse of controlled substances
- Boundary violations: nontherapeutic relationships formed between a nurse and a client in which the nurse derives a benefit at the client's expense (National Council of State Boards of Nursing, 2011)
- Sexual misconduct: inappropriate physical or sexual contact with a client
- Abuse: maltreatment of clients that is physically, mentally, or emotionally harmful
- Fraud: misrepresentation of the truth for gain or profit (usually related to credentials, time, or payment)
- Positive criminal background checks: detection of reportable criminal conduct as defined by statute (Russell, 2012, p. 39)

Consensus Model for APRN Regulation

The Consensus Model for APRN Regulation: Licensure, Accreditation, Certification & Education, also referred to as the "LACE Model," was developed by the APRN Consensus Work Group and the National Council of State Boards of Nursing (NCSBN) Advisory Committee for the purpose of defining advanced practice registered nurse (APRN) practice. This regulatory model describes roles, titles, specialties, and population foci. The model has been endorsed by more than 40 nursing organizations and provides a national baseline for APRN licensure, accreditation, certification, and education (LACE).

Licensure

Licensure and regulation work together to provide a structure and symmetry to the profession. Licensure first appeared in New Zealand in 1901 as a way to give meaning to the term "trained nurse." In 1903, North Carolina was the first state to pass a law that licensed nurses. New Jersey, New York, and Virginia followed within the same year. This new type of legislation provided protection to the public by establishing standards of practice and recognized the profession and title associated with the term "nurse." The laws from state to state differed and were inconsistently applied. The role of protection to the public was of the highest order and provided the first measurement of quality through regulation.

Starting with the admission process for entry-to-practice education, potential students must meet specific criteria that are measured in a competitive environment. Once accepted, the student will follow a rigorous curriculum, leading to the culminating effort of passing the state board licensure examination. This laborious process leads to meeting the entry-to-practice qualifications of a nurse. The educational continuum of a new licensed nurse starts with a mentored internship and progresses to advanced degrees and certifications. The practice of nursing is sometimes seen by its professional members as a right, but it is also a privilege that needs to be maintained in good standing.

Examination

As nursing students complete the final educational requirements to practice nursing, they must apply to take the National Council Licensure Examination (NCLEX). This testing procedure, which is regulated by member states and territories, provides for the ability for nurses to migrate among states. Each state and territory has a different nurse practice act (NPA) but all use the NCLEX for RNs and licensed practical nurses (LPNs). This process includes applying to the state board of nursing by filling out either the NCLEX-RN or NCLEX-PN application. Part of the application process includes a criminal background check that is reflective of all 50 U.S. states and of U.S. territories. Once students receive the authorization to take the NCLEX, they may schedule the computerized adaptive test specific to their educational preparation. If the student has information on the application that is false or misleading, or the board of nursing requests a personal appearance, the individual is notified in writing of the date and time to appear before the board members. The board decision is then based on the testimony and adherence to the disciplinary guidelines set by the governing state and its NPA. All boards of nursing disciplinary decisions are based on their primary goal of protection of the public.

Certification

Most states require APNs to take a national certification examination that measures their knowledge and skill after completion of the master's degree. This certification examination is recognized as a standard of practice for the ARPN and offers many specialty areas, such as Family Nurse Practitioner and Gerontological/Acute Care. Some states still require an ARNP to have a signed protocol from a physician, but most states allow the ARNP to work as an independent practitioner.

Endorsement

Endorsement is useful when a nurse who is licensed in one jurisdiction wants to apply for a license in another jurisdiction without the requirement of retaking the NCLEX.

The process includes an application verifying that the person has graduated from an accredited school, is proficient in English, has clinical experience, and is of good moral character. Whether criminal activity and/or disciplinary history existed in the home state is investigated. The state in which the additional jurisdiction is located provides an evaluation of education that meets or exceeds the requirement in that state based on the state's NPA.

Multistate licensure compacts (see the following section) also allow for the nurse to practice in more than one state. Nurses who work for the military or the Department of Veterans Affairs are allowed to work using their primary state license in any U.S. state or territory.

Multistate Licensure Compacts

The mutual recognition model allows RNs and LPNs to work in multiple states as long as each state is part of the compact. Nurses must be compliant with the NPA and the nursing licensure compact rules of each state. Nurses must also be in compliance with the scope of practice in the state where they are practicing. Both the home and remote states may take disciplinary action against the nurse's license, and they communicate between the state boards of nursing through the "NURSES" database, to which all 50 states as well as U.S. territories have access.

Only three states (Utah, Texas, and Iowa) have passed laws authorizing APNs to participate in a licensure compact. A separate APN licensure compact has not been implemented (NCSBN, 2011).

Professional Regulations

Professional regulation represents a social contract. Vulnerable citizens, such as the sick, infirm, young, elderly, disabled, and others who are not able to advocate for themselves, have the potential to be endangered by incompetent or unqualified practitioners. Through nursing regulation, the profession is held accountable to the public for its actions. Government oversight through boards of nursing in each state and territory provides this accountability.

Protection of the public is the paramount responsibility of the regulation proceedings. Evaluating the competence of all nursing practitioners through licensure, competency validation, and continuing education is the responsibility of the profession and the government. Boards of nursing are usually made up of members of the profession as well as consumer representation. Through legal due process, all members provide ethical decision making with the goal of protecting the public. Issues that are commonly presented at boards of nursing meetings include individual versus system accountability, standards of care, patient safety, infractions of the NPA, and requests for declaratory statements. Declaratory statements are usually made by a practitioner asking for an opinion from the board on a conflict with scope of practice or a request to advance the scope of practice to include a given procedure.

Based on state laws, state boards of nursing oversee licensure, continuing education requirements, disciplinary procedures, scope of practice issues, professional misconduct, and mandatory reporting requirements. Some boards of nursing also monitor NCLEX passing rates, educational preparation of faculty and administration in the field of nursing, clinical experience in the area of nursing specialization, and available resources of academic institutions to assist with the success of the nursing program. This quality monitoring is all part of the commitment to protect the public.

Governmental Regulations

Both state and national organizations regulate health care. The Department of Health and Human Services (HHS) is the U.S. federal government agency established to protect the health of all Americans. This department with all of its agencies regulates food and drug safety, Medicare and Medicaid programs, health-care fraud, medical research, technology standards, Native American tribal matters, privacy, and civil rights. HHS serves as the umbrella organization for the Centers for Disease Control and Prevention, the Centers for Medicare & Medicaid Services (CMS), the Food and Drug Administration, and the Office of Civil Rights. The Office of Inspector General provides accountability and integrity to all of the programs based on monitoring guidelines (U.S. Department of Health and Human Services, 2014).

The CMS provides health-care programs for qualified individuals. Medicare is the federally funded program that is available to persons aged 65 years and older and those aged under 65 years with established disabilities or end-stage renal disease. Medicaid is a program designed to address health-care issues for low-income individuals and families at the state eligibility level.

The Joint Commission

The Joint Commission (TJC) is an independent, not-for-profit organization that accredits and certifies more than 20,000 health-care organizations in the United States. The standards and survey aspect of its intensive organizational review is supported by CMS because it recognizes the intensive survey approach used by TJC. The standards for review include safety, communication among caregivers, sentinel events, quality improvement initiatives, staffing, credentialing, and nursing performance indicators (TJC, 2014). Through the TJC survey and accreditation process, patient outcomes are reviewed, recorded, and measured to improve the health and well-being of U.S. citizens. This process is considered voluntary, and the cost associated with this survey is paid by the organization. TJC's stated mission "to continuously improve health care for the public, in collaboration with other stakeholders, by evaluating health care organizations and inspiring them to excel in providing safe and effective care of the highest quality and value" (p. 1) is the foundation for the work that the organization provides in the evaluation of safe and quality health care in all settings.

Local Health Departments

Public health departments also monitor laws enacted to promote community health at the state and local levels. Emphasizing emergency preparedness, epidemiological health concerns, utilization of health-care facilities, housing, sanitation, childhood nutrition, and reporting mechanisms, they ensure that the well-being of local residents is monitored. Through state and federal funding, local health departments provide statistical reporting on communicable diseases for observing health trends at the local level.

REFLECTIONS 3.3 **Regulation**

As an APN and active member of the nursing profession, what are your thoughts about the governance of your profession? Do you feel comfortable about regulatory actions that your state legislature or board of nursing has determined to be within the scope of practice for nursing?

LEADERSHIP IN DEVELOPMENT AND IMPLEMENTATION OF INTERNATIONAL, FEDERAL, STATE, AND INSTITUTIONAL HEALTH POLICY

Globalization is the interdependence of the world's citizens based on international effects on the economy, government, culture, and technology. Health-care services as well as the associated professions may be considered as commodities on the international market. Individuals looking for health-care services soon realize that payment for services, care delivery systems, and demonstrated health-care outcomes have wide ranges of benefits to the health-care consumer. As the health-care market becomes smaller as a result of easier access to multiple health-care sources, many countries are expressing an interest in mutual agreements for health-care professionals to practice in multiple countries.

The shortage of health-care personnel has influenced the global health-care agenda. "Today, nearly all nations face a nursing shortage brought about by increasing demand and diminished supply, an aging nursing workforce, shortage of other professional and ancillary staff, increasing acuity of illness, a poor image of nursing, and continuing health sector reform" (Mason et al., 2011, p. 715). There are two types of nursing shortages, a real shortage and a pseudoshortage. The pseudoshortage occurs when the number of nurses in a country is enough to meet the societal needs, but there is limited funding for the posted positions or nurses are not willing to work under poor conditions (World Health Organization, 2014). For example, in South Africa there were 31,000 reported vacancies and 35,000 unemployed nurses. Because of low salaries, poor benefits, unhealthy work environments, diminished supplies and equipment, inadequate nurse/patient ratios, limited professional development opportunities, lack of family-friendly policies, and a limited professional voice for decision making, these unemployed nurses remain in the position of not contributing to societal health-care needs and their profession (International Council of Nurses, 2013a, 2013b, 2013c).

The imbalance of health-care personnel gravely affects the morbidity and mortality rates of the country. Organizations such as the World Health Organization (WHO), International Council for Nurses (ICN), International Centre for Human Resources in Nursing, and the International Confederation of Midwives have worked together since 2006 to host a biennial meeting to address recruitment, retention, regulation, and advocacy (ICN 2013a; WHO, 2014). These key global health-care issues require consistent ideologies across countries to minimize migration based on code of practice. Some national nursing organizations, such as the National League for Nursing (NLN), ICN, and ANA, to list a few, have committed white papers, publications, and position statements to address their stand on globalization, diversity, nurse retention and migration, international trade agreements, ethical nurse recruitment, and scope of practice.

Analyzing nursing and health policies on a global scale calls for a model that provides a comprehensive evaluation of all cultures and countries involved. The Milstead Model (Milstead, 2013) provides this structure for nurse researchers involved in analyzing and evaluating international health-care systems. The components of the international health-care model address international settings, identification of the problem, policy concerns, sociocultural systems, economic and political factors, and evaluation of the health-care system. Using a comparison approach between and among countries, the Milstead Model provides a framework to address complex health-care issues.

International Council of Nursing

The ICN is a federation of national nurse associations representing nurses from more than 130 counties. Nurse-operated since 1898 and located in Geneva, Switzerland, the organization strives to ensure high-quality nursing care and sound global health-care policies, as well as the acknowledgment of a competent nursing profession. The ICN's "mission is to represent nursing worldwide, advancing the profession and influencing health policy" (ICN, 2013e, p. 1). Based on its three stated goals and five core values, the ICN is committed to the improvement of the worldwide view of nursing as a profession. See Table 3.1.

TABLE 3.1   International Council of Nurses Goals and Values

Goals	Values
Bring nursing together worldwide	Visionary leadership
Advance nurses and nursing worldwide	Inclusiveness
Influence health policy	Innovativeness
	Partnership
	Transparency

Source: International Council of Nurses. (2013d). Position statement on scope of nursing practice (p. 1). Retrieved from http://www.icn.ch/publications/position-statements/

The ICN states, "The ICN's Code for Nurses is the foundation for ethical nursing practice throughout the world. ICN standards, guidelines and policies for nursing practice, education, management, research and socio-economic welfare are accepted globally as the basis of nursing policy" (ICN, 2013d, p. 1). Publications such as position statements and the ICN's professional peer-reviewed journal provide the latest information on how nurses and nursing compare on a worldwide stage (ICN, 2013e). See Table 3.2.

National Council of State Boards of Nursing

Founded in 1978 as an independent, 501(c)(3) not-for-profit organization, the NCSBN can trace its roots to the ANA Council on State Boards of Nursing. Based on the premise of public safety, this organization determined that the regulation of nurses needed to be a separate entity from the organization representing professional nurses. Through its commitment to ensure public safety, a determination of effective care by competent licensed nurses is measured through testing, licensure, policy, and regulations. "NCSBN is the vehicle through which boards of nursing act and counsel together on matters of common interest. The member boards are charged with the responsibility of providing regulatory excellence for public health, safety and welfare" (NCSBN, 2011, p. 1). To meet that goal of competent licensed nurses, NCSBN is devoted to developing a psychometrically sound and legally defensible nurse licensure examination consistent with current nursing practice. NCSBN became the first organization to implement computerized adaptive testing (CAT) for nationwide licensure examinations in 1994. In addition to the NCLEX-RN and NCLEX-PN examinations, NCSBN also develops and administers the largest competency evaluation for nurse aides known as the National Nurse Aide Assessment Program. The ongoing assessment of these examinations includes research and data collection that contributes to the tests' currency with the evolving health-care environment. See Table 3.3. Since 1994, more than 2.4 million U.S. candidates for nurse licensure have taken the NCLEX via CAT (NCSBN, 2011).

The Delegate Assembly, NCSBN's voting body, convenes once a year at the organization's annual meeting. The meeting's highlights include discussion and elections for key NCSBN leadership positions. The committee and special committees made up of representatives of member nursing boards address timely regulation and governance issues that affect U.S. state and territory boards of nursing.

State Boards of Nursing

All states and territories in the United States have a state board of nursing that is made up of nondisciplined nurses with a current active license and includes consumer representation. State boards of nursing also address national and international nursing concerns by participating with NCSBN and the ICN. Through NCSBN, each state reports data and outcomes to compare themselves to other states and territories. Their meetings are formal with all actions related to the meeting formally recorded. All communications from state boards of nursing are usually in written format and served via registered mail for proof of receipt. Boards of nursing recognize that to guard the safety of the public is to ensure that nurses entering the workforce have the necessary knowledge and skills to practice.

TABLE 3.2 **International Council of Nurses Code for Nursing**

Professional Nursing Practice	Nursing Regulations	Welfare for Nurses (Socioeconomics)
International Classification for Nursing Practice (ICNP)	Regulations and credentialing	Occupational health and safety
E-health	Code of ethics, standards, and competencies	Human resources planning and policy
Telenursing	Continuing education	Remuneration
Connecting nurses		Career development
Advanced nursing practice		International trade in professional services
Entrepreneurship		
HIV/AIDS, tuberculosis, and malaria		
Women's health		
Primary health care		
Family health		
Safe water		

Source: International Council of Nurses. (2013d). Position statement on scope of nursing practice (p. 1). Retrieved from http://www.icn.ch/publications/position-statements/

TABLE 3.3 **National Council of State Boards of Nursing Mission, Vision, and Values**

Mission	Vision	Values
To provide education, service, and research through collaborative leadership to promote evidence-based regulatory excellence for patient safety and public protection	Advance regulatory excellence worldwide	**Collaboration:** Forging solutions through respect, diversity, and the collective strength of all stakeholders. **Excellence:** Striving to be and do the best. **Innovation:** Embracing change as an opportunity to better all organizational endeavors and turning new ideas into action. **Integrity:** Doing the right thing for the right reason through honest, informed, open, and ethical dialogue. **Transparency:** Demonstrating and expecting openness, clear communication, and accountability of processes and outcomes.

Source: National Council of State Boards of Nursing. (2011). About NCSBN (p. 2). Retrieved from https://www.ncsbn.org/about.htm

LEADING TO INFLUENCE OTHERS: NURSING ORGANIZATIONS WITH A POLITICAL VOICE

Many professional nursing organizations provide a venue for political action. As members of a professional organization, nurses are provided a political voice through lobbying efforts; power in numbers; and national, state, and local recognition. The benefit to joining a national professional organization is that it provides a platform for nurses from all practice settings to share, discuss, and debate issues that have a potential effect on the profession and health care.

American Association of Colleges of Nursing

The AACN is a recognized professional organization with a national voice in the areas of nursing education, research, advocacy, and publications. The AACN's quality standards for nursing education are internationally recognized and contribute to the nursing profession's influence on improved health care by providing a structure for ongoing evaluation. The essentials document that provides curriculum standards uses a consensus-based process that provides competency benchmarks for baccalaureate, MSN, and DNP programs. Through the AACN's accreditation program, nursing programs can ensure the public that they adhere to the highest standards of nursing education (AACN, 2013b). Other publications from the AACN include quality indicators, white papers, and guidelines outlining clinical resources for nursing education, research, and practice, all emphasizing the impact of educational preparation on nursing and health care.

As an advocacy voice for nursing, the AACN is active in its oversight of public policy related to nursing education, research, and practice. Organization members benefit from the AACN's innovative approach to nursing education legislation, regulatory policies, continuing education for faculty development, and funding for nursing students' financial support. National meetings, webinars, and conferences provide ongoing resources for best practices and address current issues affecting nursing education programs. Through the organization's grant funding, special projects addressing current nursing education issues promote advancing the science of nursing education.

American Nurses Association

The PAC of the ANA is a bipartisan approach to support regulatory actions that align with the goals of the ANA. The ANA-PAC also seeks funding for endorsed candidates who demonstrate support for legislation and regulatory actions to improve health care.

The ANA's organizational goals include providing for the nursing profession's needs and establishing the following:

- *Code of Ethics for Nurses with Interpretive Statements*
- *Nursing's Social Policy Statement*
- *Nursing: Scope and Standards of Practice* (ANA, 2013c)

The power of one voice is seen through its 21 nursing organizations' affiliations that monitor and provide education to its numerous membership nationally, which include the American Association of Critical-Care Nurses; the American Association of Nurse Anesthetists; the American Psychiatric Nurses Association; the American Association of periOperative Registered Nurses; the Association of Women's Health, Obstetrics and Neonatal Nurses; the Emergency Nurses Association; the Association of Rehabilitation Nurses; the National Association of Orthopaedic Nurses; and the Oncology Nursing Society (ANA, 2013a). Through their ANA membership and the membership of the affiliate nursing organizations, nurses are exposed to current and future issues affecting the profession, research, and professional guideline references.

American Organization of Nurse Executives

The American Organization of Nurse Executives (AONE) is an organization that gives a nurse leadership voice to health care by providing leadership, professional development, advocacy, and research to advance nursing practice and patient care; promote nursing leadership excellence; and shape public policy for health care nationwide. AONE is a subsidiary of the American Hospital Association and has been in existence since 1967 for the purpose of shaping health care through innovative and expert nursing leadership (AONE, 2013). See Table 3.4.

TABLE 3.4 **American Organization of Nurse Executives Mission, Vision, and Values**

Mission	Vision	Values
To shape health care through innovative and expert nursing leadership	Global Nursing Leadership–One Voice Advancing Health	Providing vision and actions for nursing leadership to meet the health-care needs of society. Influencing legislation and public policy related to nursing and patient-care issues. Offering member services that support and enhance the management, leadership, educational, and professional development of nursing leaders. Facilitating and supporting research and development efforts that advance nursing administration practice and quality patient care.

Source: American Organization of Nurse Executives. (2012). AONE advocacy (p. 1). Retrieved from http://www.aone.org/advocacy/index.shtml

AONE also values state perspectives on nursing leadership issues. Through its state affiliations, networks of nurse leaders meet to address state and local issues. At its annual conference, all state affiliations convene to address national and international issues facing our nurse leaders including legislation, research, and practice. As a national nursing organization, AONE also provides its members with access to the ongoing committees and task forces that are addressing current nursing and health-care issues (Box 3.2).

National League for Nursing

The NLN is dedicated to excellence in nursing education and to supporting nurse faculty and leaders. As members of this organization, nurses are offered opportunities in program development, nursing research grants, public policy initiatives, and networking. Delivering improved, enhanced, and expanded services to its 33,000 individual and 1,200 institutional members is the NLN's philosophy. "Founded in 1893, under the name The American Society of Superintendents of Training Schools of Nursing, the NLN was the first nursing organization in the United States" (NLN, 2013b, p. 1).

The organization encourages all nurses to become active members and to use their voice and actions to support nursing. The NLN's Government Affairs Action Center

---

BOX 3.2 AONE 2013 Committees and Task Forces

Abstract Review Task Force

Bylaws Committee

Diversity on Board Task Force

Early Career Professionals Task Force

Education Committee

Foundation Education Committee

Foundation Research Committee

Health Care Worker Safety Taskforce

Industry Partner Taskforce

International Committee

Membership Committee

Nominations Committee

Political Action Committee

Publications Committee

Strategic Planning Committee

Technology Committee

Value of Nursing Task Force (AONE, 2013, p. 2)

---

provides an avenue for nurses to review proposed legislative bills and projected hearing schedules. The NLN encourages nurses to provide feedback on legislative issues related to current nursing education and political perspectives. Through the organization's commitment to the advancement of nursing education, the NLN will be a voice to shape and influence the future of nursing and tomorrow's health-care system.

Specialty Nursing Organizations

Many nurses feel a connection to their nursing specialty group or practice setting. Based on policies and standards set by these specialty nursing organizations, nurses are able to connect on a national, state, or local level with nurses who work in the same environment. Sharing the issues that face the nurse, health care, and patient populations provides networking opportunities that are based on evidence-based practice initiatives, research, and policy making. Many of the more than 100 specialty nursing organizations offer education, advocacy, and research opportunities for their members.

Nursing Organizations Alliance

Internships and fellowships provide a valuable service to the politically minded nurse advocate. By providing active learning opportunities, they mentor the nurse through the political process. Networking is another valuable skill that this hands-on approach provides. By being exposed to individuals who are active in the political process, interns or fellows begin to establish professional and personal relationships that will be invaluable in their political future. The Nurse in Washington Internship is a great example of a Nursing Organizations Alliance (NOA) program that is designed to facilitate politically minded nurses to develop dialogue on policy. Topics included in this internship span most aspects of the political process, including legislation, influencing policy and politics, working with legislative staff, networking with nursing organizations on common political issues, economic factors affecting policy, and special interest groups and their effects on society (NOA, 2013).

REFLECTIONS 3.4 **Political Action**

Professional membership in nursing organizations has many benefits. Based on your personal political action history, provide a trajectory of political action over the past 5 years outlining the issues with which you have been involved and the action steps you have taken.

CONCLUSION

APNs have an opportunity to be a voice of reason. Prepared for multiple roles, the APN has been educated as a direct care provider, researcher, consultant, educator, administrator, and advocate (Milstead, 2013). A study that interviewed nurses who were considered politically active confirmed that political skills such as persuasion, effective use of power, addressing barriers, and mobilizing support are all skills that can be learned and are invaluable (Gebbie, Wakefield, & Kerfoot, 2000). Being exposed to the political process as early as possible, believing in oneself, preparing educationally, having role models, and being mentored all provide the foundation for political activism. APNs should be knowledgeable about current legislative efforts and should know how to make their opinions known.

According to the AACN's Essentials of Doctoral Education for Advanced Nursing Practice, doctoral candidates should use their advanced knowledge of the profession of nursing to advocate for health-care access, quality, and reform:

> Political activism and a commitment to policy development are central elements of professional nursing practice, and the DNP graduate has the ability to assume a broad leadership role on behalf of the public as well as the nursing profession. (AACN, 2006, p.13)

Most state legislative Web sites list representatives by zip code. Get to know your legislators through individual or professional organization contacts because they are vital when support is needed for your political agenda. Do not be afraid to be the voice for your profession, community, or a particular cause. You may even consider running for office—believe that you can make a difference!

References

Accreditation Commission for Education in Nursing. (2013). Mission/purpose/goals. Retrieved from http://acenursing.org/mission-purpose-goals/

American Association of Colleges of Nursing. (2013a). AACN mission and values. Retrieved from http://www.aacn.nche.edu/about-aacn/vision-mission

American Association of Colleges of Nursing. (2013b). CCNE accreditation. Retrieved from http://www.aacn.nche.edu/ccne-accreditation

American Nurses Association. (2010). *Nursing: Scope and standards of practice* (2nd ed.). Silver Springs, MD: Nursesbooks.org.

American Nurses Association. (2011). *Nursing administration: Scope and standards of practice* (2nd ed.). Silver Springs, MD: Nursesbooks.org.

American Nurses Association. (2013a). Advocacy—Becoming more effective. Retrieved from http://www.nursingworld.org/AdvocacyResourcesTools

American Nurses Association. (2013b). Policy & advocacy. Retrieved from http://www.nursingworld.org/MainMenuCategories/Policy-Advocacy

American Nurses Association. (2013c). About ANA. http://www.nursingworld.org/FunctionalMenuCategories/AboutANA

American Nurses Association. (2014). *Guide to code of ethics for nurses: Interpretation and application* (3rd ed.). Silver Springs: Nursesbooks.org.

American Organization of Nurse Executives. (2012). AONE advocacy. Retrieved from http://www.aone.org/advocacy/index.shtml

Anderson, J. (2006). *Public policymaking: An introduction* (6th ed.). Boston, MA: Houghton Mifflin.

Coalition for Patient Rights. (2015) Advocacy and legislation. Retrieved from http://www.patientsrightscoalition.org/Main-Menu/Advocacy-Legislation Gallup

Gebbie, K. M., Wakefield, M., & Kerfoot, K. (2000). Nursing and health policy. *Journal of Nursing Scholarship, 32*(3), 307–315.

Institute of Medicine. (2010). *The future of nursing: Leading the charge, advancing health.* Retrieved from http://www.iom.edu/Reports/2010/The-future-of-nursing-leading-change-advancing-health.aspx

International Council of Nurses. (2013a). Position statement on ethical nurse recruitment. Retrieved from http://www.icn.ch/publications/position-statements/

International Council of Nurses. (2013b). Position statement on international trade agreements. Retrieved from http://www.icn.ch/images/stories/documents/publications/position_statements.pdf

International Council of Nurses. (2013c). Position statement on nurse retention and migration. Retrieved from http://www.icn.ch/publications/position-statements/

International Council of Nurses. (2013d). Position statement on scope of nursing practice. Retrieved from http://www.icn.ch/images/stories/documents/publications/position_statements/B07_Scope_Nsg_Practice.pdf

International Council of Nurses. (2013e). Who We Are. Retrieved from http://www.icn.ch/who-we-are/who-we-are/

The Joint Commission. (2014). About The Joint Commission. Retrieved from www.jointcommission.org/about_us/about_the_joint_commission_main.aspx

Katz, M. H. (2009). Structural interventions for addressing chronic health problems. *JAMA, 302*(6), 683–685.

Kocher, R., Emanual, E. J., & DeParle, N. A., (2010). The Affordable Care Act and the future of clinical medicine: The opportunities and challenges. *Annals of Internal Medicine, 153*(8), 536–539.

Lewenson, S. B., & Truglio-Londrigan, M. (2015). *Decision-making in nursing: Thoughtful approaches for leadership* (2nd ed.). Sudbury, MA: Jones & Bartlett.

Mason, D. J., Leavitt, J. K., & Chaffee, M. W. (2011). *Policy & politics in nursing and health care* (6th ed.). St Louis, MO: Elsevier Saunders.

Milstead, J. A. (2013). *Health policy and politics: A nurse's guide* (4th ed.). Burlington, MA: Jones & Bartlett.

National Council of State Boards of Nursing. (2011). About NCSBN. Retrieved from https://www.ncsbn.org/about.htm

National League for Nurses. (2013a). *Global diversity initiative.* Retrieved from http://www.nln.org/centers-for-nursing-education/nln-center-for-diversity-and-global-initiatives

National League for Nurses. (2013b). About NLN. Retrieved from http://www.nln.org/aboutnln/index.htm

National Student Nurse Association. (2013). NSNA: About us. Retrieved from http://www.nsna.org/AboutUs.aspx

Nursing Organizations Alliance. (2013). About us. Retrieved from http://www.nursing-alliance.org/About-Us

Porter-O'Grady, T., & Malloch, K. (2013). *Leadership in nursing practice.* Burlington, MA: Jones & Bartlett.

Rossi, P. H., & Freeman, H. E. (1995). *Evaluations: A systematic approach* (5th ed.). Beverly Hills, CA: Sage.

Russell, K. (2012). Nurse practice acts guide and govern nursing practice. *Journal of Nursing Regulations, 3*(3), 36–40.

U.S. Department of Education. (2014). Mission. Retrieved from http://www2.ed.gov/about/overview/mission/mission.html?src=ted

U.S. Department of Health and Human Services. (2014.) About HHS. Retrieved from http://www.hhs.gov/about/

U.S. Department of Health and Human Services. (2016). Health insurance coverage and the Affordable Care Act, 2010–2016. Retrieved from http://www.hhs.gov/programs/health-insurance/index.html

World Health Organization. (2014). About WHO. Retrieved from http://www.who.int/about/en/

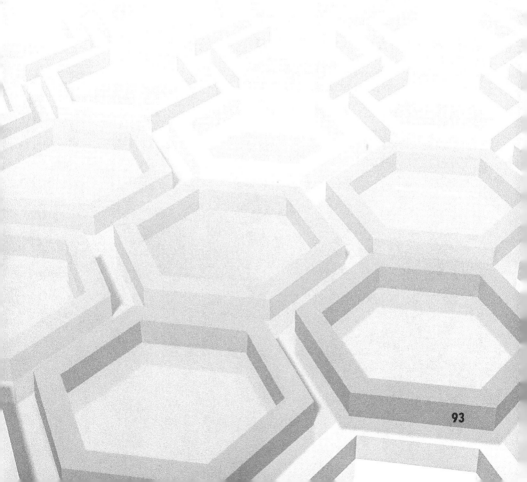

II

Leading the Business of Health Care

4

Economic and Fiscal Leadership

Remember the saying, "There's no such thing as a free lunch"? This statement holds especially true when discussing health-care economics and finance. Economics and finance are not interchangeable concepts. *Economics* is the social science that seeks to describe the factors that determine the production, distribution, and consumption of goods and services. *Finance* is a branch of economics concerned with resource allocation as well as resource management, acquisitions, and investment (investor-words, 2016; Wikipedia, 2016). The American Organization of Nurse Executives (AONE) Nurse Executive Competencies identify health-care economics as an essential component of nurse executives' knowledge of the health-care environment (AONE, 2005). Health-care leaders must seek to defend the individual patient's health while simultaneously recognizing the limits of health-care resources and the increasing expenses related to health-care delivery (Millonis, 2013).

The nurse leader is ultimately responsible for ensuring the economic and fiscal stability of nursing's contribution to the organization. In an editorial for *Nursing Economic$*, Dr. Donna Nickitas (2011) wrote that "every nurse who brings more efficiency, improves patient satisfaction, innovates and focuses on evidence-based practice using metrics to measure performance and control the cost of care is a nurse economist" (p. 229). Nurses at all levels must be exposed to quality, safety, and financial data and participate in translating data to make meaningful nursing decisions. However, although many nurses may participate in the discussion of structure, process, and outcomes, leaders set the culture, create the strategies, and motivate others. It is the nurse leader who must recognize, measure, monitor, and execute the solutions needed to make adjustments in the complex, ever-changing landscape of health care. It is the leader who must conceive and articulate goals that unite people in pursuit of objectives worthy of their best efforts (Ajami, Costa, & Kulik, 2014; Gardner, 1990; Goetz, Janney, & Ramsey, 2011).

HEALTH-CARE ECONOMICS

Health care is now one of the largest industry segments in the United States. The U.S. Census Bureau's 2015 data reported annual revenue for the health-care industry at

$1.668 trillion, with 784,626 health-care companies registered in the United States. These companies reported a total of 16,792,074 employees.

Milstead (2015) frames health-care economics discussions around three concepts: *access, cost,* and *quality and safety.* These concepts are discussed in the following sections.

Access

The U.S. Census Bureau solicits information on health insurance coverage during the Census. The Census Bureau classifies health insurance as private coverage or government coverage. Government health insurance includes Medicare, Medicaid, military health care, the Children's Health Insurance Program (CHIP), and individual state health plans. Table 4.1 depicts highlights from these surveys. Federal, state, and local government programs provide more than half of all health insurance.

Medicare

Medicare is a national social insurance program, guaranteeing access to health insurance for Americans aged 65 years and older who have worked and paid into the system, younger people with disabilities, and those with end-stage renal disease or amyotrophic lateral sclerosis. Medicare spreads the financial risk associated with illness across society to protect everyone and thus has a somewhat different social role from for-profit private insurers, which manage their risk portfolio by adjusting their pricing according to perceived risk. Enacted in 1965, Medicare has been funded through two trust fund accounts held by the U.S. Department of the Treasury. The Hospital Insurance Trust Fund is funded by payroll taxes, income taxes paid on social security benefits, and Medicare Part A (hospital) premiums. The Supplementary Medical Insurance (SMI) Trust Fund is authorized by Congress to support Medicare services. The SMI also receives funds from people enrolled in Medicare Part B (medical insurance) and Medicare Part D (prescription drug coverage) (Centers for Medicare & Medicaid Services, 2014a).

Medicaid

Medicaid is the largest funding source for health-related services for low-income Americans. The federal government and state governments jointly fund Medicaid. States are not required to participate in the Medicaid program and have broad leeway in determining eligibility of participants. The Patient Protection and Affordable Care Act (PPACA) expanded the eligibility for and federal funding of Medicaid. Under the current law, all U.S. citizens and legal residents with income up to 133% of the poverty line, including adults without dependent children, would qualify for coverage in any state that participated in the Medicaid program. The U.S. Supreme Court ruled in *National Federation of Independent Business v Sebelius* (Case Brief Summary, 2016) that states do not have to agree to this expansion in order to continue to receive previously established levels of Medicaid funding, and many states have chosen to continue with pre-PPACA funding levels and eligibility standards (Centers for Medicare & Medicaid Services, 2014b).

Veterans Health Administration

The Veterans Health Administration (VA) is the largest integrated health-care system in the United States. The VA serves 8.76 million veterans annually, providing care at more than 1,700 sites (U.S. Department of Veterans Affairs, 2014).

TABLE 4.1 Health Insurance Coverage in the United States, 2011–2014

Coverage	2011 Census	2012 Census	2014 Census
Without health insurance	15.7%	15.4%	10.4%
With health insurance	84.0%	84.6%	89.6%
Covered by government health insurance	32.2%	32.6%	34%
Covered by private health insurance	63.9%	63.9%	66.0%
Covered by employment based health insurance	54.9%	54.9%	55.4%
Covered by Medicaid	16.4%	16.4%	19.5%
Covered by Medicare	15.2% 46.9 million	15.7% 48.9 million	16.0%

Adapted from: DeNavas-Walt, C., Proctor, B., & Smith, J. (2013). *Income, poverty, and health insurance coverage in the United States: 2013*. United States Census Bureau. Washington, DC: U.S. Government Printing Office. Retrieved from http://www.census.gov/prod/2013pubs/p60-245.pdf; Smith, J. C. & Carla, M. (2014). U.S. Census Bureau, Current Population Reports, P60-253, Health Insurance Coverage in the United States: U.S. Government Printing Office, Washington, DC, 2015. Retrieved from https://www.census.gov/content/dam/Census/library/publications/2015/demo/p60-253.pdf

Department of Defense

Effective October 2013, the Department of Defense Military Health System (the Civilian Health and Medical Program of the Uniformed Services) was discontinued, and TRICARE was established. This program provides civilian health benefits for military personnel, military retirees, and their dependents. This program contracts with health insurance and managed care companies to provide health care and administrative services (TRICARE, 2014).

Children's Health Insurance Program

CHIP provides health coverage to children in families with incomes too high to qualify for Medicaid but who cannot afford private coverage. Signed into law in 1997, CHIP provides federal matching funds to states to pay for this coverage. The PPACA also has provided more than $40 million in additional funding to promote enrollment in Medicaid and CHIP (Centers for Medicare & Medicaid Services, 2014a).

Patient Protection and Affordable Care Act

PPACA, also called the Affordable Care Act (ACA), or "Obamacare," is a U.S. federal statute signed into law by President Barack Obama on March 23, 2010. The goals of the PPACA include increasing the quality and affordability of health insurance, expanding public and private insurance coverage, and reducing health-care costs for both individuals and the government.

Affordable Care Act Reforms

The PPACA is slated to enact provisions between 2010 and 2020. Significant reforms include the following (The White House, 2014):

- Insurers are prohibited from denying coverage to individuals because of preexisting conditions. A community rating requires insurers to offer the same premium price to all applicants of the same age and geographic location without regard to gender or most preexisting conditions (excluding tobacco use). Minimum standards are set for health insurance policies.
- All individuals not covered by an employer-sponsored health plan, Medicaid, Medicare, or other public insurance program must secure an approved private-insurance policy or pay a penalty. Provisions are included for individuals with financial hardship and members of a recognized religious sect exempted by the Internal Revenue Service. The law includes subsidies to help people with low incomes comply with the mandate. Medicaid eligibility was expanded to include individuals and families with incomes up to 133% of the federal poverty level, including adults without disabilities and without dependent children.
- Health insurance marketplaces operate through which individuals and small businesses in every state can compare policies and buy insurance (with a government subsidy if eligible). Low-income individuals and families whose incomes are between 100% and 400% of the federal poverty level will receive federal subsidies on a sliding scale if they purchase insurance via an exchange.

Providing health insurance to millions of previously uninsured Americans is not the only change brought about by the PPACA. The new "Patient's Bill of Rights" provides Americans with the increased stability and flexibility necessary to make informed health-care choices. Key components of this Bill of Rights are described in Box 4.1 (The White House, 2014).

Affordable Care Act Outcomes

A 2014 study from Pellegrini, Monguio, and Qian revealed that during recessions public payer sources (Medicare and Medicaid) become a larger component of the U.S. health insurance system. At the same time that labor force participation declined, public health-care spending increased and private health-care spending decreased. Worsening health status, increased risk of mortality, and decreased access to cost-effective prevention and health-promotion services were self-reported. This study

BOX 4.1 PPACA Patient's Bill of Rights

- Ends preexisting condition exclusions for children under age 19 years

- Keeps young adults under age 26 years covered under a parent's health plan

- Ends arbitrary cancellation of coverage

- Guarantees right to appeal

- Ends lifetime limits on insurance coverage

- Covers recommended preventive care at no cost or co-pay

- Allows selection of primary care physician from plan network

- Removes barriers to emergency services

- Requires insurance companies to publicly justify unreasonable rate hikes

Retrieved from: https://www.cms.gov/cciio/Resources/Fact-Sheets-and-FAQs/index.html#Patient%E2%80%99s
Bill of Rights

collected data from 50 states and the District of Columbia for a decade using data from the Bureau of Labor Statistics, Centers for Disease Control and Prevention, and Centers for Medicare & Medicaid Services (CMS).

The 2012 Supreme Court's ruling in *National Federation of Independent Business v Sebelius* upheld the constitutionality of the PPACA, which had been disputed by those opposed to the bill. The one exception was to allow individual states to opt out of Medicaid expansion without loss of existing federal funding. This exception was the result of the suit brought by 26 states arguing that mandating Medicaid expansion placed a large burden on state budgets.

By the end of open enrollment in 2015, 16.4 million people had signed up for private insurance in the various health insurance marketplaces. This number includes 11.4 million people enrolled in federal and state plans, 10 million on Medicaid, and 3 million young adults enrolled through their parents' plan. Health-care costs are growing at the slowest level since 1960. Health-care costs for 2020 are predicted to be $180 billion lower than they were in 2010 as a result of reduced premiums and Medicaid costs ("Obamacare Facts," n.d.; The White House, 2014).

The Future of the Affordable Care Act
The PPACA has faced repeated opposition. In 2012, the Supreme Court released an opinion on *National Federation of Independent Business v Sebelius*, the two main provisions of which were the individual mandate and the Medicaid expansion. Under the individual mandate, most Americans must purchase "minimum essential" insurance coverage or face a penalty in the form of a tax assessment. Under the Medicaid expansion, state Medicaid programs must cover most individuals below 133% of the federal poverty level. States that do not comply with the Medicaid expansion could lose all of their federal Medicaid funding.

The plaintiffs in *National Federation of Independent Business v Sebelius* alleged that both the individual mandate and the Medicaid expansion exceeded the federal government's power. The federal government claimed that the individual mandate was justified by three of its enumerated powers: the Commerce Clause, the Taxing and Spending Clause, and the Necessary and Proper Clause. A majority of the Court ruled that the federal government does not have the authority to force people to buy a product under the Commerce Clause or the Necessary and Proper Clause. However, a majority of the Court upheld the mandate under the Taxing and Spending Clause insofar as the sole consequence for failing to purchase insurance is a tax; in other words, the PPACA can be read as taxing people who fail to buy insurance, which is within the authority of the federal government.

A majority of the Court also ruled that threatening states with the loss of all Medicaid funding if they do not comply with the Medicaid expansion is unconstitutional. According to the Court, the potential loss of such a large sum of federal money essentially deprives states of the option not to comply with the expansion. The Court ruled that states that do not comply with the Medicaid expansion would only lose the matching funds for the newly eligible population; existing Medicaid funding would not be affected. States that elect to proceed with the Medicaid expansion would presumably be unaffected by the ruling (Case Brief Summary, 2016).

The next threat to the PPACA came in the form of *King v Burwell,* which questioned the constitutionality of income-based subsidies/federal tax credits for the estimated 6.4 million Americans living in the 34 states that do not have their own state health-care exchanges. These income-based subsidies are crucial to the success of the PPACA, making health insurance affordable and ultimately reducing the number of uninsured Americans; striking down the subsidies would have had disastrous effects for the health-care market and the health-care reform law. But on June 25, 2015, the Supreme Court, in a 6–3 decision, ruled that PPACA authorizing federal tax credits for eligible Americans living not only in states with their own exchanges but also in the 34 states with federal marketplaces *is* constitutional. Chief Justice Roberts and Justices Kagan, Ginsburg, Breyer, and Sotomayor supported the reasoning that Congress acted within its authority to tax when it enacted the law.

The decision confirms that, despite the president and congressional Democrats specifically disclaiming that the law was being enacted under the tax authority, the health-care reform law is a tax. Second, the decision acts as a reminder to Americans that this law was passed by the administration that a majority of Americans elected. Third, the Court put an end to the inexhaustible authority of Congress under the Commerce Clause. Two of the president's Court appointees would have upheld the act as valid under this authority, as would the other Democratic appointees. This decision means that the next president cannot undo federal exchanges, but that it will take an act of Congress and a president willing to sign it to change or eliminate the PPACA (Leonard, 2015).

Unfortunately, this decision contradicts President Obama's pledge not to raise taxes on families making less than $250,000. Families of four making $72,000 or less and individuals making $35,400 or less will bear nearly half of the mandate tax.

Cost

The 2013 *Economic Report of the President* (Council of Economic Advisors, 2013) demonstrates that health-care expenditures are currently about 17.2% of the gross domestic product. By 2050, Medicare payroll collections and premiums are estimated to cover only 53% of Medicare expenditures. Medicaid expenditures are also estimated to increase faster than the rate of inflation (Fuchs, 2013).

Contributing to these increases are such factors as demands for increased services associated with an aging population and with an unhealthy lifestyle (obesity, tobacco use, sedentary lifestyle). Increases in costs are also related to medical malpractice claims, health-care company profits (insurance, pharmaceuticals, providers), billing fraud, and advances in technology such as adoption of electronic health records and use of innovative and complex equipment (Wendel, O'Donohue, & Serratt, 2014).

Controlling Cost

With the passage of the ACA of 2010, the previous substantial profit margins to hospitals and providers ended. Exceptionally thin hospital profit margins are now the rule. The ACA's emphasis on incentive-based inpatient and outpatient reimbursements has called for a change in the payment model from fee-for-service (FFS) to value-based purchasing (VBP). This pressure to reduce costs and prove quality outcomes is calling for a shift in the strategies previously used to manage reimbursement and risk. The shift will continue to become less focused on event-driven reimbursement and more focused on utilization trends and proactive, long-term management of health (Aldhizer & Juras, 2015; Cassatly, 2012).

Health-care leaders must be on the forefront of developing strategies that will (1) manage care across the continuum with a team-based integrated model, (2) reduce readmissions for all diagnoses, (3) build and support a patient-centered medical home (PCMH) model, and (4) achieve clinical integration through aligning incentives and governance structures across previously independent practices (Jacquin, 2014). Currently, consumers make purchasing decisions for every other commodity based on transparent price and quality information. Should not the same criteria be taken into consideration for health-care decisions (Emery & Brantes, 2015)?

The legacy of FFS gave providers the incentive to deliver as many examinations, tests, and procedures and fill as many beds as possible. A decade of publications from the Institute of Medicine Quality Chasm Reports (National Academies Press, 2015) has demonstrated that more services do not equal high-quality, safe, and effective care. The current VBP focus holds providers more accountable for the cost and quality of charges that exceed the allowable amount for a diagnosis.

Value-Based Purchasing Models

Organizations must now manage variations in cost and quality as they demonstrate the economic and clinical value they are providing to the populations served. VBP is a broad set of performance-based payment strategies linking financial incentives to performance. Early pay-for-performance models (P4P) emerged more than a decade ago. Today, the most common VBP models are accountable care organizations (ACOs) and bundled payments (Sackman & Buseman, 2015).

Pay-for-Performance

P4P strategies are payment arrangements in which providers receive bonuses or reductions in payments based on pre-established benchmarks targeting quality and/or efficiency. Today, the Integrated Healthcare Association (IHA) is the largest nongovernmental physician incentive program in the United States. After 9 years of the P4P program, IHA services more than 35,000 physicians with more than 200 physician groups and provides care for 10 million health maintenance organization/point-of-service members. This P4P program rewards performance attainment and improvement, focusing on a common set of performance measures, a public report card, health plan incentive payments, and public recognition. IHA has identified six priority clinical areas—cardiovascular, diabetes, maternity, musculoskeletal, prevention, and respiratory—along with the following seven types of measures with data and benchmarks for each measure (IHA, 2012):

- Prevention/risk factors
- Care processes
- Appropriateness of care
- Utilization
- Resource use
- Patient experience
- Outcomes

Accountable Care Organizations

Section 3022 of the ACA (p. 313) defines an ACO as a "group of providers who are accountable for quality, cost, and overall care of patients" (McCanne, 2015). Projected to save the U.S. health-care system $4.9 billion during the first 10 years of implementation, ACOs will transition from an FFS model to a model of population management. Chronic disease accounts for an estimated 78% of the annual expenditure for health care. The goal of the ACO is to coordinate care and ensure that patients, especially the chronically ill, receive the right care at the right time while avoiding unnecessary duplication of services and preventing medical errors.

Both the CMS and commercial health-care providers support ACO programs. Since 2011, the number of CMS-sponsored ACOs has grown from 23 pioneer organizations to more than 300. Growth continues for both CMS and private insurers (Macfarlane, 2014). Successful ACOs providing services for CMS will share in the savings it achieves for the Medicare program. Although different ACO models exist, in most ACOs the health insurer will designate a block of members for whose health care the ACO will assume complete risk.

Criteria for private ACOs are much less stringent than those set by CMS for the Medicare market. Wang and Maniccia (2013) state, "At its core, an ACO is a health care delivery system that has partnered with a payer or purchaser of health care to develop arrangements that align financial interests with the delivery of effective and quality care for a specific population" (p. 15).

Based on the criteria set forth in the ACA, some of the options for qualifying as an ACO include the following:

- Group practices
- Individual practices forming a network
- Partnerships between professionals and hospitals
- Hospitals employing professionals
- Other providers deemed appropriate by the secretary of the U.S. Department of Health and Human Services (HHS)

ACOs, especially those not associated with CMS, are still in their infancy. Members of Medicare ACOs must participate for no less than 3 years while demonstrating the criteria in Box 4.2.

BOX 4.2 **Criteria Needed to Participate in Centers for Medicare & Medicaid Accountable Care Organizations**

- Trust and transparency across all partners including governance, leadership, material investment, and long-term commitment

- Care coordination across entire care continuum

- Ample primary care providers to treat the defined beneficiary population

- Demonstrated mechanisms to promote evidence-based medicine

- Organizational culture of teamwork and partnerships

- Information technology infrastructure for population management and care coordination

- Resources for patient education and support

- Dissemination of best practices with established lineages to public health and community resources

- Processes in place for monitoring, managing, and reporting quality and cost measures

- Participation in regional health information exchanges focusing on improving the health of the community

Source: Panning, R. (2014). Accountable Care Organizations: An integrated model of patient care objectives. *Clinical Laboratory Science, 27*(2), 112–118; Wang, I., & Maniccia, M. (2013). Accountable Care Organizations–an employer POV primer. *Benefits Quarterly, 29*(4), 14–19.

Currently, CMS ACOs must report on 33 quality metrics divided among four health domains (Box 4.3).

The at-risk population domain includes measures that center on five chronic conditions: diabetes, hypertension, ischemic vascular disease, heart failure, and coronary artery disease.

There are at least three advantages to forming an ACO: First, with a variety of options available for forming an ACO, one of these options may work better and be less costly than maintaining existing arrangements. Second, by forming a Medicare Shared Savings Program, the ACO is rewarded through withholding a percentage of the hospital's diagnosis-related group (DRG) payments and sharing in incentives. The ACO is guaranteed at least the standard Medicare reimbursement for beneficiaries within the plan. Last, and most important, if the ACO performs as intended, quality will improve and costs will decrease (Bennett, 2012; Panning, 2014).

Bundled Payments

Bundled payments for care improvements (BPCIs) are payments to providers based on the expected costs for a clinically defined episode or bundle or related services. First introduced by CMS in 2013, 100 health-care organizations were selected by CMS

BOX 4.3 **Centers for Medicare & Medicaid Quality Metrics for Accountable Care Organizations**

- Patient/caregiver experience
  - Getting timely care, appointments, and information
  - How well your providers communicate
  - Patient rating of provider
  - Access to specialists
  - Health promotion and education
  - Shared decision making
  - Health status/functional status

- Care coordination/patient safety
  - Risk-standardized all-condition readmission
  - Ambulatory sensitive conditions admissions: COPD or asthma in older adults
  - Ambulatory sensitive conditions admissions: Heart failure
  - Percent of primary care physicians who successfully quality for an EHR program incentive payment
  - Care coordination and patient safety practice reported measures

- Preventive care
  - Preventive care measures
  - Breast cancer screening
  - Colorectal cancer screening
  - Preventive care and screening: Influenza immunization
  - Pneumonia vaccination status for older adults
  - Preventive care and screening: BMI and follow-up
  - Preventive care and screening: Tobacco use and cessation intervention
  - Preventive care and screening: Hypertension and follow-up
  - Preventive care and screening: Depression and follow-up

- At-risk population
  - Coronary artery disease measures
  - Diabetes measures
  - Heart failure measures
  - Hypertension measures
  - Ischemic vascular disease measures

Retrieved from: https://www.cms.gov/Medicare/Medicare-Fee-for-Service-Payment/sharedsavingsprogram/Downloads/ACO-Shared-Savings-Program-Quality-Measures.pdf

to participate in the BPCI initiative for 3 years. Four models were introduced (CMS, 2013):

- Model 1: Inpatient stay only with physician payment separately
- Model 2: Inpatient stay plus post–acute care and all related services

- Model 3: Post–acute care only
- Model 4: Acute care hospital stay all services

Currently, widespread data on use of BPCIs in the private sector are not available. However, examples of smaller programs, such as the following two, have demonstrated their effectiveness:

> *Knee-replacement surgery.* CaroMont Health and North Carolina's largest health insurer, Blue Cross and Blue Shield of North Carolina (BCBSNC), implemented a bundled payment arrangement that includes the presurgical period of 30 days prior to hospitalization, the surgery itself, and most follow-up care within 180 days after discharge from the hospital. In a 1-year pilot, BCBSNC saved about 8% to 10% per-episode cost.
>
> *Coronary artery bypass graft surgery (CABG).* Geisinger Health System implemented a unique performance-based bundled payment system called ProvenCare, which achieved a 10% reduction in readmissions, shorter average length of stay, and reduced hospital charges.

CMS continues to expand its use of this payment model with the 2013 BPCI initiative. To date, Medicare has saved $42.3 million on CABG patients treated in the BPCI demonstration hospitals.

Bundled payment models are not for everyone—not every system will be equipped to participate in this type of arrangement and not every service will be the best fit for this model. For instance, academic health centers, which emphasize research, teaching, and new technologies, may be disadvantaged by this system. Physicians might hospitalize patients unnecessarily or seek to avoid patients for whom reimbursement may be inadequate. Hospitals may seek to maximize profit by limiting access to specialists during inpatient stays (Reynolds, 2011).

Current State of the Value-Based Purchasing Model

VBP models are recent developments in our health-care system, and they continue to be implemented and tested in a variety of models. In 2014, the Catalyst for Payment Reform started to measure VBP progress in the private sector, including the prevalence of specific payment methods. The report showed that the vast majority of payment (89%) was still tied up in FFS. Of the remaining 11% of supposedly "value-oriented" payments, 43% of them give providers financial incentives by offering a potential bonus or added payment to support higher quality and more affordable care, such as FFS with shared savings, whereas the other 57% put providers at financial risk for their performance if they do not meet certain quality and cost goals, such as bundled payment (Delbanco, 2014, 2015).

Value-Based Nursing Care

The shift from FFS to a value-based program affords health-care leaders opportunities to translate VBP into value-based care (VBC) delivery models fostering high-quality, coordinated, collaborative, lower-cost, patient-centered care (Aroh, Colella, Douglas, & Eddings, 2015). Aroh et al. (2015) describe their experience in developing systems that would improve scores on Hospital Consumer Assessment of Healthcare Providers and Systems (HCAHPS), National Database of Nursing Quality Indicators, and Press Ganey patient experience assessments; improve institutional and patient-care processes; and foster development of new processes to improve outcomes. Key components of this project included the following:

- *Implementing a value-based advanced practice nurse (APN) nurse practitioner position:* Requiring skills in collaboration, coaching, mentoring, direct patient care, leadership, research, ethics, and process improvement
- *Having Lean Six Sigma nurses on all levels:* Staff, APNs, and nurse managers to streamline and improve team performance
- *Value-based policy integrating operations, quality, and clinical practice:* Integrates data-driven, quality improvement methods for evaluating process inputs and outputs for effectiveness and efficiency, as well as customer, hospital, and regulatory expectations

Examples of nurse-led value-based care projects include an early patient mobility protocol, a vaccine protocol, and advancement of diet for the medically managed patient with diverticulitis. Gardner (2013) called value-based purchasing a "game changer." This mandate to do things differently via a lean construct provides the right timing for nursing as direct caregivers to change nursing care to a value-based financial model.

Visionary leadership is critical as health-care organizations transition to VBP models. What should a nurse leader focus on to survive and thrive in the new payment era? Box 4.4 outlines suggestions for leaders to survive and thrive in this new financial climate (Edmondson, 2015).

Quality and Safety

Quality and safety issues are inextricably entwined with economic and fiscal issues. The focus of current health reform legislation is primarily on cost savings to the government

---

BOX 4.4 Visionary Leadership

- Focus on a community-wide orientation including beneficiaries who may not be active participants in your system.
- Seek out those with chronic diseases and actively engage them in disease management programs.
- Build a continuum of care using low-cost approaches and settings.
- Partner proactively with physicians to develop creative strategies related to the challenges of value-based purchasing.
- Rebuild infrastructure to manage, assess, monitor, and influence quality and fiscal control.
- Embrace the concept of a broad range of services.
- Collaborate with payers to develop products that demonstrate value and appeal for consumers.

Adapted from: Edmondson, W. (2015). The per capita payment model. *Population Health, 60*(1), 14–16.

through improving care. Measuring the overall value of an individual life is not really possible; however, quality-adjusted life year (QALY) measurements can offer approximate economic estimates. Using the Institute of Medicine (IOM) figure of 98,000 preventable deaths each year with an estimate of 10 lost years of life at $75,000 to $100,000 per year, the loss for those deaths conservatively is $73.5 billion to $98 billion in QALYs. This figure neither includes direct costs associated with errors, nor does it take into account that preventable death is actually 10 times the IOM estimate at a cost of $735 billion to $980 billion (Andel, Davidow, Hollander, & Moreno, 2012).

The following discussion reveals that health reform and quality form a much broader concept than preventable readmissions, medical errors, and facility-acquired conditions. In addition to providing better care, the national mandates for improving quality will continue to force providers to focus on efficiency and quality. Hospitals providing poor quality care will start to lose Medicare reimbursements, and, with the already low estimated operating profit margin of 5%, they will eventually go out of business as a result.

Because information about quality care is public, eventually consumers with private insurance will eschew poorly rated facilities. Beginning in 2015, physicians will be included in the individual performance reports published on the CMS Web site (CMS, 2015b).

Patient-Centered Medical Homes

The patient-centered medical home (PCMH) was originally introduced by the American Academy of Pediatrics in the early 21st century as a coordinated-care model for children with complex medical problems as part of the ACA. PCMHs differ from the traditional care delivery model. In order to apply for recognition as a PCMH, the organization must meet five key domains as outlined by the Agency for Healthcare Research and Quality (AHRQ) in 2015:

1. *Comprehensive care:* providing a primary care workforce in a team approach to meet the majority of a patient's physical and mental health-care needs
2. *Patient-centered care:* respect for culture, unique needs, preferences, and values through a partnership with patients and families
3. *Coordinated care:* across all of the health-care system—specialty care, hospitals, home care, and community services with an emphasis on efficient care transitions
4. *Accessible services:* focus on accessibility through minimal wait times, enhanced office hours, and after-hours access using a variety of methods
5. *Quality and safety:* use of clinical decision-support tools, evidence-based practices, shared decision making, performance measurement, and population health management with the goal of providing safe, high-quality services

The AHRQ currently coordinates a catalog of federal PCMH activities in order to disseminate information and avoid duplication. AHRQ provides resources, webinars, papers, guides, and case studies for health-care providers interested in becoming a PCMH. Further information on how to apply to become a PCMH is available on their website: https://pcmh.ahrq.gov/page/defining-pcmh

The ACA has provided an avenue for the creation and testing of this innovative health-care practice. Preliminary evidence from demonstration projects has shown favorable results in cost reduction, improved care coordination, and timely patient access. Criteria for recognition as a PCMH have been developed by several agencies listed in Box 4.5.

Among the challenges for this new model are the variations in how the PCMH is organized; the differences in resources between small and large providers seeking to become PCMHs; variations in accreditation standards and benchmarks for improvement; and the lengthy process for team development, technological implementation, and financial stability. However, the ACA and meaningful use initiatives discussed further in this chapter are creating a favorable environment to continue testing PCMHs. Although the process is labor intensive and involves many parties, the model may represent the future vision as described by the ACA and others (Klein, Laugesen, & Liu, 2013; Milstead, 2013).

Hospital Consumer Assessment of Healthcare Providers and Systems Survey

The CMS and the AHRQ jointly developed the HCAHPS survey, a standardized instrument administered to a random sample of patients continually throughout the year. The CMS collects the data; cleans, adjusts, and analyzes the data; and then publicly reports the results. Collecting these data nationally has created the ability for the CMS to make valid comparisons across hospitals. The public reporting of this data has also served to enhance transparency and public accountability to consumers. Data are reported on the Medicare Web site (www.medicare.gov/hospitalcompare/) four times a year.

The 11 items in the HCAHPS are listed in Table 4.2.

The survey is available in English, Spanish, Chinese, Russian, and Vietnamese via U.S. mail as well as in English and Spanish by telephone and interactive voice-response formats. Hospitals may add customized hospital-specific items. Patients who are aged 18 years or older at time of admission, have at least one overnight stay, have a nonpsychiatric DRG principal diagnosis, and are alive at time of discharge are included in the population who will be randomly sampled for the quarter. Patients discharged to hospice care, nursing homes, or skilled nursing facilities; prisoners; and patients with a foreign home address are excluded from the sample population.

Although voluntary reporting began in 2006, mandatory HCAHPS scoring began in 2008. Inpatient prospective pay systems (IPPS) hospitals must collect, submit, and publicly report data in order to receive full IPPS payments (CMS, 2015a).

BOX 4.5 **National Recognition and Accreditation Patient-Centered Medical Home Programs**

Accreditation Association for Ambulatory Health Care (AAAHC)

National Committee for Quality Assurance (NCQA)

The Joint Commission (TJC)

Utilization Review Accreditation Commission (URAC)

TABLE 4.2 **Hospital Consumer Assessment of Healthcare Providers and Systems Survey**

Composite Topics	Individual Topics	Global Topics

Nurse communication
Doctor communication
Responsiveness of hospital
    staff
Pain management
Communication about
    medicines
Discharge information
Care transition
	Cleanliness of hospital
	    environment
	Quietness of hospital
	    environment
		Overall rating of
		    hospital
		Willingness to recom-
		    mend hospital

Retrieved from: http://www.hcahpsonline.org/home.aspx

Clinical Quality Measures

A variety of clinical quality measures (CQMs) exist that health-care facilities can use to track and measure the quality of their services. The Joint Commission (TJC) began as early as 1999 to solicit input from a wide variety of stakeholders regarding initial core measurement areas for hospitals. At the same time, TJC was working with CMS to align the core measures that were common to both organizations. Beginning in November 2003, they created one common set of measure specifications documented in the *Specifications Manual for National Hospital Inpatient Quality Measures* found at https://www.jointcommission.org/specifications_manual_for_national_hospital_inpatient_quality_measures.aspx (TJC, 2016).

Beginning in 2014, TJC began reclassifying some of the core measures into accountability measures. Information on accountability measures can be found at https://www.jointcommission.org/accountability_measures.aspx. In order to be reclassified, a core measure must meet the following four criteria:

1. *Research:* Strong scientific evidence exists demonstrating that compliance with a given process of care improves health-care outcomes (either directly or by reducing the risk of adverse outcomes).
2. *Proximity:* The process being measured is closely connected to the outcome it impacts; there are relatively few clinical processes that occur after the one that is measured and before the improved outcome occurs.
3. *Accuracy:* The measure accurately assesses whether the evidence-based process has actually been provided. That is, the measure should be capable of judging whether the process has been delivered with sufficient effectiveness to make improved outcomes likely. If it is not, then the measure is a poor measure of quality, likely to be subject to workarounds

that induce unproductive work instead of work that directly improves quality of care.

4. *Adverse Effects:* The measure construct is designed to minimize or eliminate unintended adverse effects (TJC, 2016).

Many aspects of care can be measured using CQMs (Box 4.6). The requirements for tracking and reporting may change each year, but providers can refer to the CMS Web site for current requirements (www.cms.gov/Medicare/Quality-Initiatives-Patient-Assessment-Instruments/QualityMeasures/CMS-Measures-Inventory.html).

National Quality Strategy Domains

Closely aligned with CMS and TJC CQMs are the six National Quality Strategy (NQS) domains, representing the HHS NQS priorities for health-care quality improvement and mandated by the ACA. The NQS received input from more than 300 groups, organizations, and individuals to establish three aims, six priorities, and nine levers (core business functions, resources, or actions), as shown in Table 4.3.

The six NQS domains are listed in Box 4.7. For 2016, reporting the CQMs selected must cover at least three of the six NQS domains and at least one lever.

Institute for Healthcare Improvement Triple Aim

Officially founded in 1991, the Institute for Healthcare Improvement (IHI) began work in the late 1980s as part of the National Demonstration Project on Quality Improvement in Health Care. IHI's vision is for everyone to have the best care and health possible with a mission to improve health and health care worldwide (IHI, 2015). With a growing community of leaders, practitioners, and visionaries around the globe, IHI developed an organizing "Triple Aim" framework. Currently used by the HHS and

---

BOX 4.6 Aspects of Care Measured by Clinical Quality Measures

- Health outcomes
- Clinical processes
- Patient safety
- Efficient use of health-care resources
- Care coordination
- Patient engagements
- Population and public health
- Adherence to clinical guidelines

Retrieved from: https://www.cms.gov/regulations-and-guidance/legislation/ehrincentiveprograms/clinicalqualitymeasures.html

TABLE 4.3 **National Quality Strategy Aims, Priorities, and Levers**

Three Aims	Six Priorities	Nine Levers
1. Better Care: Improve the overall quality by making health care more patient-centered, reliable, accessible, and safe.	1. Making care safer by reducing harm caused in the delivery of care.	1. Measurement and Feedback: Provide performance feedback to plans and providers to improve care.
2. Healthy People/ Healthy Communities: Improve the health of the U.S. population by supporting proven interventions to address behavioral, social, and environmental determinants of health in addition to delivering higher-quality care.	2. Ensuring that each person and family is engaged as partners in their care.	2. Public Reporting: Compare treatment results, costs, and patient experience for consumers.
3. Affordable Care: Reduce the cost of quality health care for individuals, families, employers, and government.	3. Promoting effective communication and coordination of care.	3. Learning and Technical Assistance: Foster learning environments that offer training, resources, tools, and guidance to help organizations achieve quality improvement goals.
	4. Promoting the most effective prevention and treatment practices for the leading causes of mortality, starting with cardiovascular disease.	4. Certification, Accreditation, and Regulation: Adopt or adhere to approaches to meet safety and quality standards.

Continued

TABLE 4.3 **National Quality Strategy Aims, Priorities and Levers–cont'd**

Three Aims	Six Priorities	Nine Levers
	5. Working with communities to promote wide use of best practices to enable healthy living.	5. Consumer Incentives and Benefit Designs: Help consumers adopt healthy behaviors and make informed decisions.
	6. Making quality care more affordable for individuals, families, employers, and governments by developing and spreading new health-care delivery models.	6. Payment: Reward and incentivize providers to deliver high-quality, patient-centered care.
		7. Health Information Technology: Improve communication, transparency, and efficiency for better coordinated health and health care.
		8. Innovation and Diffusion: Foster innovation in health-care quality improvement and facilitate rapid adoption within and across organizations and communities.
		9. Workforce Development: Invest in people to prepare the next generation of health-care professionals and support lifelong learning for providers.

Adapted from: National Quality Strategy. (2015). About the National Quality Strategy (NQS). Retrieved from http://www.ahrq.gov/workingforquality/about.htm

BOX 4.7 **National Quality Strategy Domains**

- Patient and Family Engagement
- Patient Safety
- Care Coordination
- Population/Public Health
- Efficient Use of Healthcare Resources
- Clinical Process/Effectiveness

Retrieved from: https://www.pqrspro.com/measures/nqsdomains/

the CMS, this three-pronged framework focuses on improving the health of populations and the experience of care while reducing the per capita cost of care. Currently, more than 100 organizations around the world are in one of six phases of pilot testing this framework (IHI, 2015).

The Triple Aim continues the focus on managing access, cost, and quality, including the measurement principles that will support these processes. The IHI describes these key principles as follows (Stiefel & Nolan, 2012):

- Need for a defined population
- Need for data over time
- Need to distinguish between outcome and process measures and between population and project measures
- Value of benchmark/comparison data

Table 4.4 describes a few of the recommended outcome measures for the IHI Triple Aim framework. Each organization will select measures based on data availability, resource constraints, and the overall objectives set by the organization.

Regardless of where an organization is in the quest for managing access, cost, and quality, the IHI has tools and publications that will provide information and guidance. Review the extensive IHI Web site (www.ihi.org/) to read about organizations and people all over the world from a variety of entities that have initiated the IHI Triple Aim framework and improved the health and well-being of their communities.

Meaningful Use

Meaningful Use is using certified electronic health record (EHR) technology to improve quality, safety, and efficiency and reduce health disparities; engage patients and families; improve care coordination and population and public health; and maintain the privacy and security of patient health information (Office of the National Coordinator for Health Information Technology, 2015).

The 2009 Health Information Technology for Economic and Clinical Health Act component of the ACA focuses on the use of EHRs as a means of creating a more efficient,

TABLE 4.4 **Institute for Healthcare Improvement Triple Aim Recommended Outcome Measures**

Dimension	Outcome Measure
Population Health	**Health Outcomes** Mortality: life expectancy; years of potential life lost; standardized mortality rates Health and Functional Status assessments Health Life Expectancy: combining life expectancy and health status into a single measure reflecting remaining years of life in good health **Disease Burden** Incidence and/or prevalence of major disease conditions **Behavioral and Physiological Factors** Behavioral: smoking, alcohol use, exercise, and diet Physiological: blood pressure, body mass index, cholesterol, blood glucose, health risk assessment score
Experience of Care	Standard questions from patient **surveys** such as HCAHPS or How's Your Health surveys Likelihood to recommend Measurement based on **key dimensions** of the IOM's six aims: safe, effective, timely, efficient, equitable, and patient centered
Per Capita Cost	**Total cost** per member of the population per month Hospital and emergency department **utilization rates and/or costs**

Adapted from: Stiefel, M., & Nolan, K. A. (2012). *A guide to measuring the triple aim: Population health, experience of care and per capita cost.* IHI Innovation Series white paper. Cambridge, MA: Institute for Healthcare Improvement.

patient-centered system and that compliance with Meaningful Use criteria will demonstrate improved clinical and population health outcomes and supply a rich source of research data for ongoing quality improvement. The three main components of Meaningful Use are (1) use of a certified EHR in a meaningful manner such as e-prescribing, (2) use of certified EHR technology for electronic exchange of health information, and (3) use of certified EHR technology to submit CQMs and other reports required by HHS (CMS, 2015a).

From 2009 to 2014, implementation of the EHR has increased dramatically. Through the federal government's EHR Incentive Program, $23.7 billion in Medicaid or Medicare payments have been distributed to hospitals and eligible professionals meeting the Meaningful Use criteria or the requirements for adoption, implementation, or upgrade of a certified EHR system (McQuade-Jones, Murphy, Novak, & Sarnowski, 2014). Full implementation of Meaningful Use will take place in three stages from 2011 to 2016. Table 4.5 summarizes the criteria for each stage of Meaningful Use implementation.

Participants may progress to stage 2 after meeting 2 years of stage 1 criteria. The CMS has established a set of core objectives that all providers must meet in order to demonstrate Meaningful Use. In addition, providers can select from a list of established

TABLE 4.5 Criteria Focus of Meaningful Use

Stage 1: 2011–2012	Stage 2: 2014	Stage 3: 2016
Electronically capturing health information in a standardized format	More rigorous health information exchange	Improving quality, safety, and efficiency, leading to improved health outcomes
Using that information to track key clinical conditions	Increased requirements for e-prescribing and incorporating laboratory results	Decision support for national high-priority conditions
Communicating that information for care-coordination processes	Electronic transmission of patient-care summaries across multiple settings	Patient access to self-management tools
Initiating the reporting of clinical quality measures and public health information	More patient-controlled data	Access to comprehensive patient data through patient-centered health information exchange
Using information to engage patients and their families in their care		Improving population health

Adapted from: Office of the National Coordinator for Health Information Technology. (2015b). *How to attain meaningful use*. Retrieved from http://www.healthit.gov/providers-professionals/how-attain-meaningful-use

menu objectives. For stage 1, eligible hospitals must meet 14 core objectives and 5 menu objectives selected from a total list of 10. Eligible providers must meet 15 core objectives and 5 menu objectives selected from a list of 10. Stage 2 retains the stage 1 core and menu structure with additional new objectives added. Stage 3 is scheduled to begin in 2016. Policy and standards committees are developing recommendations to continue to expand Meaningful Use objectives to improve health-care outcomes for stage 3. Current Meaningful Use regulations 2015–2017 are found at http://www.himss.org/library/meaningful-use/stage-3-final-rules

MEASURING NURSING

More than 1.5 million registered nurses contribute to the inpatient nursing labor expenditures on an annual basis, yet inpatient nursing care is often billed as a daily per diem charge. Welton and Harper (2015) ask the following question: "If value is the function of quality and cost, what is the contribution of each nurse to patient care?" (p. 14). In other settings, nursing care is included within procedure codes, bundled payments, or FFS reimbursement. Although nursing often uses such indicators as patient classification systems or patient diagnoses to indicate acuity, there is no alignment among nursing direct-care time and costs, billing for nursing services, and payment for nursing care. This begs the following question: How can a leader control costs when the data and information used to calculate those costs are based on an unknown (and probably nonexistent) "average" patient?

The discussion of nursing care value-based financial models is still in its infancy. The 2013 invitational conference Nursing Knowledge: Big Data Research for Transforming Health Care, held at the University of Minnesota, brought together a national representation of informaticists, economists, nurse leaders, software vendors, and representatives of nursing professional organizations and other health-care professions to begin this discussion. As discussions move forward related to nursing care value-based financial models, challenges will include the following:

- Identification of nursing care value in all settings
- Incorporating nursing care into existing and new payment models such as ACOs and bundled payments
- Identification of how nurses can be linked in electronic data sets to individual patients, many patients, and aggregates (Welton & Harper, 2015)

Understanding the environments where nurses work has been identified as an important step in achieving quality targets. Previously, studies have looked at nurses' work environments and/or the financial and human costs associated with patient safety, citing unit characteristics identified in Box 4.8 as factors contributing to meeting quality measures (Brewer & Verran, 2013; Warburton, 2009). Other studies have identified the relationship between patient trust and patient satisfaction scores (Dwyer, Liu, & Rizzo, 2012; Rutherford, 2014; Snellman & Gedda, 2012).

Sheingold and Sheingold (2013) introduced the concept of social capital as a framework to enhance measurement of the nursing work environment. The researchers define social capital as focusing on improving productive capacity by examining relationships and networks (p. 790). By focusing on relationships and networks available to individuals and organizations, the theory states that those with more social capital have greater productivity and are more able to confront vulnerability, crisis, conflict, and new

BOX 4.8 **Unit Characteristics Contributing to Meeting Quality Measures for Nursing**

Nursing Culture. Control over practice, staff satisfaction, nursing communication

Team Culture. Collaborative relationships, team communication, self-regulation

Staffing. Skill mix, nursing hours, registered nurse workload

Turbulence. Support service response, uncertainty, accessibility, distance, size (patients/day)

Adapted from: Brewer, B., & Verran, J. (2013). Measuring nursing unit environments with four composite measures. *Nursing Economic$, 31*(5), 241–248.

opportunities. Adapting the World Bank Social Capital Integrated Questionnaire, the researchers tested a survey measuring the following aspects of social capital:

Groups and networks. Nature and extent of participation in informal network and social associations as well as the contributions one gives and receives within them

Trust and solidarity. Identified as essential to meaningful participation with individual, institutions, and community

Collective action and cooperation. How community members participate with others on projects or in response to crises

Information and communication. Exploration of the communication infrastructure

Social cohesion and inclusion. Exploration of social relations, conflict, and inclusion

Empowerment and political action. Relation to how much control individuals have over processes that directly affect their well-being (Sheingold & Sheingold, 2013, p. 792)

One concept not considered in the various models suggested for measuring nursing is the concept of caring. However, as early as 2011, Nelson identified 41 studies completed by the Caring International Research Collaborative of Sigma Theta Tau International that described measuring caring and associated outcomes. These studies were completed by a variety of professions within and outside of health care. The researchers shared a belief that caring is healing and that caring behaviors have the potential to contribute positively to nursing's return on investment (Nelson, 2011). The challenge facing nursing is to create a common, comprehensive data model to guide extraction of existing EHR data applicable in many settings that will meet the IHI Triple Aim objectives (Welton & Harper, 2015).

LEADER RESPONSIBILITIES

Effective nursing leaders develop relationships with other leaders within the organization and community, appreciating the financial constraints and outcomes impacting all health-care decisions. Through strong leadership partnerships, these leaders will provide evidence that nursing is an indispensable key component of a quality health-care system (Kavanugh, Cimiotti, Abusalem, & Coty, 2014; Valentine, Kirby, & Wolf, 2011).

Nurse leaders need to be at the forefront of innovative strategies promoting nurse-led interprofessional collaborative models of care that can demonstrate improved outcomes and decreased costs. Team-building initiatives, mentoring, and positive role modeling are imperative in developing a new shared culture of fiscal responsibility. Nurse leaders must know how to ask the questions and conceptualize the models that will help drive the processes necessary to predict optimal outcomes. Evidence will become much more important than experience, opinions, or intuition (Douglas, 2014).

In 2003, the IHI and the Robert Wood Johnson Foundation (RWJF) launched the national program Transforming Care at the Bedside (TCAB) to create a framework for change on inpatient units. The goals of this joint effort are to (Needleman et al., 2007):

- Improve the quality and safety of patient care on medical and surgical units,
- Increase the vitality and retention of nurses,
- Engage and improve the patient's and family members' experience of care, and
- Improve the effectiveness of the entire care team.

For the initial phase, three hospitals were selected to develop and test innovative processes on medical-surgical units. In phases II and III, 13 sites were selected to improve performance related to the above themes with the addition of transformational leadership. Currently, more than 200 hospitals in the United States and Canada are participating in TCAB programs. The TCAB method consists of the nine steps listed in Box 4.9. The TCAB toolkit, developed by RWJF and IHI, provides assistance to

---

BOX 4.9 **TCAB Nine Steps**

1. Storytelling: describing an experience that impacted a unit

2. Brainstorming: deep diving or snorkeling ideas for change

3. Prioritizing: innovations to test

4. Hypotheses: using plan-do-study-act cycles

5. Testing: carrying out small tests of change

6. Evaluation: evaluating outcomes

7. Decision making: determining whether an innovation should be abandoned, adapted, or adopted

8. Testing: performing rapid-cycle testing to modify the innovation

9. Dissemination: spreading results

Source: Lavoie-Tremblay, M., et al. (2014). The effect of transforming care at the bedside initiative on healthcare teams' work environments. *Evidence-Based Nursing, 11*(1), 16–25.

hospitals interested in adopting the TCAB model. (The toolkit can be found at inno-vations.ahrq.gov/qualitytools/transforming-care-bedside-toolkit.) The IHI Web site (www.ihi.org/Engage/Initiatives/Completed/TCAB/Pages/default.aspx) contains many resources, guidelines, and articles related to this effort.

Overall, studies have demonstrated improvements in safe and reliable care out-comes, increased empowerment of frontline staff, and an increase in multiprofessional teams. Current recommendations for research include determining whether using TCAB leadership principles makes managers more effective as well as further research investigating how to engage patients and frontline staff in the redesigning of care (Dearmon et al., 2013; Lavoie-Tremblay et al., 2013).

CONCLUSION

The new paradigm of health care puts an economic value on patient care and describes nursing care in terms of access, cost, and quality. The introduction of this data era is transforming the health-care organization's culture and capabilities. Through initia-tives such as TCAB, nursing leaders are imagining the possibilities for nursing's influence to use data to make better decisions, more accurate predictions, and more precise interventions (Douglas, 2014). The 2004 report from the IOM stated, "How well we are cared for by nurses affects our health, and sometimes can be a matter of life or death" (p. 2). It is our responsibility as leaders to embrace these changes and continually inspire others.

References

Agency for Healthcare Research and Quality. (2015). Patient centered medical home. Retrieved from https://www.pcmh.ahrq.gov/

Ajami, M., Costa, L., & Kulick, S. (2014). Gap analysis: Synergies and opportunities for effective nursing leadership. *Nursing Economic$, 32*(1), 17–25.

Aldhizer, G., & Juras, P. (2015, January). Improving the effectiveness and efficiency of healthcare delivery systems. *The CPA Journal*, 66–71.

American Organization of Nurse Executives. (2005). *The AONE Nurse Executive Competencies.* Washington, DC: Author.

Andel, C., Davidow, S., Hollander, M., & Moreno, D. (2012). The economics of health care quality and medical errors. *Journal of Health Care Finance, 39*(1), 1–15. Retrieved from www.wolter-skluwerlb.com/health/resource-center/articles/2012/10/economics-health-care-quality-and-medical-errors

Aroh, D., Colella, J., Douglas, C., & Eddings, A. (2015). An example of translating value-based purchasing into value-based care. *Urologic Nursing, 35*(2), 61–74.

Bennett, A. (2012). Accountable Care Organizations: Principles and implications for hospital administrators. *Journal of Healthcare Management, 57*(4,) 244–254.

Brewer, B., & Verran, J. (2013). Measuring nursing unit environments with four composite measures. *Nursing Economic$, 31*(5), 241–249.

Case Brief Summary (2016), *National Federation of Businesses vs. Sebelius.* Retrieved from: http://www.casebriefsummary.com/national-federation-of-independent-business-v-sebelius/

Cassatly, M. (2012). The four critical drivers of healthcare reform. Retrieved from http://www.medachieve.com/MedAchieve/Publications_files/CRITICALDRIVERS.pdf

Centers for Medicare & Medicaid Services. (2013). Bundled Payments for Care Improvement (BPCI) initiative: General information. Retrieved from http://innovation.cms.gov/initiatives/bundled-payments

Centers for Medicare & Medicaid Services. (2014a). Medicare program—general information. Retrieved from www.cms.gov

Centers for Medicare & Medicare Services. (2014b). Medicaid—keeping America healthy. Retrieved from www.medicaid.gov

Centers for Medicare & Medicaid Services. (2015a). CAHPS hospital survey. Retrieved from http://www.hcahpsonline.org

Centers for Medicare & Medicaid Services. (2015b). Physician Quality Reporting System. Retrieved from http://www.cms.gov/Medicare/Quality-Initiatives-Patient-Assessment-Instruments/PQRS/index.html?redirect=/PQRS/

Council of Economic Advisors. (2013). Economic report of the president. Retrieved from https://www.whitehouse.gov/administration/eop/cea/economic-report-of-the-President/2013

Dearmon, V., Roussel, L., Buckner, E., Mulekar, M., Pomrenke, B., Salas, S., . . . Brown, A. (2013). Transforming care at the bedside (TCAB): Enhancing direct care and value-added care. *Journal of Nursing Management, 21,* 668–678.

Delbanco, S. (2014). The payment reform landscape: Bundled payment. *Health Affairs.* Retrieved from http://healthaffairs.org/blog/2014/07/02/the-payment-reform-landscape-bundled-payment/

Delbanco, S. (2015). The payment reform landscape. *Health Affairs* [Web log]. Retrieved from http://healthaffairs.org/blog/index.php?s=%22The+Payment+Reform+Landscape%22&submit=Go

DeNavas-Walt, C., Proctor, B., & Smith, J. (2013). *Income, poverty, and health insurance coverage in the United States: 2013.* United States Census Bureau. Washington, DC: U.S. Government Printing Office. Retrieved from http://www.census.gov/prod/2013pubs/p60-245.pdf

Douglas, K. (2014). How data is changing our world. *Nurse Leader, 13*(5), 37–39, 67.

Dwyer, D., Liu, H., & Rizzo, J. (2012). Does patient trust promote better care? Applied *Economics, 44,* 2283–2295.

Edmondson, W. (2015). The per capita payment model. *Population Health, 60*(1), 14–16.

Emery, D., & Brantes, F. (2015, February). Curing an ill healthcare system. *Healthcare Financial Management,* 80–83.

Fuchs, V. R. (2013). The gross domestic product and health care spending. *New England Journal of Medicine, 269,* 107–109.

Gardner, D. (2013). ACA implementation: A vulnerable and misunderstood endeavor. *Health Policy and Politics, 31*(6), 307–308.

Gardner, J. (1990). *On leadership.* New York, NY: Simon & Shuster.

Goetz, K., Janney, M., & Ramsey, K. (2011). When nursing takes ownership of financial outcomes: Achieving exceptional financial performance through leadership, strategy, and execution. *Nursing Economic$, 29*(4), 173–182.

Institute for Healthcare Improvement. (2015). *Transforming care at the bedside.* Retrieved from http://www.ihi.org/Engage/Initiatives/Completed/TCAB/Pages/default.aspx

Integrated Healthcare Association. (2012). *IHA Pay for Performance Measure Set Strategy: 2012–2015.* Oakland, CA: Author.

Investorwords. (2016). *Finance.* Retrieved from http://www.investorwords.com/1940/finance.html

Jacquin, L. (2014, April). A strategic approach to healthcare transformation. *Healthcare Financial Management,* 74–79.

The Joint Commission. (2015). Joint Commission FAQ page: What are "Accountability Measures?" [*sic*]. Retrieved from http://www.jointcommission.org/about/JointCommissionFaqs.aspx#174

Kavanagh, D., Cimiotti, J., Abusalem, S., & Coty, M. (2012). Moving healthcare quality forward with nursing-sensitive value-based purchasing. *Journal of Nursing Scholarship, 44*(4), 385–395.

Klein, D., Laugesen, M., & Liu, N. (2013). The patient-centered medical home: A future standard for American Health care? *Public Administration Review, 73*(Suppl. 1), S582–S592.

Lavoie-Tremblay, M., O'Conner, P., Harripaul, N., Biron, A., Ritchie, J., Lavigne, G., . . . Sourdif, J. (2013). The effect of transforming care at the bedside initiative on healthcare teams' work environments. *Worldviews on Evidence-Based Nursing, 11*(1), 16–25.

Leonard, K. (2015). Supreme court upholds Obama subsidies. *U.S. News*. Retrieved from http://www.usnews.com/news/articles/2015/06/25/supreme-court-upholds-obamacare-subsidies-in-king-v-burwell

Macfarlane, M. (2014). Sustainable competitive advantage for accountable care organizations. *Journal of Healthcare Management, 59*(4), 263–271.

McCanne, D. (2015). Medicare "Accountable Care Organizations." Retrieved from http://pnhp.org/blog/2010/10/28/how-does-the-affordable-care-act-define-ac

McQuade-Jones, B., Murphy, J., Novak, T., & Sarnowski, L. (2014). Nurse practitioners and meaningful use: Transforming health care. *The Journal for Nurse Practitioners, 10*(10), 763–768.

Millonis, C. (2013). Provision of healthcare in the context of financial crisis: Approaches to the Greek health system and international implications. *Nursing Philosophy, 14*, 17–27.

Milstead, J. (2015). *Health policy and politics: A nurse's guide* (5th ed.). Burlington, MA: Jones & Bartlett.

National Academies Press. (2015). *Quality chasm series: Health care quality reports from the Institute of Medicine.* Retrieved from http://www.nap.edu/catalog/12610/quality-chasm-series-health-care-quality-reports-from-the-institute

National Quality Strategy. (2015). About the national quality strategy (NQS). Retrieved from http://www.ahrq.gov/workingforquality/about.htm

Needleman, J., Pearson, M., Parkerton, P., Upenieks, V., Soban, L., Bakas, A., & Yee, T. (2007). *Transforming care at the bedside: Lessons from Phase II.* Los Angeles, CA: University of California.

Nelson, J. (2011). Measuring caring—the next frontier in understanding workforce performance and patient outcomes. *Nursing Economic$, 29*(4), 215–219.

Nickitas, D. (2011). Every nurse is a nurse economist. *Nursing Economic$, 29*(5), 229–231.

Obamacare Facts: Affordable Care Act, Health Insurance Marketplace. (n.d.). Retrieved from http://obamacarefacts.com/sign-ups/Obamacare-enrollment-numbers/

Office of the National Coordinator for Health Information Technology. (2015a). Meaningful use definition and objectives. Retrieved from https://www.healthit.gov/providers-professionals/meaningful-use-definition-objectives

Office of the National Coordinator for Health Information Technology. (2015b). *How to attain meaningful use.* Retrieved from http://www.healthit.gov/providers-professionals/how-attain-meaningful-use

Panning, R. (2014). Accountable care organizations: An integrated model of patient care objectives. *Clinical Laboratory Science, 27*(2), 112–118.

Pear, R. (2015, June 17). G.O.P. is wary about winning on health law. *The New York Times*.

Pellegrini, L., Rodriguez-Monguio, R., & Qian, J. (2014). The US healthcare workforce and the labor market effect on healthcare spending and health outcomes. *International Journal of Health Care Finance Economics, 14*, 127–141.

Reynolds, M. (2011). Medicare bundled payment program: Meaningful risk and limited reward. *Healthcare Financial Management, 65*(10), 50–54.

Rutherford, M. (2014). The value of trust in nursing. *Nursing Economic$, 32*(6), 283–288.

Sackman, J., & Buseman, C. (2015, March). Payment reform: A primer for taking on risk. *Healthcare Financial Management, 69*(3), 50–53.

Sheingold, B., & Sheingold, S. (2013). Using a social capital framework to enhance measurement of the nursing work environment. *Journal of Nursing Management, 21*, 790–801.

Smith, J. C., & Carla, M. (2014). U.S. Census Bureau, Current Population Reports, P60-253, Health Insurance Coverage in the United States: U.S. Government Printing Office, Washington, DC, 2015. Retrieved from https://www.census.gov/content/dam/Census/library/publications/2015/demo/p60-253.pdf

Snellman, I., & Gedda, K. (2012). The value ground of nursing. *Nursing Ethics, 19*(6), 714–726.

Statistic Brain. (2015). Health care industry statistics. Retrieved from http://statisticbrain.com/health-care-industry-statistics/

Stiefel, M., & Nolan, K. (2012). *A guide to measuring the triple aim: Population health, experience of care and per capita cost.* IHI Innovation Series white paper. Cambridge, MA: Institute for Healthcare Improvement.

TRICARE. (2014). TRICARE home page. Retrieved from www.tricare.mil

U.S. Department of Veterans Affairs. (2014). Veterans Health Administration. Retrieved from www.va.gov/health/

Valentine, N., Kirby, K., & Wolf, K. (2011). The CNO/CFO partnership: Navigating the changing landscape. *Nursing Economic$, 29*(4), 201–210.

Wang, I., & Maniccia, M. (2013). Accountable care organizations–an employer POV primer. *Benefits Quarterly, 29*(4), 14–19.

Warburton, R. (2009). Improving patient safety: An economic perspective on the role of nurses. *Journal of Nursing Management, 17,* 223–229.

Welton, J., & Harper, E. (2015). Nursing care value-based financial models. *Nursing Economic$, 33*(1), 14–25.

Wendel, J., O'Donohue, W., & Serratt, T. (2014). *Understanding healthcare economics.* Boca Raton, FL: CRC Press.

The White House, Office of the Press Secretary. (2014). Fact sheet: Affordable care act by the numbers. Retrieved from http://www.whitehouse.gov/the-press-office/2014/04/17/fact-sheet-affordable-care-act-numbers

Wikipedia (2016). *Finance.* Retrieved from https://en.wikipedia.org/wiki/Finance

5

Leading With a Culture of Quality and Safety

Nurse leaders are called upon to evaluate patient care on a regular basis. As part of their all-encompassing job, they continually balance the best possible care with reasonable and affordable costs. Health care in the United States in 2014 cost approximately $3.8 trillion with less than stellar outcomes (Forbes, 2014). Although the U.S. health-care consumers of today expect high quality for their expenditures in the U.S. health-care system, in relation to other countries, the United States spends 50% more per capita without providing acceptable health-care outcomes. James (2013) states the numbers may range between 210,000 and 440,000 patients each year who go to the hospital for care and suffer some type of preventable harm that contributes to their death. The Institute of Medicine (IOM) reported that approximately 42% of Americans have received substandard medical care (IOM, 2006).

Nurses are in a unique position as patient-care advocates to minimize medical error and enhance patient safety. As the coordinators of health care on a 24-hour basis, they are the first line of defense through their assessments to initiate, enhance, and/or modify the plan of care. As the profession of nursing monitors itself through standards of care, risk management, and continuous quality management, it becomes the champion of quality and safety for patients and employees (Friesen, Farquhar, & Hughes, 2005).

Quality management is not just a concept, but also a philosophy and an organizational expectation. This philosophical approach should be customer driven, decentralized, and empowering. Interprofessional teams are essential to the success of quality management and should be built on open, trusting, cooperative relationships. Successful customer relations should be a by-product of the quality approach and the foundation of education and training, technology, product reliability, and flexibility for continuous improvement (Koch, 2013).

RISK ASSESSMENT

Health-care environments need to provide an effective system for patients, visitors, and employees for patient safety and to avert or decrease loss to the institution (Pozgar, 2007). Identification and evaluation of actual or potential negative outcomes is the focus of risk assessment. By determining trends and patterns in health-care processes and then controlling or eliminating the causative factors, nurses can minimize risk. Risk management in most health-care institutions focuses resources on loss reduction and prevention, claims management, financial risk, safety, regulatory adherence, policy and procedure compliance, and reporting of sentinel events. "Sentinel events" are defined by TJC as unexpected, unwanted occurrences involving death or serious physical injury that call for immediate attention occurrences involving death or serious physical injury that call for immediate attention (TJC, 2014).

Nursing leadership roles focus on the monitoring of patient and employee safety. With rapid patient turnover, gaps in communication, increased interruptions, and continuous technology changes, the possibility of error increases. As the largest group of health-care providers, nurses are in key positions to prevent and identify system errors.

Communication is the key to risk management and risk reduction. Good communication and rapport between providers and patients as well as safety measures are essential in mitigating risk claims. As consumers of health care become less trusting and forgiving of possible mistakes, they are more prone to seek litigation as a possible response to an unexpected outcome (Sollecito & Johnson, 2013). Documentation as a form of communication establishes timing and sequencing that provides for a realistic portrayal of events.

As we look to improved documentation systems, such as electronic health records that provide a user-friendly approach while ensuring patient anonymity, we promote timely reporting, prompt investigation, and corrective action. Through safety educational preparation and technology advances we offer our health-care providers a safe and effective environment to provide care. These safe work environments are based on a foundation of open communication, properly prepared employees, adequate human and material resources, and an infrastructure in which communication concerning safety is everyone's responsibility.

Safety and Quality Communication

As nurse leaders, the quality agenda must be planned and communicated clearly to all members of the organization for a culture of safety to exist (Hendrich et al., 2007). All employees must be familiar with the mission, vision, and goals of the organization and understand their role in accomplishing the expected outcomes. Safety and quality communication should start with the employment interview and extend throughout the years of service. As an organization becomes more safety driven, the threads of quality management are integrated into communications including newsletters, meeting minutes, data sharing, and evaluations.

Being available for informal and formal communication with staff during rounds and office time provides for additional insights on the daily operations of the nursing unit. As an observer of the daily activities of a unit or department, nurse leaders are involved in current practices while introducing best-practice changes for continuous improvement. As best practices are introduced and initiated, they should be benchmarked for outcome comparison with similar health-care institutions.

Best-Practice Strategies for Managing Events

Ongoing quality analysis tools such as Failure Mode and Effects Analysis (FMEA) and Root Cause Analysis (RCA) inform nurse leaders to evaluate either potential or real-time errors.

Failure Mode and Effects Analysis

FMEA is an ongoing quality improvement process that is carried out in health-care organizations by an interdisciplinary team. FMEA is a proactive process that acknowledges that errors are inevitable but also predictable. It anticipates errors and designs a system that will minimize their impact. Corrective actions from FMEA include the determination that the error is tolerable or that specific steps must be put in place to address potential errors with significant impact. The Joint Commission (TJC) does not require FMEAs under its patient safety standards, but it is imperative that proactive evaluation of potentially dangerous processes and medical devices are routinely examined (TJC, 2014). The purpose of the FMEA is to do the following:

- Identify potential failures.
- Prioritize their significance.
- Investigate where the potential causes for the failure originate.
- Propose potential solutions.
- Create a forum to ensure potential solutions are implemented.
- Assess the effectiveness of the solution (TJC, 2014).

Root Cause Analysis

RCA is a quality-monitoring tool used to address an error that is complex in nature. RCA investigates the multifaceted processes leading up to the event carried out retrospectively in response to a sentinel event. RCA uses a framework for the continual improvement of health care known as *building and applying*. An alternating sequence of "what" and "why" questions are asked repeatedly to get to the "root cause" of the event. Members of the RCA team include individuals from all roles who were present at the event. This interprofessional team provides different views of the same event, preferably within 72 hours of the event. The process includes doing the following:

- Review the event.
- Understand the process failure.
- Develop action plans.
- Plan implementation.
- Evaluate corrections (Nash & Goldfarb, 2006).

The outcome of RCA is an action plan with delineated dates for implementation and effectiveness measurement. Strategies that have potential impact on structure, process, and outcomes surrounding the event are measured over time in an organizational plan to address the error. Many external groups require the RCA evaluation process including TJC, state regulators, the American Hospital Association, the National Committee for Quality Healthcare, and the National Association of Health Data Organizations. By reporting sentinel events to organizations that gather and analyze health-care quality data, nurse leaders hope to achieve improvements in the health status of clients and reduce unnecessary use of health-care services.

Just Culture

Moving from a culture of blame to a just culture begins with identifying errors and initiating measures to protect those served (Dearmon, 2013). In 2000, during testimony before Congress, a member of the Committee on Quality of Health Care in America at the IOM made a statement about the approaches to error reporting. It was within this testimony that Dr. Lucian Leape stated, "Approaches that focus on punishing individuals instead of changing systems provide strong incentives for people to report only those errors they cannot hide" (Leape, 2000). As an alternative to a punitive approach, the Just Culture Model seeks to provide an environment that encourages individuals to report potential and actual errors for the purpose of a proactive system investigation (Marx, 2001). The just culture concept was introduced in a report regarding patient safety presented to the Agency for Healthcare Research and Quality (AHRQ) in 2001.

Error reporting in the area of health care has traditionally held individuals responsible for negative patient outcomes. The just culture environment, by contrast, recognizes that individuals should not be held responsible for system failings. It also recognizes active errors and opposes a "no-blame culture" by not tolerating conscious disregard of or gross misconduct toward a patient (Marx, 2001).

For nurse leaders and administrators, the Just Culture Model represents a commitment to improving care delivery models, continuous quality improvement, and system work culture improvements for employees. This commitment to just culture was validated when the American Nurses Association (ANA) endorsed this concept. By developing its position statement, the ANA (2010) outlined the following recommendations for nursing:

- Collaborate with state government, boards of nursing, all health-care professional associations, and hospital and long-term care associations in the development and implementation of the Just Culture Model.
- Encourage continued research into the effectiveness of the just culture concept in improving patient safety and employee performance outcomes.
- Nurse administrators, at any level of oversight, act in their dual role as representatives of nursing and stewards of the organization to promote safe systems in the spirit of a just culture to promote safe patient outcomes and protect employees from failure.
- Direct-care registered nurses advocate for the use of the just culture concept in their practice settings.
- Educators incorporate just culture concepts into nursing curricula at every level and adhere to just culture concepts in the academic setting.
- Collaborate with other health-care professionals to develop just culture joint statements.
- Encourage all health-care organizations to implement a zero-tolerance policy related to disruptive behavior, including a professional code of conduct and educational and behavioral interventions to assist nurses in addressing disruptive behavior (ANA, 2010).

The concept has proved effective in error reduction and safety improvements in many fields. In health care, where errors have serious consequences, the just culture concept will promote error recognition, risk management, and quality improvement. By promoting system improvements over individual punishment, a just culture in health care has the potential to improve patient safety, reduce errors, and give nurses and other health-care workers a major stake in the improvement process (ANA, 2010).

QUALITY IMPROVEMENT THROUGH DATA ANALYSIS AND BENCHMARKING

The principles of quality management should be a fundamental goal of all disciplines in health. Starting in the 1960s, nursing quality assurance (QA) programs, mostly hospital based, determined that there was a need to self-evaluate processes through audits. The QA leaders, however, quickly determined that health-care quality could not be ensured through audits. TJC determined that continuous improvement must be executed to ensure quality health care. Quality management became synonymous with quality improvement, continuous quality improvement, and performance improvement, which was based on benchmarking similar organizations for comparison. These terms have evolved and tend to be used interchangeably. Their focus is on the activities that organizations use to direct, control, and coordinate quality initiatives (praxiom.com/iso-definition.htm#). During the mid-1960s, many organizations invested in the assessment and improvement of quality in health-care organizations and set out to measure themselves against organizations that were exhibiting excellent quality outcomes or "best practices." The IOM started to publish evidence-based information with stated health outcomes with the intent that like organizations would measure their quality outcomes.

At the same time, quality leaders outside the field of health care, such as Deming, Juran, Crosby, and Donabedian (Koch, 2013), offered structures and processes for analyzing quality. Through their quality theories, they proposed for the first time that 80% to 85% of an organization's problems stemmed from a systems origin and that 15% to 20% were worker-related errors. Based on this information, quality action teams or circles were integrated into the quality management process, the premise being that participatory management, through the use of statistical analysis, can make improvements.

Three types of QA tools provide graphic in-depth reports of outcomes to compare with best practices: decision-making tools (e.g., brainstorming, multivoting, and nominal voting technique), data analysis charts (e.g., control charts and process flowcharts), and relational charts (e.g., bar charts, histograms, Pareto charts, and fishbone cause-and-effect diagrams).

Brainstorming

Brainstorming is an approach to problem-solving that starts with the generation of free-flowing ideas (Fig. 5.1). This first step creates excitement, promotes involvement, and produces original solutions to issues. The ground rules established for this idea-generating process include passing no judgment, accepting all ideas, and not measuring ideas by worth or feasibility. Brainstorming works well in situations in which a list of possible ideas is needed and is usually followed by multivoting or a cause-and-effect diagram.

Multivoting

Multivoting is a method to determine the most popular item from a list based on individual opinion (Fig. 5.2). This method includes a series of voting opportunities that pares down the list of items to be considered. This method usually follows brainstorming to prioritize key items for a group.

Topic: Diabetes Education			
1. not enough equipment	7. get food service delivery to notify when en route to unit	13. patient doesn't check sugar at home like we do	19.
2. not enough staff	8. place a glucometer in every room	14.	20.
3. patient won't use the call bell	9. ask patients to bring their own glucometer	15.	21.
4. family member thinks they can handle	10. ask patients to notify staff of room service request times	16.	22.
5. invent a continuous glucose monitor	11. nursing assistants are not comfortable notifying nurse quickly	17.	23.
6. teach food service delivery to test blood sugars	12. invent a catch phrase for low blood sugar	18.	24.

FIGURE 5.1 Brainstorming.

	Person 1	Person 2	Person 3
Place a glucometer in every room	✖		
Teach nursing assistants communication skills		✖	
Ask family member to perform glucose check			✖
Teach food service delivery to test sugars			

FIGURE 5.2 Multivoting.

Nominal Group Technique

Nominal group technique is a group decision-making process that starts with individual work (Fig. 5.3). The technique is effective when individuals are unfamiliar with one another or have diverging opinions and goals. The process provides structure that allows prioritization from a large group of items.

Control Chart

A control chart is a run chart in which control limits have been placed above and below the mean (Fig. 5.4). The upper and lower control limits are statistically placed by

Item	Participants				Total	Ranking
	1	2	3	4		
A						
B						
C						
D						
E						
F						
G						

FIGURE 5.3 Nominal Group Technique.

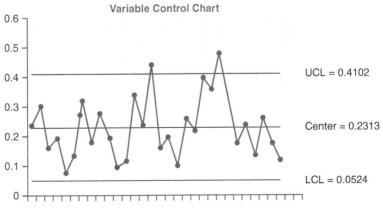

FIGURE 5.4 Control Chart.

adding and subtracting three standard deviations from the mean. With a normal distribution, the majority of the data points should fall within the upper and lower control limits. Variances within the control limits should be considered common occurrences and should not affect the process.

Process Flowchart

A process flowchart is a graphic display of a process familiar to frontline members of the team (Fig. 5.5). The chart outlines the sequence of the process including key individuals who interact in the process. As the team evaluates the flowchart, members should focus on the structure, activities, and outcomes of the process.

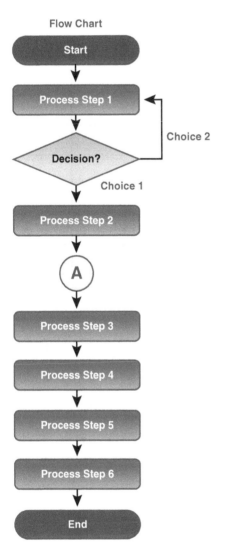

FIGURE 5.5 Process Flowchart.

Bar Charts

Bar charts are graphic displays that show the distribution of values for each variable (Fig. 5.6). Based on the data available, a bar chart can represent separate variables as individual bars (up to 12 values) or with larger data sets organized in categories.

Histogram

A histogram is a graph that displays frequency distribution presenting the measurement scale of values along the x-axis and a frequency scale along the y-axis (Fig. 5.7). The x-axis consists of discrete categories, and each bar represents different groups. The graph is used to show data distribution whether the data is symmetric or skewed.

Pareto Chart

Based on the Pareto principle that 80% of problems or effects come from 20% of the cause, this chart displays a series of bar graphs that prioritizes from tallest (most frequent) to shortest (least frequent), as shown in Figure 5.8. The bars appear in descending

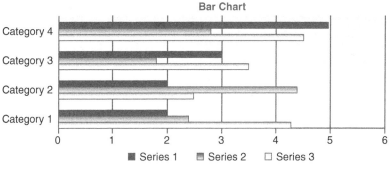

FIGURE 5.6 Bar Chart.

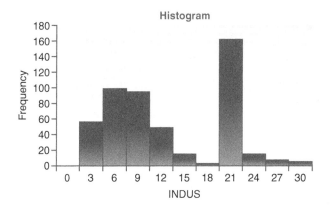

FIGURE 5.7 Histogram.

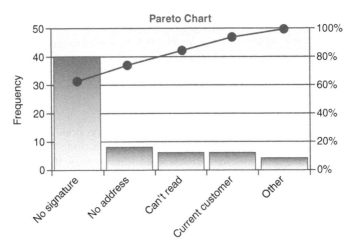

FIGURE 5.8 Pareto Chart.

heights. The graphic display readily conveys the most frequent contributing causes or factors.

Fishbone Cause-and-Effect Diagram

A cause-and-effect diagram is used to analyze potential causes of a process so that a root cause may be identified (Fig. 5.9). The "bones" of the fishbone diagram represent either the four Ms of manpower, methods, machines, and materials or the five Ps that are delineated as patrons, people, provisions, place, and procedure. This method graphically displays for the team how each of the main bones of the fish has an effect on the others and the whole process.

USING DATA FOR DECISION MAKING

Once problems are identified, action plans should be developed to address the situation. When competing issues arise, the team must prioritize them based on safety concerns. Critical problems regarding patient care are always addressed first with a quick turnaround time to implement the change. Influencing factors may be severity and frequency of the problem, cost-effectiveness of the proposed solutions, risks and benefits of proposed solutions, and accreditations and achievements that reflect the quality of the organization. An action plan can then be based on data and directed by goals that are specific, measurable, achievable, realistic, and time bound in order to project positive outcomes.

Data collection and analysis form the foundation for the decision-making process. The use of data provides sound principles for addressing the low-volume and high-risk practices in health care that pose the greatest risk to the organization and the people that it serves. The analysis of data guides decision making based on actual performance, rather than on one incident or anecdotal experiences. Thus, data should be a component

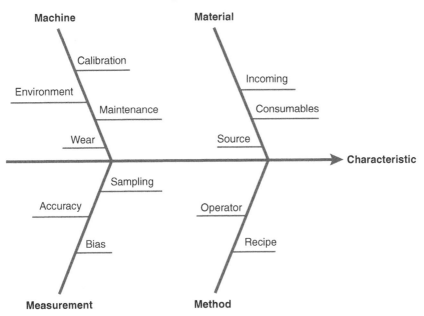

FIGURE 5.9 Fishbone Cause-and-Effect Diagram.

of any quality initiative so that a comparison can be made for pre- and postintervention performance. The tool, known as an A3, demonstrates how these data can be documented in one location to chronicle the improvement efforts and outcomes (see Fig. 5-10 on Davis*Plus* at http://davisplus.fadavis.com). Quality management is a continuous process that calls for nursing leaders to be vigilant in their planning, intervention, and evaluation of quality.

QUALITY MONITORING MEETING REGULATORY STANDARDS

Accreditation as it relates to health-care organizations is one important strategy that provides for continuous measurement and improvement in quality and safety. Accreditation has been defined as a "formal declaration by a designated authority that the organization, system, service or individual has demonstrated competency, authority and/or credibility to meet a predetermined set of standards" (Sollecito & Johnson, 2013, p. 514). This measurable process provides external stakeholders with reassurance that quality and safety standards have been met and that quality improvement initiatives are continually monitored and compared with national benchmarks. Since the 1970s, the United States and other countries have sought a mechanism of regulatory oversight and accreditation to control societal risk. Health-care organizations are accredited based on the type of services offered, professional standards, patient outcomes, and how the organization self-governs its own standards.

External organizations are currently driving the quality agenda in the field of health care in both the private sector and public sector. Establishing standards of measurement for health-care organizations provides the structure for implementing regulatory mandates, accreditation procedures, benchmarking, data gathering, and data analysis (Sadeghi, Barzi, Mikhail, & Shabot, 2013).

Governmental Quality Organizations

Some of the key U.S. governmental agencies that play a part in quality management include the following:

- U.S. Department of Health and Human Services (HHS)
- Centers for Medicare & Medicaid Services (CMS)
- Agency for Healthcare Research and Quality (AHRQ)
- National Quality Measures Clearinghouse (NQMC)
- U.S. Department of Veterans Affairs (VA)

U.S. Department of Health and Human Services

HHS monitors and controls public reimbursement for health-care services; regulates health-care systems' quality performance; and provides the public with individual hospitals, health-care systems, and nationally trended data as a component of transparency for the informed health-care consumer (U.S. Department of Health and Human Services, 2014). HHS also provides valuable funds to support research that provides evidence-based advancement in health-care quality monitoring; HHS includes CMS and AHRQ under its umbrella of services.

Centers for Medicare & Medicaid Services

The federal government currently sets health-care policy through legislation, funding, data reporting, and reimbursement through the many regulatory mandates and programs under CMS oversight. CMS has also created a set of outcome measures called Outcome-Based Quality Improvement through the Medicare Quality Monitoring System (MQMS) in an effort to provide continual monitoring and improvement in the quality of care delivered to Medicare beneficiaries (CMS, 2014a). Highlights of the MQMS include the establishment of quality outcomes benchmarks for Medicare patients, quality outcomes measures based on utilization of services provided, and national and state quality outcomes.

In 2002, CMS launched the CMS Quality Initiative in combination with the Nursing Home Quality Initiative. Services continued to be expanded; in 2004 CMS added the End-Stage Renal Disease Quality Initiative and in 2005 it added the Physician Voluntary Reporting Program. CMS also plays a role in monitoring patient safety and experiences, health disparities, and the use of health information technology.

Agency for Healthcare Research and Quality

AHRQ provides four quality indicators (QIs) for different providers and administrators of health-care settings. These QIs provide a reporting structure for trends such as data over time by placing them in a comparative database for measurement of national, regional, and state benchmarks. The four AHRQ quality measures include inpatient quality indicators, prevention quality indicators, patient safety indicators, and pediatric quality indicators (Bott, 2010).

This agency also maintains the Healthcare Cost and Utilization Project database, which provides a reliable source to access health statistics and information on inpatient and emergency utilization of services, and the Consumer Assessment of Healthcare Providers and Systems. Through its National Healthcare Quality Report and the National Healthcare Disparities Report, AHRQ provides useful information on national trends and supports the National Quality Measures Clearinghouse.

National Quality Measures Clearinghouse

NQMC is a dedicated Web site (guidelines.gov) and database providing educational and quality benchmark data information. NQMC establishes the quality measure conformity and rigorous evaluation criteria that are used by the health-care community. The clearinghouse of health-care data submitted by numerous third-party entities provides a data repository that is a resource for quality management.

U.S. Department of Veterans Affairs

The VA provides health-care services to veterans and their families. As part of a culture of patient safety, the VA established the National Center for Patient Safety whose goal is to prevent or reduce inadvertent patient-care harm through the adoption of established safety initiatives from fields such as aviation, nuclear energy, and safety engineering. With the emphasis on patient safety, this federally funded health-care system is one of the leaders in safety measurement and supports research studies and interventions that make a difference in the daily lives of patient and caregivers (U.S. Department of Veterans Affairs, 2014).

Nonprofit Quality Organizations

Although governmental agencies provide oversight of health-care quality, health care is also influenced by nonprofit and independent organizations. Sometimes these agencies have provided timely and influential observations on the quality of health care by providing a different view. Some of the more prominent nonprofit organizations are:

- The Institute of Medicine (IOM)
- National Association for Healthcare Quality
- The Joint Commission (TJC)
- Institute for Healthcare Improvement
- Hospital Quality Alliance
- National Quality Forum
- National Committee for Quality Assurance
- The Leapfrog Group
- American Nurses Association, American Nurses Credentialing Center (ANCC) (Magnet Designation)

Institute of Medicine

Through its efforts on quality management, the IOM has spearheaded change regarding health-care quality and performance. Emphasizing the political and strategic aspects, the IOM has provided alarming and influential reports on the state of health-care quality. With a lens focused on the importance of providing health-care quality education to the public, the IOM has generated many reports outlining quality issues in health care:

- *Statement on Quality of Care:* National Roundtable on Health Care Quality. The Urgent Need to Improve Health Care Quality, January 1998
- *Measuring the Quality of Health Care,* February 1999
- *Crossing the Quality Chasm: A New Health System for the 21st Century,* March 2001
- *Envisioning the National Health Care Quality Report,* March 2001
- *Leadership by Example: Coordinating Government Roles in Improving Health Care Quality,* October 2002
- *Priority Areas for National Actions: Transforming Health Care Quality,* January 2003
- *Patient Safety: Achieving a New Standard for Care,* November 2003
- *Medicare's Quality Improvement Organization Programs: Maximizing Potential,* March 2006
- *Preventing Medication Errors: Quality Chasm Series,* July 2006
- *The Future of Nursing: Leading Change, Advancing Health,* October 2010 (IOM, 2014)

The IOM has defined quality and health care as well as six quality aims, also referred to as "dimensions of quality," for achieving a high-quality health-care system. The IOM defines quality as "the degree to which health services for individuals and populations increase the likelihood of desired health outcomes and are consistent with current professional knowledge" (IOM, 2001, p. 1).

The IOM's six aims are safety, effectiveness, patient centeredness, timeliness, efficiency, and equitability (IOM, 2001). These aims provide a comprehensive framework that outlines what quality is, but they do not address specific quality measures. From its original charter in 1970 as a component of the National Academy of Sciences, this private, nonprofit organization provides evidence-based advice on matters of biomedical science, medicine, and health (IOM, 2006).

The Joint Commission

TJC, formerly known as the Joint Commission on Accreditation of Healthcare Organizations, is the best known quality program because of its delegated authority from CMS as a requirement for reimbursement. Based on this delegated authority, health-care organizations must report core measures of quality to the TJC, including acute myocardial infarctions, heart failure, pneumonia, the surgical care improvement project, and pregnancy (TJC, 2014).

TJC's quality-monitoring database is called ORYX. It provides performance measurement and data reporting by health-care organizations and is mandatory for maintaining accreditation. This nonprofit accreditation organization also measures risk adjustment using its Risk Adjusted Guide as a statistical process that identifies variations in quality patient outcomes based on risk factors and patient characteristics. The premise of the Risk Adjusted Guide is that different outcomes may result regardless of the quality of care received from health-care providers based on the presence of patient risk factors. The comparison of patient outcomes across organizations without the inclusion of patient risk factors would be misleading when analyzing interorganizational data trends.

In the United States, TJC accredits more than 4,000 organizations, or 82% of the country's health-care organizations. This voluntary accreditation process, overseen by an international, independent, not-for-profit, nongovernmental health-care accreditation agency, provides a measurement process with trained peer reviewers who make up their surveyor workforce. Written documentation and site visit components provide a 360-degree view of the organization.

Magnet Designation

The American Nurses Credentialing Center (ANCC) has developed a Magnet Recognition Program that focuses on helping health-care organizations to achieve outstanding performance using measurable outcomes. As the largest and most prestigious nursing credentialing organization in the United States, the program is "designed to provide people and organizations in the nursing profession with the tools they need on their journey to excellence" (ANCC, 2013). Through the rigorous evaluation process, appraisers—who are expert nurses in organizational functioning—evaluate documents, conduct site visits, and produce a final report delineating the organization's outcomes. The Magnet Model has five components:

1. Transformational Leadership
2. Structural Empowerment
3. Exemplary Professional Practice
4. New Knowledge, Innovation, and Improvements
5. Empirical Outcomes (ANCC, 2014)

Academic Accreditation

Quality monitoring of the profession of nursing starts with how we educate our future nurses. Student outcomes such as clinical achievement, employer satisfaction with graduates, and licensure rates are measures of quality and safety and monitored by academic accreditation bodies. Accreditation for schools of nursing provides an outside evaluation of the educational programs, faculty, students, and resources to meet and or exceed quality measurements. Based on a set of standards, the academic institution provides proof in the form of a written document that addresses how they measured against national nursing benchmarks. As schools or colleges of nursing determine their curricular focus, they look to national organizations that oversee the principles of nursing education.

Accreditation Commission for Education in Nursing

The Accreditation Commission for Education in Nursing (ACEN) is committed to the accreditation process. Accreditation as stated by ACEN "is a voluntary, self-regulatory process by which non-governmental associations recognize educational institutions or programs that have been found to meet or exceed standards and criteria for educational quality" (ACEN, 2013, p. 1). Through the accreditation process, ACEN believes that continual improvement related to resources development, process monitoring, and state licensing examination results assists with the preparation for the profession. ACEN's specialized nursing education accreditation process can be applied to both postsecondary and higher degree programs that provide certificates; diplomas; or professional degrees including master's degrees, post–master's degrees, and clinical doctorates.

ACEN's philosophy is founded on the concept that specialized accreditation contributes to public perception of nursing quality. Through self-assessment, planning, and continual improvement, accreditation reassures the general public and the educational community that a nursing program has met and maintained a level of acceptable quality standards set by the profession of nursing (ACEN, 2013, p. 2). Accreditation agencies as well as faculty and clinicians in the practice setting share in the responsibility to ensure that the U.S. accreditation process includes a regular review of standards.

Commission on Collegiate Nursing Education

The Commission on Collegiate Nursing Education (CCNE) is a nursing accreditation agency whose mission and purpose are to contribute to the public's health by ensuring the quality of baccalaureate, graduate, and residency nursing programs (AACN, 2013). CCNE accreditation activities are predicated on a statement of principles or values. See Box 5.1.

The accreditation program is based on a self-regulatory, voluntary, nongovernmental peer-review process whereby nursing programs are measured on standards ("essentials") specific to the individual nursing educational degree. Through the accreditation process, approved CCNE reviewers evaluate written documentation and make a site visit to determine whether the educational program meets the stated essentials. This accreditation process is grounded in the continual quality assessment and improvement that are focused on benchmarking against similar educational programs. The site visit component of the accreditation program includes the feedback of students, faculty, administrators, and community stakeholders. If the nursing educational program has a clinical component, communication in the form of meetings is established with the stakeholder groups. CCNE is in accordance with nationally recognized nursing accreditation processes in the United States.

CCNE has five general purposes:

1. To hold nursing programs accountable to the community of interest—the nursing profession, consumers, employers, institutions of higher education, students and their families, nurse residents—and to one another by ensuring that these programs have mission statements, goals, and outcomes that are appropriate to prepare individuals to fulfill their expected roles.
2. To evaluate the success of a nursing program in achieving its mission, goals, and expected outcomes.
3. To assess the extent to which a nursing program meets accreditation standards.
4. To inform the public of the purposes and values of accreditation and to identify nursing programs that meet accreditation standards.
5. To foster continuing improvement in nursing programs—and, thereby, in professional practice (CCNE, 2013, p. 1).

U.S. Department of Education

The U.S. Congress established the U.S. Department of Education on May 4, 1980, with the Department of Education Organization Act (Public Law 96-88 of October 1979). The Department of Education's mission is to promote student achievement and preparation

BOX 5.1 CCNE Commission Values

1. Foster trust in the process, in CCNE, and in the professional community.

2. Focus on stimulating and supporting continuous quality improvement in nursing education programs and their outcomes.

3. Be inclusive in the implementation of its activities and maintain an openness to the diverse institutional and individual issues and opinions of the interested community.

4. Rely on review and oversight by peers from the community of interest.

5. Maintain integrity through a consistent, fair, and honest accreditation process.

6. Value and foster innovation in both the accreditation process and the programs to be accredited.

7. Facilitate and engage in self-assessment.

8. Foster an educational climate that supports program students, graduates, and faculty in their pursuit of lifelong learning.

9. Maintain a high level of accountability to the public served by the process, including consumers, students, employers, programs, and institutions of higher education.

10. Maintain a process that is both cost effective and cost accountable.

11. Encourage programs to develop graduates who are effective professionals and socially responsible citizens.

12. Assure autonomy and due process in its deliberations and decision-making processes.

Source: AACN, 2013, p. 2) http://www.aacn.nche.edu/ccne-accreditation

for global competitiveness by fostering educational excellence and ensuring equal access. Its aims are to do the following:

- Strengthen the federal commitment to assuring access to equal educational opportunity for every individual.
- Supplement and complement the efforts of states, the local school systems, other instrumentalities of the states, the private sector, public and private nonprofit educational research institutions, community-based organizations, parents, and students to improve the quality of education.
- Encourage the increased involvement of the public, parents, and students in federal education programs.

- Promote improvements in the quality and usefulness of education through federally supported research, evaluation, and sharing of information.
- Improve the coordination of federal education programs.
- Improve the management of federal education activities.
- Increase the accountability of federal education programs to the president, Congress, and the public (U.S. Department of Education, 2014, p. 1).

To monitor the national view of education, the U.S. Department of Education uses data-driven trends to compare the United States with other countries. As the overseer of financial funding, policy, and research for educational initiatives in the United States, this federal agency has an annual budget of $69 million in discretionary funds. With two-thirds of the funding going to student financial aid and special education, the agency is instrumental in providing affordable education assistance. The U.S. Department of Education's policy initiatives include the American Recovery and Reinvestment Act and No Child Left Behind. Based on the 10th Amendment to the U.S. Constitution, most education policy is decided at the state and local levels. See Box 5.2.

USING EVIDENCE TO MAKE PRACTICE DECISIONS

The health-care community credits Dr. Archie Cochrane with developing the concept of evidence-based practice (EBP) in the 1970s, yet nurses know that Florence Nightingale used data to change practice in the 1860s. Nevertheless, EBP encourages the use of data to drive decisions based on sound clinical research. Sackett further posited that EBP is the integration of clinical expertise, patient values, and the best research evidence into the decision-making process for patient care. Clinical expertise refers to the clinician's cumulated experience, education, and clinical skills. The patient brings to the encounter his or her own personal preferences and unique concerns, expectations, and values. The best research evidence is usually found in clinically relevant research that has been conducted using sound methodology (Sackett, Strauss, Richardson, Rosenberg, & Haynes, 2000).

The learning curve on EBP is not steep, but it is wide. With 3.2 million nurses at various stages of embracing the process and principles of EBP, there has been some movement, but not enough to improve health-care quality quickly with data-driven decisions. The formal introduction of EBP began with Stetler's Model of Research Utilization, a staple of graduate programs in the 1980s. Added to this were Dobbins's and Funk's teams' frameworks for dissemination of nursing research. Subsequent refinements to EBP models included the Johns Hopkins Nursing Evidence-Based Practice Model, the IOWA

BOX 5.2 **Accreditation Is an Involved Process**

Based on your educational preparation as a student, nurse leader (practice and academic), and community stakeholder, do you value accreditations and designations from nursing or federal organizations, agencies, or departments? What has been your role in this process? What would you suggest to improve this process?

Model, the ACE-STAR Model for Knowledge Transformation, Rosswurm and Larrabee's EBP Change Model, and the Advancing Research through Close Clinical Collaboration Model (White & Dudley-Brown, 2012). Extensive information on each model is available, but is beyond the scope of this chapter.

Important, however, is the comparison of the EBP process to quality processes (Seidl & Newhouse, 2012). It is generally agreed that there are five key steps to the EBP process: ask, acquire, appraise, apply, and assess. These are the five As. When compared with quality methodologies such as Plan-Do-Check-Act, Six Sigma, Lean, RCA, and FMEA, there are misalignments with the EBP process, suggesting that the EBP process is a more comprehensive view of how to drive changes into practice than with quality methodologies alone.

Further description of the five As includes the following:

- Ask important questions about the care of individuals, communities, or populations.
- Acquire the best available evidence regarding the question.
- Critically appraise the evidence for validity and applicability to the problem at hand.
- Apply the evidence by engaging in collaborative health decision making with the affected individual(s) and/or group(s). Appropriate decision making integrates the context, values, and preferences of the care recipient as well as available resources, including professional expertise.
- Assess the outcome and disseminate the results.

This can be accomplished using PICO (an acronym for patient population or problem, intervention, comparison to nothing or another intervention, and outcome [adding setting or time is optional]) to reflect the isolated clinical issue that requires specific data and standards to affirm existing practice or to develop a practice recommendation to improve quality and safety.

PICO allows for identification of key terms for a comprehensive literature search, selection of appropriate studies, appraisal of findings from those studies, recommendations for practice, and recommendations for filling gaps in practice. Numerous appraisal criteria are available. One that allows for inclusion of single observational studies, which are very common in nursing, is the GRADE method (Guyatt et al., 2011). The GRADE method allows for labeling a study as either a strong or weak recommendation based on its use of one of four values, high, moderate, low, or very-low quality evidence. The use of three consistent characteristics for appraisal yields one of the eight possible evaluations. The method is very easy to use in combination with a matrix of literature findings to organize multiple studies for moving to recommendations.

Even with effective quality improvement methodologies, use of findings from the current body of knowledge is necessary to support data-driven decisions to improve care. The quality or EBP methodology alone is insufficient for sustainable outcomes; therefore, a new science has emerged to support implementation.

Implementation Science

Translation of evidence into practice can take up to 17 years, owing to differences in the thought processes of scientists from that of administrators, owing to insufficient evidence from poorly constructed studies, and finally owing to traditionalist thinking in spite of a changing environment. Implementation science is the study of methods to promote the integration of research findings and evidence into health-care policy and practice (Fogarty International Center, 2014). Implementation science seeks to understand the behavior of health-care professionals and other stakeholders as the key variable in the sustainable uptake, adoption, and implementation of evidence-based interventions.

Because implementation science is a newly emerging field, its definition and the type of research it encompasses may vary according to the setting and sponsor. However, the intent of implementation science and related research is to investigate and address major bottlenecks (e.g., social, behavioral, economic, management) that impede effective implementation, to test new approaches to improve health programming, and to determine a causal relationship between the intervention and its impact.

This rapidly evolving adjunct to the quality field has a growing body of knowledge worldwide. Originally referred to as T2, the implementation phase of the research process should precede T3, the dissemination phase. This way, dissemination of effective implementation strategies can be shared. Without knowing what is implemented, how it is implemented, and the effect of implementation, all those who read original research, known as T1, know only results without application. Centers for Implementation Science, formal courses, and a dedicated online journal, in its ninth year, have emerged to accelerate the implementation of meaningful findings. In order for health-care professionals to improve health-care quality, we must know how to adopt, implement, and sustain evidence-based interventions.

QUALITY MANAGEMENT THROUGH INFORMATION MANAGEMENT SYSTEMS

CMS (2014b) developed an Electronic Health Record (EHR) Incentive program to provide financial incentives to organizations for the meaningful use of EHR (certified) technology to improve patient care. This allowed for adoption, implementation, or upgrade of EHR technology. After demonstration that the EHR is being used meaningfully and is able to extract documentation that meets certain thresholds, incentive payments are made to organizations. The investment in the EHR is hefty, and the incentives do not offset the purchase and implementation costs, but they are geared to motivate the resulting improvements.

The program was rolled out in two stages with compliance milestones available at the CMS Web site (CMS, 2014b). Stage 1 required hospitals to meet 11 core and 5 elective objectives. Upon completion of stage 1, 20 additional core objectives are added:

1. Use computerized provider order entry for medication orders (stage 1).
2. Implement drug-drug and drug-allergy interaction checks (stage 1).
3. Maintain an up-to-date problem list of current and active diagnoses (stage 1).
4. Maintain an active medication list (stage 1).
5. Maintain an active medication allergy list (stage 1).
6. Record all items: preferred language, gender, race, ethnicity, date of birth, and date and preliminary cause of death in the event of mortality (stage 1).
7. Record initial and changes in vital signs: height, weight, blood pressure, body mass index for adults, and growth charts for children (stage 1).

8. Record smoking status for patients aged 13 years or older (stage 1).
9. Implement one clinical decision support rule related to a high-priority hospital condition (stage 1).
10. Provide patients the ability to view online, download, and transmit information about a hospital admission (stage 1).
11. Protect EHR created or maintained by the certified EHR technology through the implementation of appropriate technical capabilities (stage 1).
12. Incorporate laboratory results into EHR technology (stage 2).
13. Generate lists of patients for quality improvement, research, and outreach (stage 2).
14. Use EHR technology to generate patient-specific patient education (stage 2).
15. Upon transfer from another setting of care, perform medication reconciliation (stage 2).
16. When transferring to another setting of care, provide a summary care record (stage 2).
17. Demonstrate capability to submit immunization data to immunization registries (stage 2).
18. Demonstrate capability to submit laboratory data to public health bodies (stage 2).
19. Demonstrate capability to submit syndromic surveillance data to public health bodies (stage 2).
20. Automatically track medications from order to administration (stage 2).

This extensive list of objectives provides insight into how the electronic record supports the use of the data that are collected and documented by various providers in the organization. Currently, participating organizations are reconciling their performance on these objectives using a variety of indicators to support each one. Reconciliation is necessary insofar as previous measurement methods may not align with the data that result from EHR-generated reports without fine-tuning.

Big Data

"Big data" is a popular term used to describe the exponential growth and availability of data, both structured and unstructured. Because more data lead to increasingly accurate analyses, the concept of big data has grown to be important to both business and society. Although political views differ on the value of big data as being intrusive or informative, it is clear that more data leading to more accurate analyses lead to better decision making, resulting in reduced risk, greater efficiencies, and satisfying cost reductions. Most can agree that these three outcomes are vital to today's health-care market.

As far back as 2001, Laney developed the now-mainstream definition of big data as the three Vs: volume, velocity, and variety. *Volume* has increased owing to the ability to store more data, integrate more data systems, and develop analytics that can create value from the stored data. *Velocity* refers to the speed with which data are fed to systems, at a torrential pace, requiring real-time analysis rather than any kind of retrospective review. *Variety* describes the exponentially increasing platforms and data points that make up multiple data sources, types, and possibilities.

Two important considerations about big data are variability and complexity, much like what was cited in the foregoing section on the EHR. Data flow and consistency vary and, in fact, can confound findings because of slow, blocked, or crashing flow. As emphasized in the EHR section, consistency in terms and their connectivity are critical to the ability to extract necessary data later. A common definition of each term used by all stakeholders is necessary for any data point to have meaning when the data come from multiple sources. Cleansing and matching the data coming from multiple systems is time consuming but required to discover relationships or causality, with one analysis often taking hours to process on very large, integrated systems.

A simple example of an innovative approach to examining patterns comes from a tracking site for currency, started for fun, found at http://www.wheresgeorge.com/#url. More than 250,000,000 U.S. currency bills have been entered and are being tracked as they move about the United States and the globe. This grassroots activity has now become a means of predicting the spread of disease based on the big data showing how items we handle are spread throughout the world. A shift in how political campaigns are now managed has occurred because of the analysis of big data (Isenberg, 2012).

What, then, does big data have to do with quality? Data available from the Centers for Disease Control and Prevention or the CMS are examples of the input and analysis of big data. Data sets are available from these sites to allow further exploration into new relationships and, in turn, explanations of how and why things work. CMS is the largest single payer for health care in the United States and thus generates huge amounts of data. Like many organizations, CMS has experienced technological challenges, primarily based on privacy concerns and volume, yet has made rapid progress providing new capabilities to use data in new and innovative ways (Brennan, Oelschlaeger, Cox, & Tavenner, 2014). Examples of different types of CMS data used both internally and externally are fee-for-service claims; assessment data from patient assessment instruments; various surveys, such as the Medicare Current Beneficiary Survey, the Health Outcomes Survey, and the Healthcare Effectiveness Data and Information Set; quality through the value-based purchasing programs; Medicare Advantage encounters; and Medicare Part D prescription drug events. Some resulting innovations are tracking readmission rates, monitoring beneficiaries' health status, and predictive modeling. CMS outcomes include the ability to detect fraud and provide data to all its stakeholders (providers, beneficiaries, and researchers) more quickly.

The progression of big data promises to guide health-care quality with clear evidence to promote the best decisions. Although every health-care stakeholder will not perform analysis, all will surely benefit from the use of advanced analytics.

Sharing Data With Stakeholders

Making data accessible to stakeholders is important to the daily decision making driving patient care across the nation. When data are shared with frontline staff and managers, the intent is both to inform and to guide practice. Data sources, such as the National Database for Nursing Quality Indicators (NDNQI), provide a common forum for the measurement of outcomes of patient-care coordination. Although trained individuals at participating hospitals submit the data, the analysis that emerges is intended for the use of direct care staff and their leadership. Presenting the data the way that they are reported by the source organization may not be in the form that is easiest for the end users to comprehend and apply to their practice. It is recommended that rounding with staff to seek their understanding of graphs and tables be conducted regularly. Often there is an incomplete or incorrect interpretation of the graphic depiction of the data because of lack of clarity of definitions, data collection methods, the graph or table labels (or lack thereof), and the desirable targets.

Organizations set targets that might not match benchmarks set by the source organization. The organization's targets may be at a higher level, driving the organization's stakeholders to optimal performance. Therefore, rather than performance at the median, or 50th percentile, where half the participating organizations perform below the median and half perform above it, high-performing organizations might set targets at the 75th percentile, indicating a performance better than 75% of all other participating organizations. Benchmarking allows comparison with similar organizations and encourages the sharing of best practices to achieve that performance. Setting that benchmark is the responsibility of the source organization and, in the example of NDNQI, is currently the mean or the median performance of all participating subscribers.

During rounding, quality leaders can ask stakeholders for an explanation of the graph in order to collect input on the usability of the graph, for necessary information to help staff understand the implications of the findings, and to learn of best practices to share with others. Often a minor modification to the graph, such as adding an arrow to show whether a higher number means better or worse performance, can make the difference in accurate interpretations. Use of color, an effective range of performance, clear data labels, and actual numbers in addition to percentages can help draw a visual image of the complex relationship of all the data points represented. Leadership can also write notes of encouragement and points of emphasis on the graphs so that staff members' roles in improvement are recognized. Trending the data over time also demonstrates a diminishing or improved approach to the outcome, providing additional information to motivate continued attention to the outcome. Finally, helping staff know the difference in reporting periods is helpful. Whether weekly, quarterly, or annually, these must be labeled clearly to differentiate calendar periods (e.g., January to December) from fiscal periods (e.g., 13 four-week periods from July to June).

Data should be transparent, timely, and effective. They should be shared in publications and live discussions, such as unit/department staff meetings and organizational town hall meetings. Those presenting them should have a thorough understanding of the data and be prepared to field questions from those viewing the data. Ideas that result from understanding the data should be shared with leadership and other stakeholders so that all ideas are considered equally.

SYSTEMS APPROACH TO QUALITY

A systems approach to quality management is based on the premise that 80% to 85% of problems arise from the system and 15% to 20% from the workers. Continuing this thought process, managers use statistical methods to look for variation in activities and pinpoint causes. Variation is a concept that makes a statistical measurement of routine processes and addresses the cause. Understanding that system management looks for causes while proposing system solutions provides the manager an opportunity for improvement and quality. Managers need to provide an open communication process that is bidirectional to address potential positive or negative effects to the up- or downstream processes related to the system change. Different theories are used to analyze quality by combining statistics, consistency, cultural change, and innovation, all with the desired outcome of improving quality overtime.

Chaos Theory

The modern study of chaos (Gleick, 1987) began with mathematical analysis resulting from how tiny differences in input quickly become overwhelming differences in output. This suggests a phenomenon involving sensitive dependence on initial conditions. Chaos theory also suggests that the bell-shaped curve (normal distribution) does not occur in nature or in business very often, but that symmetry does result from examination of multiple patterns emerging from massive data sets. One of the premises of chaos theory is that standard logic, once the foundation of mathematics education, can be replaced with logistic difference equations and now with many other new statistical processes. This provides the varied and necessary strategies needed to explain the current health-care world. When faced with a practice problem to improve quality, staff often state, "It doesn't make any sense . . . we've tried this or that." Therefore, we must ask for additional analyses that offer different views of the data and thus other possible explanations. An example is the up and down movement of patient satisfaction scores. An immediate reaction might be to report something like, "We're doing great!" or "Oh no, what went wrong?" or, "It's OK; we're back on the rise." Yet, stabilization occurs with sustained efforts and not reactive adjustments to short-term shifts in the data. Consistent upward trending over time is far more important than weekly fluctuations.

When the results of analysis countermand the nurse leader's own thoughts about reasonable behavior, then one of four rationales can be offered:

1. A mistake has been made in the formal mathematical development
2. The starting assumptions are incorrect or constitute a too-drastic oversimplification
3. The nurse leader's own intuition about the biological field is inadequately developed
4. A penetrating new principle has been discovered

Finally, management thought leader Peters (1987), when developing the title for his provocative *Thriving on Chaos*, considered how management and chaos could interrelate effectively. Knowing that competition creates (and will continue to create) *chaos*, he wanted to word the title appropriately. Knowing that *thriving* was an imperative, he considered both *amidst* and *on* as the precise term to connect the terms. Peters discounted the use of *amidst*, as it implied coping or coming to grips with, and *on* suggested the leaders of tomorrow will deal proactively with chaos. Most leaders would agree that Peters was right.

General System Theory

General System Theory (GST) originates from Bertalanffy (1969), a biologist. The term evolved into a pseudoscience with little resemblance to the original intent. GST was focused on a new way of thinking about science and its paradigms in order to delineate the interdependence of relationships as they evolve in organizations. A central topic of systems theory is self-regulating systems, meaning that the system will self-correct through feedback. A core concept of quality management is constant feedback, yet in health care we remain challenged to achieve the self-correction. The advent of multiple systems offering guidance or guidelines has deferred self-regulation for external regulation, making it difficult for the relationships to guide performance. Self-regulating systems are found in nature and in society, leaving us to consider what is the best approach to nurture self-regulation.

Current leadership strategies are focused on building relationships within organizations (Baptist Leadership Group, 2011). Rounding by leadership affords the opportunity to see the total organization and detect patterns that are not visible when leaders work in silos. Helping disciplines and levels of staff to make connections and embrace their similarities and common goals for patient-centered care is the output of leader rounding. Work by Kuczmarski and Kuczmarski (2007) suggests that leaders must possess six new qualities in order to move organizations: humility, compassion, transparency, inclusiveness, collaboration, and values-based decisiveness. These qualities make up their success model and thus serve as a new leadership paradigm. In terms of quality, transparency and values-based decisiveness are self-explanatory, yet the concepts of humility and compassion require a new approach by many leaders who believe change will happen, not that change must be nurtured. As inclusiveness is about accepting differences and collaboration is about building relationships, this model contributes to how GST guides quality endeavors and supports implementation science.

Social Physics

Pentland (2014) has popularized a new area for systems to consider, *social physics*. This is a quantitative social science examining patterns of behavior, data, and societies. It tracks connections between idea flow and information, reflecting on human behavior. It builds on social learning and how the flow of ideas shapes societal norms, business productivity, and creative output. Social physics offers predictive output and pathways for communication. The core concept of social physics is the flow of ideas that can serve to provide timely information to create efficient systems and thus drive behavior change and innovation.

The mathematic focus of social physics can limit group thinking, a common outcome of social networks. It can diffuse some of the emotion associated with decision making and offer suggestions about how to pace the spread of information. Although social physics has its origins in the early 1800s, during the time of Newton, people resist having their responses likened to that of a machine. Yet the current application of analysis of human communication and movement has demonstrated patterns aligned with economic indicators. The use of massive data can guide the necessary changes to social interactions and communication in order to improve quality of health care.

CONCLUSION

Quality management programs call for planning, analysis of current processes through the use of data collection, development of new processes, allocation of resources, and evaluation. These quality programs are the cornerstone of measuring and maintaining quality standards and health-care delivery systems that strive for improvement. Nursing quality management programs should be based on EBP projects and research studies that are grounded in the clinical setting. Improvement of patient outcomes through the acquisition of new knowledge is the pinnacle of success for nursing.

References

Accreditation Commission for Education in Nursing. (2013). *Mission, purpose and goals.* Retrieved from http://acenursing.org/mission-purpose-goals/

Agency for Health Care Research and Quality. (2011). *About us.* Retrieved from http://www.ahrq.gov

American Association of Colleges of Nursing. (2013). *CCNE accreditation.* Retrieved from http://www.aacn.nche.edu/ccne-accreditation

American Nurses Association. (2010). *Just culture position statement* (pp. 1–13). Silver Spring, MD: Author.

American Nurses Credentialing Center. (2013). *2014 Magnet Application manual.* Silver Spring, MD: Author.

Baptist Leadership Group. (2011). *The HCAHPS imperative for creating a patient-centered experience.* Pensacola, FL: Author.

Batalden, P. B., & Stoltz, P. K. (1993). A framework for the continual improvement of health care: Building and applying professional and improvement knowledge to test changes in daily work. *Joint Commission Journal on Quality Improvement, 19*(10), 424–427.

Bertalanffy, L. von. (1969). *General System Theory* (pp. 39–40). New York, NY: George Braziller.

Bott, J. (2010). *Quality indicators 101: Background and introduction to the AHRQ QIs.* Washington, DC: Agency for Health Care Research and Quality.

Brennan, N., Oelschlaeger, A., Cox, C., & Tavenner, M. (2014). Leveraging the big data revolution: CMS is expanding capabilities to spur health system transformation. *Health Affairs, 33*(7), 1195–1202.

Centers for Medicare & Medicaid Services. (2014a). Quality initiatives—general information. Retrieved from http://www.cms.gov/Medicare/Quality-Initiatives-Patient-Assessment-Instruments/QualityInitiativesGenInfo/index.html

Centers for Medicare & Medicaid Services. (2014b). EHR incentive program. Retrieved from http://www.cms.gov/Regulations-and-Guidance/Legislation/EHRIncentivePrograms/index Chassin, M.R. & Galvin, R.W. (1998). The urgent need to improve health care quality: Institute of medicine national roundtable on health care. , *280*(11), 1000-1005.Dearmon, V. (2013). Risk management and legal issues. In L. Roussell (Ed.), *Management and leadership for nurse administrators* (6th ed., pp. 568–617). Burlington, MA: Jones & Bartlett.

Fogarty International Center. (2014). Implementation science information and resources. Retrieved from http://www.fic.nih.gov/researchtopics/pages/implementationscience.aspx

Forbes. (2014). Cost of health care in the U.S. Retrieved from www.forbes.com/sites/danmauro/2014/02/02/annual-u-s-healthcare-spending-hits-3-8-trillion/#257a6b9b313d

Friesen, M. A., Farquhar, M. B., & Hughes, R. (2005). *The nurse's role in promoting a culture of patient safety.* Silver Spring, MD: American Nurses Association Continuing Education, Center for American Nurses.

Gleick, J. (1987). *Chaos: Making a new science.* New York, NY: Penguin.

Guyatt, G., Oxman, A. D., Akl, E. A., Kunz, R., Vist, G., Brozek, J., & Schunemann, H. J. (2011). GRADE guidelines: 1. Introduction—GRADE evidence profiles and summary of findings tables. *Journal of Clinical Epidemiology, 64*, 383–394.

Hendrich, A., Tersigni, A., Jeffcoat, S., Barnett, C., Brideau, L., & Pryor, D. (2007). The Ascension health journey to zero: Lessons and leadership perspectives. *Joint Commission Journal on Quality and Safety, 33*, 739–749.

Institute of Medicine. (2001). *Crossing the quality chasm: A new health system for the 21st century.* Committee on Quality of Health Care in America, Institute of Medicine. Washington, DC: National Academies Press.

Institute of Medicine. (2006). *Performance measurement: Accelerating improvement—pathways to quality health care.* Washington, DC: National Academies Press.

Institute of Medicine. (2010). *The future of nursing: Leading change, advancing health.* Retrieved from http://www.iom.edu/Reports/2010/the-future-of-nursing-leading-change-advancing-health.aspx

Isenberg, S. (2012). How President Obama's campaign used big data to rally individual voters. *MIT Review.* Retrieved from http://www.technologyreview.com/featuredstory/509026/how-obamas-team-used-big-data-to-rally-voters/

James, J. T. (2013). A new, evidence-based estimate of patient harms associated with hospital care. *Journal of Patient Safety, 9*(3), 122–128.

The Joint Commission. (2014). *About The Joint Commission.* Retrieved from www.jointcommission.org/about_us/about_the_joint_commission_main.aspxwww.jointcommission.org/about_us/about_the_joint_commission_main.aspx

The Joint Commission. (2014). *Sentinel Events.* Retrieved from http://www.jointcommission.org/assets/1/6/CAMH_2012_Update2_24_SE.pdf

Koch, M. W. (2013). Quality management: Key to patient safety. In L. Roussell (Ed.), *Management and leadership for nurse administrators* (6th ed., pp. 619–645). Burlington, MA: Jones & Bartlett

Kuczmarski, S. S., & Kuczmarski, T. D. (2007). *Apples are square.* New York, NY: Kaplan.

Laney, D. (2001, February 6). 3D data management: Controlling data volume, velocity, and variety. *Application Delivery Strategies.* Retrieved from http://blogs.gartner.com/doug-laney/files/2012/01/ad949-3D-Data-Management-Controlling-Data-Volume-Velocity-and-Variety.pdf

Leape, L. (2000, January 25). Testimony, United States Congress, United States Senate Subcommittee on Labor, Health and Human Services, and Education.

Marx, D. (2001). *Patient safety and the "just culture": A primer for health care executives.* New York, NY: Columbia University Press.

McLaughlin, C. P., Johnson, J. K., & Sollecito, W. A. (2012). *Implementing continuous quality improvement in health care: A global casebook.* Burlington, MA: Jones & Bartlett.

Nash, D. B., & Goldfarb, N. I. (2006). *The quality solution: The stakeholder's guide to improving health care.* Sudbury, MA: Jones & Bartlett.

Pentland, A. (2014). *Social physics: How good ideas spread—the lessons from a new science.* New York, NY: Penguin.

Peters, T. (1987). *Thriving on chaos: Handbook for management revolution.* New York, NY: Knopf.

Pozgar, G. (2007). *Legal aspects of health care administration* (10th ed.). Sudbury, MA: Jones & Bartlett.

Sackett, D. L., Strauss, S. E., Richardson, W. S., Rosenberg, W., & Haynes, R. B. (2000). *Evidence-based medicine: How to practice and teach EBM* (2nd ed.). Edinburgh, Scotland: Churchill Livingstone.

Sadeghi, S., Barzi, A., Mikhail, O., & Shabot, M. (2013). *Integrating quality and strategy in health care organizations.* Burlington, MA: Jones & Bartlett.

Seidl, K., & Newhouse, R. (2012). The intersection of evidence-based practice with 5 quality improvement methodologies. *Journal of Nursing Administration, 46,* 299–304.

Sollecito, W. A., & Johnson, J. K. (2013). *McLaughlin and Kaluzny's continuous quality improvement in health care* (4th ed.). Burlington, MA: Jones & Bartlett.

White, K., & Dudley-Brown, S. (2012). *Translation of evidence into nursing and health care practice.* New York, NY: Springer.

U.S. Department of Education. (2014). *Overview and mission.* Retrieved from http://www2.ed.gov/about/overview/mission/mission.html?src=ted

U.S. Department of Health and Human Services. (2014). *About us.* Retrieved from http://www.hhs.gov/about/

U.S. Department of Veterans Affairs. (2014). *VA National Center for Patient Safety.* Retrieved from http://www.patientsafety.va.gov/

6

Leading With
a Nursing Focus

This chapter begins with assessing the organization as a whole, including its standards of practice, which, as a professional discipline, nursing looks to as measurement tools for behavior, ethics, and competencies. These standards of practice are endorsed by nursing professional organizations and are used as guides for the individual and organizations for indicators of quality. To lead the organization with a nursing focus, we must be knowledgeable about nursing standards, incorporate them into our nursing division, and commit to upholding the standards consistently. Strategic planning needs to connect to nursing standards so that the quality monitoring of the nursing division is grounded in nursing research, because the primary outcome of the nursing profession is quality patient care. This should be the central theme of the mission and strategic planning.

Next, care delivery models are examined in detail. These topics are foundational for strategic planning, the main thrust of this chapter. Strategic planning is a critical element for the success of any health-care organization today. Nurse leaders and other advanced practice nurses (APNs) have the responsibility to skillfully develop and implement plans to manage large, complex organizations (American Organization of Nurse Executives, 2014). The only effective way to do that is through a comprehensive planning process. Although many tools and methods exist that can be used to develop a strategic plan, a few simple principles are consistently present within the context of each plan: conceptual and planning frameworks; a clear mission and purpose; well-defined, inspiring vision, values, and philosophical statements; involvement of all key stakeholders in the plan; a mechanism for measurement and communication of results; and possession of the organizational will to make tough, results-oriented decisions. First and foremost, however, careful assessment of the organization's structure should be made.

ASSESSING THE ORGANIZATION

It is important for an APN in any practice setting to understand the structure of the organization in order to function effectively. Health-care providers might practice in organizational structures, care delivery, and professional practice models that can be very different. In fact, health-care delivery systems have changed dramatically over the past few years, influenced by patient demographics, technology, quality and patient safety concerns, professional scope of practice, biomedical advances, and access to care. In an environment of quality and safety, the organizational structure—whether concerning a system, division, department, service line, team, or unit—should be based on sound principles of organizational theory. That is, the organizational structure should be based on the mission, philosophy, vision, values, and objectives that include the community of interest. Assessment of the organization should be continuous and part of both the business and strategic plans.

The U.S. health-care system data on patient outcomes have not been acceptable and have therefore demanded systematic reviews of organizational structure and the associated culture to improve them. The Institute of Medicine's (IOM) report "To Err Is Human: Building a Safer Health System for the 21st Century" stated that approximately 98,000 patients who were hospitalized each year die as a result of medical error (1999). As we strive to improve our patient outcomes, we systematically address error while providing a culture of "no blame" that promotes the freedom to critically analyze root causes and, based on that knowledge, redesign systems with a quality and safety foundation. There have been critics of "no blame" cultures, especially in health care, where mistakes can be deadly. Some health-care organizations have tried to maintain a balance between no blame and individual accountability using the concept of "Just Culture." This just culture framework explores the relationship between blame and accountability in the context of safety standards. Comparing the organizational or individual act against safety standards promotes safe patient care in a culture of safety (Wachter & Pronovost, 2009). When changing or developing a new organizational structure, the latest research should be considered. Organization analysis that includes culture, practices, scope of responsibility, and communication both horizontally and vertically provides a structure for recommending and instituting change. Some recommendations based on research include the following:

- Organizations should ensure that direct care nursing staff participate in decisions related to design of work processes and workflow.
- Organizations should support and develop interdisciplinary collaboration.
- Organizations should provide the resources necessary to create a work environment for nurses to reduce errors.
- Organizations should create a culture of safety (Roussel, 2013).

STANDARDS OF PRACTICE

Nurses look to the American Nurses Association (ANA) concerning professional standards. Known for its work on standards, guidelines, and principles, the ANA provides resources to registered nurses (RNs) when deciding on a particular action such as ethics, professional standards, and staffing. As a profession and a discipline, nursing defined the values associated with their responsibilities in the 2010 ANA *Nursing: Scope and Standards of Practice*, as outlined in Table 6.1. This document describes the level of nursing care demonstrated using the "nursing process" and is significant as a resource to the profession. In 1988, Yura and Walsh defined the nursing process as an orderly systematic process to determine a health outcome. The nursing process as a decision-making model provides the structure for RNs to think critically about the care that they offer and to plan actions accordingly.

TABLE 6.1 **ANA Standards of Practice**

Standard	Description
Standard 1: Assessment	The registered nurse collects comprehensive data pertinent to the health-care consumer's health or the situation.
Standard 2: Diagnosis	The registered nurse analyzes the assessment data to determine the diagnoses or issues.
Standard 3: Outcomes Identification	The registered nurse identifies expected outcomes for a plan individualized to the health-care consumer of the situation.
Standard 4: Planning	The registered nurse develops a plan that prescribes strategies and alternatives to attain expected outcomes.
Standard 5: Implementation	The registered nurse implements the identified plan.
Standard 5A: Coordination of Care	The registered nurse coordinates care delivery.
Standard 5B: Health Teaching and Health Promotion	The registered nurse employs strategies to promote health and a safe practice environment.
Standard 5C: Consultation	The graduate-level prepared specialty nurse or advanced practice registered nurse provides consultation to influence the identified plan, enhance the abilities of others, and effect change.
Standard 5D: Prescriptive Authority and Treatment	The advanced practice registered nurse uses prescriptive authority, procedures, referrals, treatments, and therapies in accordance with state and federal laws and regulations
Standard 6: Evaluation	The registered nurse evaluates progress toward attainment of outcomes.

Source: American Nurses Association. (2010). *Nursing: Scope and standards of practice* (2nd ed., pp. 8–9). Silver Spring, MD: Nursesbooks.org.

ANA has further developed *Standards of Professional Performance* (2010), which address behavioral activities for RNs, who are "accountable for their professional actions to themselves, their healthcare consumers, their peers and ultimately to society." These standards address professional behavior and how the discipline of nursing is affected by and, in turn, affects society as a whole (pp. 9–10), as shown in Table 6.2.

By providing standards of practice for specialty areas of nursing, the ANA has also been a resource in the areas of staffing, educational requirements, legislation, and an evaluation process for measuring nursing excellence. An example of one such ANA resource is the ANA *Code of Ethics for Nurses With Interpretive Statements*. This resource can be used to address nursing responsibilities while providing quality care in an ethical manner. "The ANA believes the *Code for Nurses* is nonnegotiable and that each nurse has an obligation to uphold and adhere to the code of ethics" (2015, p. 1). Position statements, principles of nursing practice, and nursing scope and standards of practice all address issues that a nurse might confront. These resources are valuable

TABLE 6.2 ANA Standards of Professional Practice

Standard	Description
Standard 7: Ethics	The registered nurse practices ethically.
Standard 8: Education	The registered nurse attains knowledge and competency that reflects current nursing practice.
Standard 9: Evidence-Based Practice and Research	The registered nurse integrates research findings into practice.
Standard 10: Quality of Practice	The registered nurse contributes to quality nursing practice.
Standard 11: Communication	The registered nurse uses a wide variety of communication skills in a variety of formats in all areas of practice.
Standard 12: Leadership	The registered nurse demonstrates leadership in the professional practice setting and in the profession.
Standard 13: Collaboration	The registered nurse collaborates with health-care consumer, family, and others in the conduct of nursing practice.

TABLE 6.2 ANA Standards of Professional Practice–cont'd

Standard	Description
Standard 14: Professional Practice Evaluation	The registered nurse evaluates her or his own nursing practice in relation to professional practice standards and guidelines, relevant statutes, rules and regulations.
Standard 15: Resource Utilization	The registered nurse utilizes the appropriate resources to plan and provide nursing services that are safe, effective, and financially responsible.
Standard 16: Environmental Health	The registered nurse practices in an environmentally safe and healthy manner.

Source: American Nurses Association. (2010b). *ANA standards of professional performance* (2nd ed., pp. 8–19). Silver Spring, MD: Nursesbooks.org.

to the individual and organizations in providing a quality measurement that is based on evidence. Both the individual nurse and nurse leader should be familiar with these professional nursing documents and use the evidenced-based information as a foundation for good decision making.

Nurse Administration Standards of Practice

In 1991, ANA established *Standards for Organized Nursing Services and Responsibilities of Nurse Administrators Across All Settings*, subsequently renamed *Scope and Standards for Nurse Administrators* in 1995 (Table 6.3). The new document provided a resource for the transition from the traditional nurse administrator role to the new nurse executive, reflecting diversity of practice settings, scope of autonomy, qualifications, and current trends. The six standards of practice describe and guide a competent nurse administrator by reinforcing the nursing process. The nursing process depends on critical thinking and problem solving to make appropriate decisions regarding an individual's care (ANA, 2011).

Nurse Administration Standards of Professional Practice

The 16 Standards of Nursing Administration Practice describe the behaviors associated with the competent nurse administrator (Table 6.4). As an RN, the nurse administrator is expected to fully engage in activities that represent the professional role and accountability inherent in the position. By meeting these standards of practice, the nurse administrator becomes a leader, advocate, and advanced practice member of the nursing profession that influences the health-care system. As a voice for nursing

TABLE 6.3 Standards of Practice for Nursing Administration

Standard	Description
Standard 1: Assessment	The nurse administrator collects comprehensive data pertinent to the issue, situation, or trend.
Standard 2: Identifies Issues, Problems, or Trends	The nurse administrator analyzes the assessment data to determine the diagnoses or issues.
Standard 3: Outcomes Identification	The nurse administrator identifies expected outcomes for a plan individualized to the situation.
Standard 4: Planning	The nurse administrator develops a plan that prescribes strategies and alternatives to attain expected outcomes.
Standard 5: Implementation	The nurse administrator implements the identified plan.
Standard 5A: Coordination	The nurse administrator coordinates the implementation and other associated processes.
Standard 5B: Health Promotion, Health Teaching, and Education	The nurse administrator employs strategies to foster health promotion, health teaching, and the provision of other educational services.
Standard 5C: Consultation	The nurse administrator provides consultation to influence the identified plan, enhance the abilities of others, and effect change.
Standard 6: Evaluation	The registered nurse evaluates progress toward attainment of outcomes.

Source: American Nurses Association. (2011). *Nursing administration: Scope and standards of practice* (2nd ed., p. 1). Silver Spring, MD: Nursesbooks.org.

TABLE 6.4 **Standards of Professional Practice for Nursing Administration**

Standard	Description
Standard 7: Quality of Practice	The nurse administrator systematically enhances the quality and effectiveness of nursing practice, nursing service administration, and the delivery of services.
Standard 8: Education	The nurse administrator attains knowledge and competency that reflects current practice.
Standard 9: Professional Practice Evaluation	The nurse administrator evaluates own nursing practice in relation to professional practice standards and guidelines, relevant statutes, rules, and regulations.
Standard 10: Collegiality	The nurse administrator interacts and contributes to the professional development of peers and colleagues.
Standard 11: Collaboration	The nurse administrator collaborates with all levels of nursing staff, interdisciplinary teams, executive leaders, and other stakeholders.
Standard 12: Ethics	The nurse administrator integrates ethical provisions in all areas of practice.
Standard 13: Research	The nurse administrator integrates research findings into practice.
Standard 14: Resource Utilization	The nurse administrator considers factors related to safety, effectiveness, cost, and impact on practice in planning and delivery of nursing and other services.
Standard 15: Leadership	The nurse administrator provides leadership in the professional practice setting and the profession.
Standard 16: Advocacy	The nurse administrator advocates for the protections and rights of individuals, families, communities, populations, healthcare providers, nursing, and other professions and institutions and organizations, especially related to health and safety.

Source: American Nurses Association. (2011). *Nursing administration: Scope and standards of practice* (2nd ed., p. 1). Silver Spring, MD: Nursesbooks.org.

at the decision-making table, the Chief Nursing Officer (CNO) is often called upon to defend valuable human and material resources for the safety of patients and employees. Abiding by these Standards of Professional Practice, nurse administrators are grounded to their profession and discipline of nursing in areas of practice, education, collegiality, ethics, collaboration, research resource utilization, leadership, and advocacy.

AMERICAN ORGANIZATION OF NURSE EXECUTIVES COMPETENCIES

As volatile changes loom in health-care services, access to care, and care settings, nurse administrators will take a prominent seat at the decision-making table. As nurse leaders, all RNs are expected to advocate for patients, peers, and themselves. Their voice for nursing at the local, state, and national levels should confidently articulate the role of the nurse to address patient safety concerns.

The American Organization of Nurse Executives (AONE) developed nurse executive competencies that describe the role and function of nurses who have an administrative practice (Table 6.5 and Box 6.1). The competencies outline an assessment tool to identify strengths as well as opportunities for growth for the nurse leader and those who may employ them. AONE believes that nurse managers at all levels should be competent in promoting a professional nursing practice environment and implementing an effective care delivery model.

TABLE 6.5 **AONE Nurse Executive Competencies**

Competency	Description
Communication and relationship building	Effective communication Relationship management Influence of behavior Ability to work with diversity Shared decision making Community involvement Medical staff relationships Academic relationships
Knowledge of the healthcare environment	Clinical practice knowledge Patient care delivery models and work design knowledge Healthcare policy knowledge Understanding of governance Understanding of evidence-based practice Outcomes measurement

TABLE 6.5 AONE Nurse Executive Competencies–cont'd

Competency	Description
	Knowledge of and dedication to patient safety Understanding of utilization/case management Knowledge of quality improvement and metrics Knowledge of risk management
Leadership skills	Foundational thinking skills Personal journey disciplines The ability to use systems thinking Succession planning Change management
Professionalism	Personal and professional accountability Career planning Ethics Evidence-based clinical and management practices Advocacy for the clinical enterprise and for nursing practice Active membership in professional organizations
Business skills	Understanding of healthcare financing Human resource management and development Strategic management Marketing Information management and technology

Source: American Organization of Nurse Executives. (2014). *Nurse executive competencies.* Retrieved from http://www.aone.org/resources/nec.pdf>

BOX 6.1 AONE Nurse Executive Competencies: Knowledge of the Health-Care Environment

Clinical Practice Knowledge	Delivery Models/ Work Design	Maintain current knowledge of patient care systems and innovations. Articulate various delivery systems and patient care models and the advantages and disadvantages of each.

Continued

BOX 6.1 **AONE Nurse Executive Competencies: Knowledge of the Health-Care Environment–cont'd**

		Serve as a change agent when patient care work/workflow is redesigned.
		Determine when new delivery models are appropriate and then envision and develop them.
Health-Care Policy	**Governance**	Evidence-Based Practice/Outcomes Measurement
		Patient Safety
		Utilization/Case Management
		Quality Improvement Metrics
		Risk Management

Source: American Organization of Nurse Executives. (2014). *Nurse executive competencies.* Retrieved from http://www.aone.org/resources/nec.pdf

CARE DELIVERY SYSTEMS

A nursing care delivery model is the blueprint of how nursing care is delivered within a specific setting. Models of nursing care have changed over time based on challenges and trends affecting the health-care system, such as with settings, medical advances, technology, financial constraints, and patient demographics (Roussel, 2013).

Patient-care delivery models or systems help to organize and provide care to patients and families. These models exist to provide a therapeutic relationship between the patient/family and the nurse during the care episode. Patient satisfaction research reveals that the most valued aspect of care is the interpersonal skills and caring behaviors of the hospital staff. There are four elements of a care delivery model (Person, 2004):

Element 1: Nurse–patient relationship and decision making
Element 2: Work allocation and/or patient assignments
Element 3: Communication between members of the health-care team
Element 4: Management of the unit or environment of care

These elements are the building blocks of any care delivery model, in which the leadership role of the nurse manager is paramount in the creation of a culture of care, interprofessional coordination of the health-care team, relationship building with patients and families, and influencing the performance of the team.

Historically, four care delivery models have defined and operationalized the way we care for patients. The four care delivery models are Functional Nursing, Team Nursing, Primary Care, and Total Patient Care. Starting in the 1950s, Functional Nursing was common. This system divided patient care tasks among members of the health-care team with the assigning responsibility limited to the manager, head nurse, or charge nurse. For example, one nurse would be responsible for all medications, and another for all treatment. Based on the industrial model of efficiency, the focus of this model is to complete the tasks in a timely manner (Person, 2004). However, because of the number of different nurses and health-care member interactions, few meaningful nurse–patient relationships could develop.

Team Nursing started to take seed in the 1970s with the role of the nurse as the professional responsible for the most complex treatments. The nurse's role as a supervisor and delegator to the other members of the health-care team provided the RN with more autonomy. The model was based on productivity and moved the center of decision making to the point of care but did not address the nurse–patient relationship. Other models such as Total Patient Care and Primary Care in the 1960s and 1970s made the RN the focus for all direct patient care. Within these two care delivery models, the nurse is highly valued for her education and practice competency, and the nurse–patient relationship flourishes.

Relationship-Based Care (RBC) and Professional Nursing Practice are both concepts that strengthen the nurse–patient relationship. In RBC, the care delivery system supports the role of the professional nurse, promotes collegial interchange, and organizes the work product while efficiently utilizing resources and valuing the human aspect of care (Person, 2004). RBC does not exist without professional nursing practice. The two concepts are symbolic in nature and continue to develop and change as needed. Implementation of RBC and a professional practice model have been shown to improve the work environment as perceived by staff nurses (Nelson, 2003).

Professional Practice Models

In recent years, we have seen new professional practice models (PPMs) that emphasize a systems approach that is dependent on interprofessional communication and collaboration. The models use transformational leadership, empowerment, shared decision making, and research as a basis for quality improvement.

PPMs establish a conceptual framework to provide nursing care as part of an interprofessional patient-care system. The model should illustrate a connection to the mission, vision, and core values of the organization and the nursing division. Basic components of the PPM may include professional values, professional relationships, a care delivery model, governance, and professional rewards and recognition. Through the support of the professional role for nursing, the PPM includes accountability of practice, inclusion of evidence-based practice and research, and continuity of care. The American Nurses Credentialing Center (ANCC) Magnet Model and the American Association of Critical-Care Nurses (AACN) Synergy Model are examples of PPMs.

Magnet Model

When designing or redesigning care delivery systems, hospital administrations look to the ANCC's Magnet Model, with its demonstrated ability to retain well-qualified nursing staff, provide higher quality of care, decrease error rates, decrease morbidity and mortality, and improve patient/family satisfaction as well as patient outcomes (Aiken, Clarke, Sloane, Sochalski, & Silber, 2002).

The Magnet Model was developed in 2007 "based on a statistical analysis of the appraisal scores of applicants under the 2005 Magnet Recognition Program Application Manual" (ANCC, 2014, p. 3). Based on magnet principles, the model focuses on how Structural Empowerment; Transformational Leadership; Exemplary Professional Practice; and New Knowledge, Innovations, and Improvements each dynamically and synergistically contribute to Empirical Outcomes (Table 6.6).

TABLE 6.6 **Magnet Model and Definitions**

Component	Definition
Transformational Leadership	Transformational leaders stimulate and inspire followers to both achieve extraordinary outcomes and, in the process, develop their own leadership capacity. They help followers grow and develop into leaders by responding to individual followers' needs by empowering them and by aligning the objectives and goals of the individual followers, the leader, the group, and the larger organization.
Structural Empowerment	Structural empowerment encompasses organizational structure, informational flow, nursing decision-making bodies, partnerships with the community, improved patient outcomes, professional development, and recognition of nursing.
Exemplary Professional Practice	Exemplary professional practice is evidenced by effective and efficient care services, interprofessional collaboration, and high-quality patient outcomes. The overarching professional practice model is the framework for nurses and interprofessional patient care that outlines the phenomena of how nurses practice, collaborate, communicate, and develop professionally to provide the highest-quality care for those served by the organization. Professional practice models, care delivery systems, staffing, scheduling and budgeting processes, accountability competence and autonomy, ethics, privacy security and confidentiality, and culture of safety are all components of this concept.
New Knowledge, Innovations, and Improvements	In a continuous integration of evidence-based practice and research into clinical and operational processes, nurses are enabled to integrate new findings into best practices. There is a systematic review of the latest research, and nurses serve on the board that reviews proposals for research. Outreach to the community regarding research dissemination is timely. Research, evidence-based practice, and innovations are measured and monitored under this aspect of the Magnet Model.

TABLE 6.6 **Magnet Model and Definitions—cont'd**

Component	Definition
Empirical Outcomes	The measurement of quality within a Magnet-designated organization is imperative, including nurse satisfaction, nurse-sensitive clinical indicators, patient satisfaction, and nursing research. Data-driven empirical outcomes are measured over time and across like-care areas. Outcomes can be qualitative or quantitative, relative to the impact of structure and process on the patient, nursing workforce, organization, and consumer. These outcomes are dynamic and measurable and may be reported at an individual unit, department, population, or organizational level.

Source: American Nurses Credentialing Center. (2014). *2014 Magnet application manual.* Silver Spring, MD: Author.

The Magnet designation is the most prestigious credential that health-care organizations can obtain and maintain based on nursing excellence and quality patient care (ANCC, 2014). Magnet designation organizations are held to the highest standards in areas of nursing care delivery, nursing knowledge, and evidence-based quality care both nationally and internationally. This voluntary nursing excellence designation calls for systematic attention to quality that includes a written application submission; appraiser reviews; site visits; and, ultimately, Magnet recognition for a 3-year period.

Synergy Model

The AACN's Synergy Model of patient care is based on the premise that the patient's/family's needs and characteristics drive the nurse competencies for optimal patient outcomes. Synergy is accomplished when patient and family needs coupled with the clinical environment are matched with the nurse's competencies. The model lens is widened to include the practice of advanced nurses in practice or administration. The synergistic interaction between the patient/family and the nurse is based on responsive interdependence, intersubjectivity, shared commonality, and equity. Eight characteristics span a continuum of health and include resiliency, vulnerability, stability, complexity, resource availability, participation in care, participation in decision making, and predictability (Curley, 2007). These eight dimensions can be applied to the patient, nurse, or system. As with any PPM, the Synergy Model includes assumptions that guide actions. The nurse–patient relationship is individualized based on the contributions of the patient, family, nurse, and community. With the goal of nursing to restore wellness, it must always be in context and defined by the patient (Box 6.2).

The model also describes eight dimensions of nursing practice that span the continuum from competent to expert and include clinical judgment, clinical inquiry, caring practices, response to diversity, advocacy/moral agency, facilitation of learning, collaboration, and systems thinking. All of these competencies are based on an integration of knowledge, skills, experience, and attitudes needed to meet the patient's needs

BOX 6.2 Synergy Model Guiding Assumptions

Patients are biological, psychological, social, and spiritual entities who present at a particular developmental stage.

The patient, family, and community all contribute to providing a context for the nurse–patient relationship.

Similarly, nurses can be described on a number of dimensions.

A goal of nursing is to restore a patient to an optimal level of wellness as defined by the patient.

The whole patient (body, mind, and spirit) must be considered.

All characteristics are connected and contribute to one another. Characteristics cannot be looked at in isolation.

The interrelated dimensions create a profile of the nurse.

Death can be an acceptable outcome, in which the goal of nursing care is to move a patient toward a peaceful death.

Source: American Association of Critical-Care Nurses. (2014). *The AACN Synergy Model for Patient Care.* Retrieved from http://www.aacn.org/wd/certifications/content/synmodel.pcms?menu=certification

while optimizing outcomes. Optimal outcomes, according to the Synergy Model, result when the patient and nurse competencies come together for the benefit of both parties. The three levels of outcomes are divided into patient and family level, unit level, and system level (Table 6.7). Positive outcomes can be a combination of all three levels or can address one of the three. Many outcomes are a combination—a synergy. As one level is affected, there is a positive effect on another.

Resource-Driven Practice Model

Care delivery can also be addressed from a resource perspective that can include patient care, resource management, and staffing. Addressing care delivery from a resource versus a needs perspective can reduce anxiety, replacing it with a balanced acceptance of the daily workload. With the inherent premise that there is always more work than time available and that staff can do very little to change the workload, this approach provides the clinical and administrative staff with shared responsibility, authority, and accountability to give quality patient care (Manthey & Koloroutis, 2004). Examples might include a shared governance structure with councils that are the decision-making mechanism for the nursing division. These councils would evaluate current practice and professional issues and, based on objective evidence, determine changes in practice. A resource-driven practice is based on setting priorities concerning what is most important to patients and families while balancing those individual needs with the total patient population served in that setting.

Nurses are effective resource stewards with a philosophy that all patients deserve quality care. Therefore, nursing's new mind-set requires health-care staff to change their thought process from seeing work as being driven by tasks and routines to work as being driven by prioritized caring. This empowered model of care delivery puts the clinical and administrative staff in an active decision-making

TABLE 6.7 **Synergy Model: Optimal Patient Outcomes**

Outcome Level

Patient and Family–Level Outcomes	Symptoms and disease management	Improved pain, nausea, or dyspnea management
	Resolution of ethical problems	Improved end-of-life decision making
	Achievement of appropriate self-care	Patient and family learning regarding self-management
	Demonstration of health-promoting behaviors	Achievement of mutually acceptable goals
	Health-related quality of life	Improved functional health
	Rescue phenomena	Decrease impact of expected complications, earlier detection of unexpected complications, and increased length of stay.
	Patient/family perception of being well cared for	Patient/family trust in nursing staff and patient satisfaction
Unit-Level Outcomes	Shared accountability and authority for unit operations and performance	Decisions at the level of occurrence, nurses actively participating in shared governance
	More experienced nurses catalyzing the advancement of less experienced nurses	More coaching and mentoring, interest in advancing nursing education and certification, partnering to create educational offerings to support practice
System-Level Outcomes	Nurse satisfaction	Improved nurse autonomy; perception of quality of care, adequate support systems, time, professional relationships, professional role enactment
	Staffing costs	Nurse retention rates, decrease vacancy rate, less time to fill positions, shift to more hours worked per week, less absenteeism, reduce the need for per diem staff
	Resource utilization and patient charges	Less waste of supplies and services
	Multidisciplinary teamwork and satisfaction	Improved measures of collaboration
	Cross-system innovation	Improved system learning

Source: American Association of Critical-Care Nurses. (2014). *The AACN Synergy Model for Patient Care.* Retrieved from http://www.aacn.org/wd/certifications/content/synmodel.pcms?menu=certification

role. The shift in mind-set requires caregivers to think critically about care priorities instead of only tasks and routines. Three key concepts drive the Resource-Driven Practice Model:

1. Critical thinking, creative thinking, and reflection of past experience of clinicians help us find new solutions to the challenges of balancing quality and cost.
2. Financial management is an area for mutual commitment among staff, managers, and administration. Mutual commitment is based on understanding that daily decisions affect long-term financial health and that long-term strategies affect daily decisions.
3. Resource-driven care requires a proactive mindset regarding staffing and scheduling, skill mix, and professional role development for nurses. (Manthey & Koloroutis, 2004, p. 192)

Changing the mind-set of the direct caregiver relies on a new way of thinking regarding resource allocation and utilization. Through this deliberate change in thought process, the nurse is empowered to effectively distribute services and resources concerning patient care. Four key mind-set changes are needed to initiate this model:

1. The RN accepts responsibility for deciding how the resources are spent for the assigned patients and families.
2. Nurses accept that nursing work is never done until the patient leaves the unit.
3. When the workload exceeds the level of staffing, additional resources may not be the best answer.
4. Resource allocation decisions proceed from an awareness and understanding of the patient's most urgent needs (Manthey & Koloroutis, 2004, p. 203).

STRATEGIC PLANNING

In today's tumultuous health-care environment, having a well-defined pathway to assure successful goal attainment is critical. Nurse executives, nurse leaders, and APNs depend on having both a plan and a strategy for enacting that plan. A strategic plan is a systematic approach used to create a future state, resulting from the realization of a vision (Yura & Walsh, 1988). The future state becomes a reality by translation of broadly defined goals or objectives following an organized sequence of steps designed to support achievement of the vision (IOM, 2011).

Conceptual Framework

Often confused with long-term planning, a strategic plan does not begin with the current state, but rather with the desired end state. With the end state in mind, a strategic plan delivers a goal-oriented plan, a plan that actually works backward to the current state (Ackoff & Rovin, 2003). As the health-care arena is rapidly evolving, especially with the advent of the Affordable Care Act, which is complicated by ever-advancing technologies, most planning horizons in the health-care setting have a 3- to 5-year end state in mind; however, some governmental agencies continue to focus on 10- to 15-year outcomes. Regardless, the end state is the focus, not the current state, when developing a strategic plan.

Strategic planning provides direction for the future and creates the opportunity to determine allocation of capital and human resources to meet future needs (Beckham, 2004). APNs in executive and clinical settings need to possess an understanding of how to develop and execute a strategic plan. Awareness of specific planning tools and understanding effective means of measurement are essential skills for today's nurse leader. One critical aspect of strategic planning in any organization is to assure that the plan is interconnected and coordinated within and across the entire organization. The nurse executive has the responsibility to develop an area-specific plan that is well integrated in the schema of the entire organization. In cases in which the organization is a part of a larger system, integration with the system's plan into the larger system is also essential. In order to better understand the concept of strategic planning, it is important to effectively utilize and differentiate different types of tools for a planning framework (Drenkard, 2001).

Planning Framework

The Chinese philosopher Lao Tzu said, "A journey of a thousand miles begins with a single step." There is no statement truer to strategic plan development than this ancient precept. In order to move forward with the development of a comprehensive strategic plan, there needs to be a process to follow, a step-by-step template or approach to use to assure that every component of the plan is well defined and properly developed. Many organizations choose to follow a prescribed approach, using a template format that is readily available and adaptable to that organization, such as shown in Figure 6.1 (Smith-Pennington & Simms, 2011).

There are a few concepts in today's health-care arena to be considered or avoided when developing a plan and choosing a framework to follow. One nationally renowned health-care consulting organization, the Camden Group, has recommended the adoption of several fundamental principles that should be considered when beginning the strategic planning process. Visibility and engagement by top management are essential. Because delivering the plan is dependent on employee contributions to the work and outcomes, leadership must be actively engaged with the workforce; listening and considering input from the "front lines" are critical to the success of the plan. Chasing current trends or following the current "hot topics" of the health-care literature is not recommended, as they often do not stand the test of time. It is imperative that the development of the strategic plan clearly includes and considers the organization's culture and is sensitive to inclusion of plan components that address the organization's culture. When there is a clash between strategy and culture, culture will prevail 100% of the time (Masters & the Camden Group, 2006). Another key point in planning involves the commitment to financial support of the plan. As an example, assume that a CNO and her strategic planning team have developed an evidence-based goal that will increase nursing time at bedside as well as increase documentation accuracy. The proposed solution includes the addition of technology: the placement of a computer workstation at every patient bedside. The estimated capital cost for full implementation is $2.5 million, with an estimated operating expense for maintenance and upgrades calculated at more than $500,000 per year. In order for this goal to be fully realized, the CNO must assure that the organization incorporates these capital and operating expenses into the budget. It has been stated that "a brilliant strategy without financial resources is no strategy at all" (Zuckerman, 2011, p.102). Nurse leaders must understand

Strategic Planning Flow Chart

Each and every component of an organization's strategic plan is carefully developed and linked together to achieve optimum results.

Mission	Vision
Answers the question: Why or for what purpose do we exist? It is the purpose for being; the catalyst for daily operations.	Provides the strategic direction in terms of where we are heading and what we want to accomplish.

Philosophy
Explain our beliefs. Consider imbed nursing theory and professional practice model.

Core Values – Standards of Behavior
Provide guidelines for how we work and serve. Consider adoption or reference to nationally recognized nursing standards.

Pillars of Excellence
Where we organize and focus our time and attention. What do we need to accomplish in these areas?

Key Performance Indicators (KPIs)
What will we measure to know how we are successful? Consider lead measures that will drive accomplishment of lag measures

Targets
Where do we want to be? Meaningful, easy-to-understand measurement, typically structured as charts or graphs with baseline and target.

Analysis & Action Plans
What are the components that are keeping us from our targets and what steps will we take to get there? Following approval plan, this is an ongoing process to ensure targets are met.

Implementation
Implement the plan.

Reviews
Review outcomes and action plans. Modify action plans to attain results. Remember, communicate, communicate, communicate!

FIGURE 6.1 Strategic Planning Flowchart.

that strategic planning is about the willingness to make hard choices for the allocation of limited resources. We cannot say yes to every request for consideration; this simply is not possible and doing so often leads to disastrous results.

A solid, well-developed plan must be founded on an objective, quantitative analysis of the market, financial resources, and the organization's competitive position in that market. For nursing, specific consideration of future health-care resources needs to be included in this analysis in order to consider competition of other providers for limited health-care human resources, in addition to other market conditions. A thorough understanding of the analyses necessary to complete the process of strategic plan development may be compared to a "building block" structure.

Building Blocks of an Effective Strategic Plan

Much like Maslow's well-known Hierarchy of Needs, the format of a five-tier pyramid can be used to define the essential building blocks of a strategic plan (Fig. 6.2). This basic core structure should be utilized in an organized systematic approach, such as that used to build a pyramid, from a foundational layer to a finished peak.

At the initial phase of development, or first tier, of the plan are internal and external influences that need to be identified, acknowledged, and assessed in order to develop a plan. These factors include a comprehensive assessment of the situation or current state of the organization—a comprehensive identification and review of strengths, opportunities, gaps, and threats challenging the organization. Some

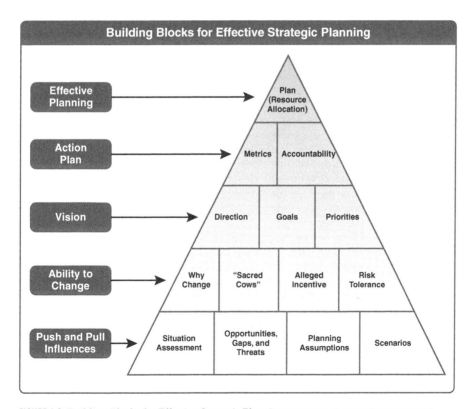

FIGURE 6.2 Building Blocks for Effective Strategic Planning. *(Courtesy of the Camden Group, 2006.)*

call this process a "SWOT" analysis, which is discussed in detail later in this chapter. The organization must identify certain planning assumptions about the future desired state of the organization. Finally, utilization of scenarios is a very helpful foundation from which a strategic plan can be developed and then flourish. A scenario is a projection of possible outcomes related to a specific plan element. Effective scenario analyses are most often utilized to improve decision making by considering potential outcomes and their implications. Using the example of placing nursing workstations at every bedside, here are a few potential scenarios that could be explored: If we place a workstation at every bedside, what are the potential problems associated with protecting patient privacy? What is the potential impact on the Information Technology department's deployment of resources on a 24/7 basis? What could be the impact on patients' sleep patterns if bedside documentation is required? What would be the impact on the nurse's time to review and assess documentation for information purposes—would it be enhanced or hindered? By exploring these potential outcomes, the planning team can decide to move forward, develop mitigating measures to minimize negative impact, or modify the plan completely.

The nurse leader must also assess the organization's ability to change in order to define the scope of the plan. A thorough understanding of the culture of the workplace is imperative. Adaptability and flexibility are important components of developing strategies that will thrive; therefore, time spent on understanding the will of the organization to change is critical. Considerations in this assessment include workforce understanding of the need to change, recognition of internal barriers that could impede progress (i.e., facility layout, pressure by staff or leadership's desire to maintain the status quo) and aligning incentives to entice or induce cooperation and active participation, and having a conscious awareness of the history of "risk tolerance" within the organization's culture (Masters and the Camden Group, 2006).

The third tier in the pyramid is devoted to reaching toward the future. It is about creation of the future state. Development of a clear, concise, and precise vision statement is perhaps the most important component of the planning process (Ackoff, 1986). Identifying the direction, the major goals, or key deliverables and defining the organization's priorities occur during this phase of development.

Once influences have been considered, the ability to change assessed, and the vision defined, the action-planning component, or fourth tier of the pyramid, commences. Too many leaders want to jump to this action-planning step prior to completion of the underpinnings of the plan. The results of moving into action planning too quickly are often disastrous, resulting in failed plans, frustrated leaders, and demotivated employees (Drucker, 1999).

The fifth and final tier of the pyramid or "actualization" of the strategic plan is when the proverbial "rubber hits the road." This phase of the planning process focuses on alignment and allocation of resources to assure plan effectiveness. Once the organizational assessment has been completed, the culture assessed, the vision defined, and the plan developed, assuring success of the plan's execution through allocation of necessary resources is a top priority. Too many grandiose plans have failed repeatedly simply owing to failure of leadership to appropriately allocate necessary resources to implement and execute the plan. Specific considerations for nurse leaders in the development of a strategic plan are described in more detail in the following sections.

Mission Statements

To inspire hope and contribute to health and well-being by providing the best care to every patient through integrated best clinical practice, education and research.

The quote is an example of a well-written mission statement from the Mayo Clinic. A strategic plan needs to begin with a focus on the mission statement. A mission statement answers the question, "For what purpose do we exist?" It is the purpose for being, the catalyst for daily operations. According to Smith-Pennington and Simms (2011), mission statements provide information, direction, and inspiration for the organization. The mission statement is not only important to the workplace itself, but also extremely important to other stakeholders, namely, the community that the organization serves. Therefore, the review process to define or redefine the purpose of the organization must include feedback and input from key stakeholders outside of the organization. This feedback is commonly sought via focus groups or open community forums. The feedback from external sources is then combined and included with feedback from internal stakeholders in the organization, from top leadership to frontline staff. The result is a defined mission statement that meets internal and external expectations.

Although asking an organization's leadership to reconsider its mission or purpose when beginning the strategic planning process may seem counterproductive, in fact, nothing could be more important. As health-care facilities become more and more dynamic and the health-care landscape changes, an organization's current purpose could have changed dramatically from what it was when the organization first opened its doors. Hospitals around the world first opened their doors to provide inpatient acute care, exclusively, and bricks, mortar, and staff were the keys to success. Today, many of those same facilities are competing in a high-tech, virtual world, and the majority of the care they provide is in the outpatient setting. As of 2012 the Agency for Healthcare Research and Quality (AHRQ), which is the latest statistics available, 9.3 million surgeries were performed as outpatient procedures. This represents 48.9 percent of all surgical procedures. Furthermore, to continue bricks-and-mortar construction in an "over-bedded" health-care society is inefficient and potentially financially disastrous (Greene, 2009).

Therefore, it is not only appropriate but indeed absolutely necessary to review and redefine the purpose of the organization as a foundation and springboard for the strategic planning process. As most strategic plans in health care now cover a 3- to 5-year time frame, after the initial plan has been developed, the process of tweaking the purpose becomes easier with each update cycle.

When reviewing and redefining the purpose statement, also remember that interconnectedness among the system, organization, division, and department is needed. Sharing of purpose statements between and across departments within a system or organization creates the synergy needed to develop plans that are cohesive and mutually supportive.

Vision Statements

Inspired by our healing Mission and guided by our Core Values, we will be the Southeastern leader for compassionate, high quality, accessible, cost-effective, innovative, adult healthcare.

The quote is the vision statement adopted by Saint Joseph's Hospital of Atlanta, Emory Healthcare. The vision of the organization is the key component driving the strategic plan. The vision defines where it is heading and what it wants to accomplish. Simply stated, the mission defines why the organization exists, and the vision describes what the organization is focused on becoming or delivering to the community it serves.

In their 2003 groundbreaking business book, *Redesigning Society*, Ackoff and Rovin focused on understanding how a society adapts to change, how the future is created, and the importance of having vision without allowing the disillusionment of today's society to interfere with dreaming of a future state. This latter ability is a pivotal component of developing an effective strategic plan (Ackoff & Rovin, 2003). Other great leadership experts, such as Tom Peters and Peter Drucker, also challenge leaders to be willing to define their dream or vision for the future and then outline the steps to meet that vision, bypassing current constraints (Drucker, 1999; Peters, 1987).

Creating a vision takes courage and invites risk. Creating a vision statement also takes knowledge and will. Initially, the vision may be most important to the creator of the statement, but sharing it with others with passion and fervor can ultimately make the vision statement a driving force for the entire organization and sometimes for the larger community. The vision must reflect the mission and values of the organization as well as provide a stimulus or challenge to stakeholders to deliver a new level of accomplishment or success (AONE, 2014). In order to be effective, the vision must be clear, easily understood, and able to be repeated. Another consideration in developing the vision statement is the population being served, including diversity as a key element. Hospital Corporation of America (HCA), one of the largest healthcare entities in the United States, has a vision statement that clearly incorporates the concept of diversity inclusion: "At HCA, we will provide culturally competent care to every patient we serve. We will foster a culture of diversity and inclusion across all areas of our company that embraces and enriches our workforce, physicians, patients, partners and communities." The best vision statements consist of a few single sentences, ideally of less than 10 to 15 words, primarily because they are easy to remember and recite.

Once adopted, the vision statement needs to be regularly communicated and reinforced; therefore, the simpler, the better. According to Daft (2008, p. 12), "Follower motivation and energy are crucial to the success of any endeavor: the role of leadership is to focus everyone's energy on the same path." The best tool with which to accomplish this task is a compelling vision statement communicated frequently. People are drawn to work for organizations that provide them with the opportunity to do meaningful work. The best way to motivate those people to work is by sharing a compelling vision for the future.

Values Statements

A values statement provides standards of behavior, or guidelines, outlining how we work and serve others. Core values drive specific behaviors that are necessary to fulfill the mission or purpose of the organization. Values statements help to drive the culture of tolerance within the organization to accepted norms. Typically described as single words with simple defined behaviors, health-care organizational values usually describe behaviors in support of caring, compassion, competence, and safety. Nurse leaders are often the thought leaders in the organization who define these core values (Marshall, 2011). Values are considered the moral compass of the organization and drive the culture of the workforce.

Philosophy Statements

A comprehensive philosophy statement considers values, beliefs, expected behaviors, and outcomes of the organization. Once adopted, it drives the focus of the organization's strategic plan. For nursing services, a written statement of nursing philosophy defines specific values, concepts, and beliefs that pertain to nursing leadership and practice within the organization (Rundio & Wilson, 2013). Strategic planning shares much in common with the nursing process, insofar as it is also a systematic, orderly process. The nurse leader is positioned to emphasize the nursing process and nursing standards of care as defined by national standards—setting entities such as the ANA, AACN, AONE, and others when defining the nursing organization's philosophy (ANA, 2011).

A well-written philosophy statement should be no longer than a page and, in addition to the elements described above, should contain educational and self-learning, best clinical practice, research and evidence-based practice, attributes of leadership, and nursing's role in the organization (Daft, 2008). Compliance and support for the philosophy typically increase ethical practices within the organization. The philosophy statement is usually best supported when written by those who will be held accountable for compliance with the philosophy. Nursing services should include participants from all levels within the nursing services department. In many nursing organizations, the shared governance structure develops the philosophy for nursing. Once defined, approved, and communicated, the philosophy becomes a founding document, and unless there are significant changes in the entire organization, the philosophy statement is rarely modified. An example of a significant change could include a major revision of the nursing care delivery system, conversion from nonacademic to academic setting, requiring an enhanced focus on education of other disciplines, or possibly a major change to the type of services delivered by the institution.

DEVELOPING A NURSING-SPECIFIC STRATEGIC PLAN

A well-written and executed strategic plan contains four essential components: a clear focus; alignment within and across the organization; the organizational discipline to conduct meaningful analysis, implement effective action plans, and conduct regular reviews of progress; and integrity of the processes and the people involved (Fig. 6.3). It is imperative for the nursing strategic plan to fully support the entire organization's guiding documents. The nurse leader or APN should begin the process by reviewing the organization's mission, vision, value, and philosophical statements. These statements make up the beginning of the nursing-specific strategic plan document, with the plan itself following. The primary reason for this is to assure that the organization's allocation of resources and focus align well and support the nursing's plan. The linkage of plans assures continuity or purpose across the organization.

Key Stakeholders

The most successful strategic plans have input from all key stakeholders, both internal and external (Fig. 6.4). The nurse executive is responsible for assuring that the nursing planning timeline provides ample time to garner this input. Most nurse leaders can readily identify external stakeholders—patients, their families, physicians, vendors,

Keys for Success

Clear Focus
Critical Few vs.
Trivial Many.

Vision
All resources and activities in
sync to achieve the plan.
Establish a clear line of sight
throughout the organization.

Discipline
The "will" and "discipline" of the
organization to conduct
meaningful analysis, implement
effective action plans, and
conduct regular reviews
of progress.

Integrity
Of the Processes
and the People.

FIGURE 6.3 Keys for Success.

Identifying Customer Needs and Expectations

Customer Needs and Expectations
Who are your **CUSTOMERS?** What are their
NEEDS and **EXPECTATIONS?** What are the
products and services you provide? How do
these products and services address your
CUSTOMERS NEEDS?

Note: Give serious thought about your
internal and external customers. It is
important to understand your customer's
requirements, whether it is a report that
you provide or other service.

FIGURE 6.4 Identifying Customer Needs and Expectations.

and other agencies. However, many struggle with identifying the internal stakeholders. Staff, other departments with whom nursing interacts, supervisors, accounting, facilities, and others are sometimes omitted from the internal stakeholder list. Nevertheless, nursing needs to specifically seek input from nursing personnel at all levels, especially if the organization desires to attain ANCC Magnet status recognition (ANCC, 2011).

Once key stakeholders (or customers) are identified, the process requires that the plan considers the needs and expectations of each stakeholder group and the identification of the products or services that the nursing organization delivers to each stakeholder group. These lists should then be validated with each stakeholder group. This process supports validation of the plan and enhances support for the plan by all constituents.

Key Focus Areas

Many organizations choose to organize their plans under key focus areas (KFAs), sometimes called *key strategic directions* or "pillars of excellence" (Fig. 6.5) The most common are Quality, Service, People, Finance, and Growth, a structure that encourages alignment of goals and objectives under major performance indicators (Studer, 2003).

It is not uncommon to see a schematic drawn as a building, with the foundation of the building being the core values and the roof of the building being the vision supported by the pillars of excellence (Studer, 2003).

When organized under KFAs, the major categories are listed and the specific plan elements are articulated under each specific pillar. Each pillar defines where time and attention are organized and focused. Once the pillars are defined and listed, the process of identifying specific goals under each pillar is next: What do we need to accomplish in these areas to achieve our vision? Key performance indicators (KPIs) are then developed to measure success. Each KPI also needs a defined target. The target is based on current-state data and is set to answer the question: Where do we want to be?

Once the plan document is developed and goals set, a detailed analysis ensues. This includes a rigorous assessment of the current state, barriers, and challenges that may detract from meeting targets, as well as key strengths on which to build to support organizational success. Following the analysis, action plans to achieve results are developed, focused primarily on key strategic priorities.

Preimplementation Review, Approval, and Postimplementation Review

The final plan document requires preimplementation review by senior leadership (structure as defined by the organization); the key stakeholders who helped develop the plan (for endorsement); and, in some cases, the system leadership, which includes the organizational senior executive team and, potentially, the board of trustees or directors. Upon final approval, the plan is placed into effect, typically at the beginning of the planning period, which most often coincides with the organization's fiscal year calendar. Note that planning for the allocation of resources usually occurs during the preceding budget planning cycle, so plans that require significant allocation of financial resources (to include staffing) require prior approval through the budget-planning process.

After the plan has been developed, reviewed, and approved, and the planning cycle has commenced, communication of the plan to all stakeholders is key, to be

FY 2015 MUSC Excellence Goals for Finance & Administration

Service	Quality	People	Finance	Growth
• Customer satisfaction: score (88%) or better on "responds in a timely and effective manner."	• Customer satisfaction: score (88%) or better on "deliver quality products."	• Employee satisfaction: score (88 %) or better on "I am pleased to be working at MUSC."	• Meet 80% of the Key Process Indicators for productivity in each major Department throughout the Division by year end.	• Assess workforce professional development needs by Dec. 31, 2014.
• Customer Satisfaction: score (88%) or better on "displays a good spirit of service, cooperation and professional -ism."	• Academic Leadership assessment of F&A service satisfaction and priority of service: Move composite priority services scores up by 10% on fiscal year end reassessment survey.	• Employee satisfaction: score (88%) or better on "my division's culture values diversity."	**Range - same as last year**	**Range:** −4 = by 12/15/14 −3 = by 12/31/14 −2 = by 1/15/15 −1 = after 1/15/15
Range for all customer sat goals: −4 = 93% - 100% −3 = 88% - <93% −2 = 61% - <88% −1 = <61%		• Employee Satisfaction: score (88%) or better on "I believe I am treated respectfully by manage- ment within the Finance & Adminis- tration Division."	• Meet Budget to Actual goals for FY2015 **Range - same as last year**	• Ensure D&I enterprise wide Core training to 100% of available staff within 90 days of availability.
	Range: −4 = >10% −3 = >5% - <10% −2 = 0% - <5% −1 = <0%			**Range:** −4 = 100% −3 = 95% - <100% −2 = 90% - <95% −1 = less than 90%

FIGURE 6.5 Model of Studer Group Pillars of Excellence as Utilized by the Medical University of South Carolina. (*Courtesy of Medical University of South Carolina Nursing Administration, 2015.*)

followed by regular and consistent communication of goal-achievement status reports throughout the plan cycle. Most organizations today use a "balanced scorecard" approach to measure goal attainment. A balanced scorecard approach is easily communicated to and understood by all stakeholders (Naranjo-Gil, 2009). This method assigns a percentage to each specific goal, and the sum total adds up to 100%. For example, if a nursing plan has six discrete goals, each goal is assigned a percentage value. The determination of the value applied to a specific goal is most often based on the order and importance of strategic priorities; however, it may alternatively be driven by the organization's strategic plan. For example, a health-care system might require that each strategic plan assign a 30% value to financial goal attainment. If not, the strategic planning team identifies the order of priorities and assigns percentage values accordingly (Fig. 6.6). Balanced scorecards are most often updated monthly and compared to expected values, cumulatively adding up to year-end performance metrics.

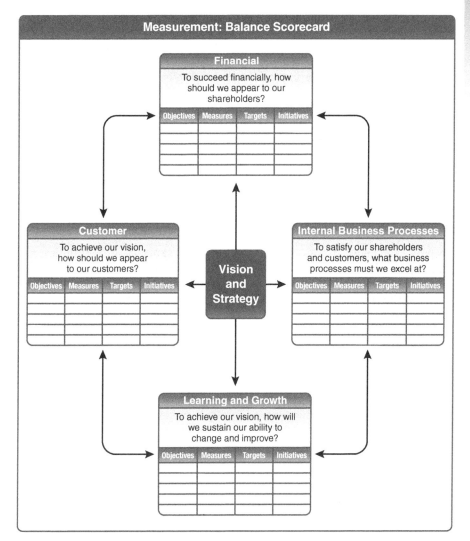

FIGURE 6.6 Measurement: Balanced Scorecard. *(Adapted from the Balanced Scorecard by Robert S. Kaplan and Dave P. Norton, Harvard Business School Press, 1996.)*

Critical to the success of the nursing-specific strategic plan is frequent postimplementation review. All too often, strategic plans are meandering, wordy documents that, once written and approved, get stashed on a bookshelf and read only by the occasional external regulator or auditor. In today's health-care environment, the most successful organizations consider their strategic plan documents to be living, breathing drivers of organizational accountability and achievement.

Perhaps one of the most challenging aspects of the plan is the assurance of involvement by all key stakeholders, both internal and external. It's not surprising that most nurse leaders can readily identify external stakeholders including patients, their families, physicians, vendors, and other agencies. However they struggle with identification of internal stakeholders. Internal stakeholders often forgotten on the list include staff, other departments with whom nursing staff members interact, supervisors, accounting, and facilities. The internal stakeholder list for nursing needs to specifically seek input from nursing personnel at all levels, especially if the organization desires to attain ANCC Magnet status recognition (ANCC, 2011).

Once key stakeholders (or customers) are identified, the process requires that the plan considers the needs and expectations of each stakeholder group, and the identification of the products or services that the nursing organization delivers to each stakeholder group. These lists should be validated with each stakeholder group, because they drive the development of action plans for goal attainment. Key here is to focus on the critical few versus the trivial many.

Strengths, Weaknesses, Opportunities, and Threats Analysis

Using a systematic approach (i.e., a strengths, weaknesses, opportunities, and threats [SWOT] analysis) to analyze the current status of the organization is critical for the development of an effective strategic plan (Fig. 6.7). This assessment encourages focus on what an organization does well and helps the planning team focus on building on strengths and identifying opportunities to mitigate weaknesses. Strengths provide a competitive or strategic advantage; weaknesses do the opposite. Opportunities, sometimes confused with weaknesses, if thoroughly evaluated can create a competitive advantage. Threats are a list of conditions or other circumstances that may have a negative impact on a strategic position. Conducting a thorough SWOT analysis puts reality up front and forces the team to face areas of focus head-on while at the same time building on strengths that provide support for goal attainment. Too often we tend to negate our strengths, focusing on weaknesses or threats, but the most important element to define and build on is the strength category.

Budget Planning

Perhaps one of the most daunting tasks in developing and attaining approval of a strategic plan is a rigorous assessment of resources required to successfully execute the plan. For instance, a new service being provided may require additional staff, facility space allocation, technology, equipment, and more. Even though there is a return on the investment in the future, the costs must be incorporated into the current fiscal year budget (Kaufman, 2011). Capital budget-planning costs can be considered more readily and easily in the operating budget than additional expenses; therefore, careful analysis and diligent negotiating may be required to gain final approval of a specific initiative in this heavily cost-constrained health-care arena. Nurse leaders need to devote time and energy to develop negotiating skills, especially when it is necessary to network and gain consensus on important strategic initiatives (Moss, 2005). This is particularly important when navigating financial challenges. One negotiating technique that helps is to spend time building good working relationships with constituents prior to presenting the plan and related costs to finance, utilizing the strengths of key stakeholders when negotiating for final approval. A detailed analysis and building a business

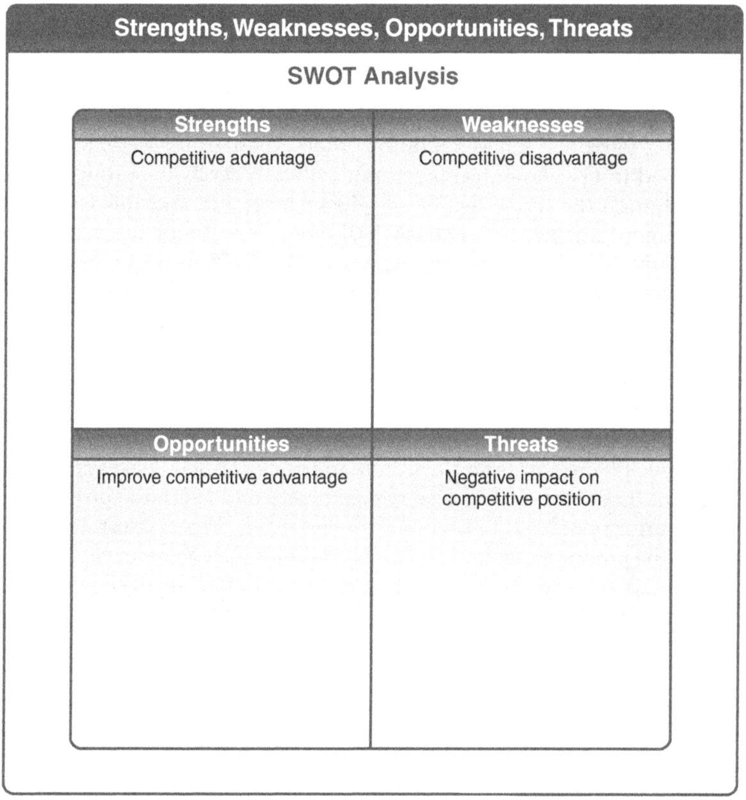

Strengths, Weaknesses, Opportunities, Threats	
SWOT Analysis	
Strengths	**Weaknesses**
Competitive advantage	Competitive disadvantage
Opportunities	**Threats**
Improve competitive advantage	Negative impact on competitive position

FIGURE 6.7 SWOT Analysis.

case for moving forward, solidified by a strong, well-thought-out strategic plan, make a big difference.

Trend Analysis

A trend analysis is an assessment of outcomes related to practices, procedures, and processes over time. Focusing on future needs when creating a vision and not getting misdirected by reacting to current issues and circumstances are important; however, it is also important to use trend analysis data to drive future vision planning and development of specific goals and objectives. Oftentimes, the trend data are used to establish a baseline or trajectory for future projections and are invaluable in this regard. The nurse leader should utilize the expertise of clinical or financial decision support departments or management engineering personnel to assist with data collection and analysis (ANA, 2011). Consideration of trend analysis data should be considered as an important assessment component for development of the strategic plan, but should not be utilized exclusively to develop the plan. Trend analysis is a consideration, not a driving force behind the plan.

Obtaining Stakeholder Input

A variety of methods should be used to gain stakeholder input as the strategic plan is developed. The time frame for the planning period is a critical factor to consider when choosing which methods will yield effective input and feedback. If the planning window is narrow, such as 3 months or less, then group feedback sessions are the best method to use. A neutral facilitator typically leads the group and receives feedback, although the nurse leader should kick off and end the session with an opening comment and closing acknowledgment. Results of the sessions should ideally be relatively anonymous (identifying the group type only), so that feedback will be unbiased and straightforward. Leaving comment cards can be helpful so that stakeholders who do not like to speak publicly can feel free to add additional feedback in writing.

Nursing organizations in which shared governance is widely practiced are well served to utilize formal council structures to provide input into all aspects of the strategic plan, from creation of the vision, development of the philosophy, all the way through to specific measures and action plans once ratified. This process can take several months, however, so it is wise to plan ahead and begin the process of review and input on an annual basis to keep information fresh. When the strategic planning cycle arrives, the process of review, feedback, and input becomes an easy one. It is also equally important to share the balanced scorecard results with all shared governance councils on a regular basis (ANCC, 2011).

Other methods include open forums, wherein preliminary plans are presented and feedback openly solicited; written feedback and input cards; wall boards for comments; online survey feedback tools; and, perhaps one of the most important methods of gaining stakeholder input, direct one-on-one interaction while actively rounding on nursing units to interact with caregivers. The nurse leader is well served by seeking input on the stakeholder's own "turf" rather than during office chats. Rounding for feedback often is self-perpetuating, with additional rounding yielding additional feedback (Moss, 2005).

Crediting key stakeholder groups with providing input once the plan is approved is vitally important, as is regularly sharing goals achieved via balanced scorecards or other methods. A monthly sharing opportunity is ideal; quarterly can be effective, but annually is grossly inadequate.

Developing Specific Goals and Objectives

Strategic planning goals tend to be long term, with specific objectives (or deliverables) defined for short-term measurement. A strategic planning goal under the category of Quality could be a 3-year goal to improve patient safety by fully implementing a specific program; however, each department, division, or facility could have a very specific objective set for a shorter horizon (1 year) to demonstrate measureable movement toward achievement of the long-term goal. Some organizations have adopted the approach of defining and adopting strategic goals that they call lag measures or lag goals and that focus the organization's annual objectives on adoption of lead measures or lead goals that are measured, reported, and responded to much more promptly and ultimately drive the strategic lag goal attainment. As an example, consider labor productivity as a goal. Perhaps an organization has defined a strategic goal of improving labor productivity over a 3-year horizon from 5.1 full-time equivalents (FTE)/per occupied bed to 4.9 FTE/per occupied bed. This is a lag measure because it is impossible to know whether the goal was met until the end of the third year. However, if every department head is challenged to support this goal by reducing worked hours by 1% per department per pay period, and reports on hours worked are produced daily by decision support to department heads, they now have a lead goal or lead measure that, if monitored and adhered to, will support accomplishment of the lag goal as defined in the strategic plan.

Every strategic plan goal must have measurable objectives written into the plan, at the department level, in support of the strategic goal. These objectives are what gets measured, reported, responded to, and revised as goals are met.

Plan Evaluation and Reevaluation

Toward the end of the current strategic plan cycle (e.g., if a 3-year plan, then at the end of year 2), the entire planning review process should begin again, planning for the next 3-year cycle. Although incomplete, if the goals were well conceived and defined, enough data exist to begin the review and feedback process to assure adequate time to develop the next strategic plan.

Most organizations include goal attainment in annual performance reviews of leadership; therefore, data should be readily available to conduct the initial analysis and begin the process of defining new KFAs. Goals that have not been met should be considered for extension, but only with a thorough analysis of the reasons the goal was not met and whether, considering current conditions, working toward that goal is still an appropriate target.

If an annual goals and objective balanced scorecard approach is used, then the process becomes routine; if the review is longer than a year or annual, then the strategic planning process can be quite cumbersome. Occasionally, changes in the health-care landscape necessitate modification or reforecasting projections in the strategic plan. The recent advent of the Affordable Care Act and Information Technology regulations have caused many organizations to rethink and refocus strategic efforts concerning investments in information systems and interconnectivity, as well as establishing alliances with providers and payers that were not even considerations when the initial plan was developed less than 4 years prior (Zuckerman, 2011). It is incumbent on nurse leaders and other health-care leaders to perpetually scan the health-care horizon to assure accurate projections. It is equally important to have an organizational structure that is nimble enough to make dynamic changes should the environment so dictate. Some organizations have included in their strategic plan the goal of becoming more proactive in and responsive to the rapidly changing landscape.

CONCLUSION

Nursing in all care delivery settings needs to provide transformational leadership in the creation of a culture of care that is based on interprofessional coordination with the purpose of safety for patients and colleagues. By defining care delivery models, standards of professional practice, and scope and standards for nurse administrators, a solid foundation for competent and effective patient care is established. Nurse leaders must be strategically positioned to influence an organization's performance. Ideally reporting to the chief executive officer, the nurse executive serves as a nurse and patient advocate and a leading clinical practitioner in patient care. The nursing mission, vision, values, and strategic plan serve as the voice of nursing and provide a foundation for quality patient care.

References

Ackoff, R. L. (1986). Our changing concept of planning. *Journal of Nursing Administration, 16*(4), 35–40.

Ackoff, R. L., & Rovin, R. (2003). *Redesigning society.* Redwood City, CA: Stanford Business Books.

Agency for Healthcare Research and Quality. (2012). Inpatient VS. outpatient surgeries in U.S. hospitals. Retrieved from https://www.hcup-us-ahrq.gov/reports/infographics/AHRQ-HCUP-Outpatient-Surgery-Inforgraphic-v06f.pdf

Aiken, L. H., Clarke, S. P., Sloane, D. M., Sochalski, J., & Silber, J. H. (2002). Hospital nurse staffing and patient mortality, nurse burnout, and job dissatisfaction. *JAMA, 288*(16), 1987–1993.

American Association of Critical-Care Nurses. (2014). *The AACN Synergy Model for Patient Care.* Retrieved from http://www.aacn.org/wd/certifications/content/synmodel.pcms?menu=certification

American Nurses Association. (2010a). *Nursing: Scope and standards of practice* (2nd ed.). Silver Spring, MD: Nursesbooks.org.

American Nurses Association. (2010b). *ANA standards of professional performance* (2nd ed.). Silver Spring, MD: Nursesbooks.org.

American Nurses Association. (2011). *Nursing administration: Scope and standards of practice* (2nd ed.). Silver Spring, MD: Nursesbooks.org.

American Nurses Association. (2015). Code of Ethics for nurses with interpretive statements Silver Spring, MD: Nursesbooks.org.

American Nurses Credentialing Center. (2011). Program overview. Retrieved from http://www.nursecredentialing.org/Magnet/ProgramOverview.aspx

American Nurses Credentialing Center. (2014). *2014 Magnet application manual.* Silver Spring, MD: Author.

American Organization of Nurse Executives. (2014). *Nurse executive competencies.* Retrieved from http://www.nurseleader.com/article/S1541-4612(05)00007-8/abstract

Beckham, J. D. (2004). Strategy: What it is, how it works, why it fails. *Health Forum Journal, 43,* 55–59.

Curley, M. (2007). *Synergy: The unique relationship between nurses and patients: The AACN Synergy Model for Patient Care.* Indianapolis, IN: Sigma Theta Tau International.

Daft, R. L. (2008). *The leadership experience* (pp. 386–383). Mason, OH: Thomson South-Western.

Drenkard, K. N. (2001). Creating a future worth experiencing: Nursing strategic planning in an integrated health delivery system. *Journal of Nursing Administration, 31*(7/8), 362–376.

Drucker, P. F. (1999). *Management challenges for the 21st century* (pp. 43–44). New York, NY: HarperCollins.

Greene, J. (2009). The new pace of strategic planning. *Trustee, 62*(8), 6–10. Retrieved from http:www.ncbi.nlm.nih.gov/pubmed/19960793

Institute of Medicine. (1999). To err is human: Building a safer health system for the 21st century. Retrieved from http://www.nationalacademies.org/hmd/-/media/Files/Report Files/1999/To-Err-is-Human/To Err is Human 1999 report brief.pdf

Institute of Medicine. (2011). *The future of nursing: Leading the charge, advancing health.* Retrieved from http://www.nationalacademies.org/hmd/Reports/2010/The-Future-of-Nursing-Change-Advancing-Health.aspx

Kaplan, R. S., & Norton, R. P. (1996). Measurement: Balanced scorecard. *Harvard Business School Press*.

Kaufman, N. S. (2011). Three brutal facts that provide strategic direction for healthcare delivery systems: Preparing for the end of the healthcare bubble. *Journal of Healthcare Management, 56*(3), 163–168.

Manthey, M., & Koloroutis, M. (2004). Resource-driven practice. In *Relationship-based care: A model for transforming practice* (pp. 183–214). Minneapolis, MN: Creative Healthcare Management.

Marshall, E. S. (2011). *Transformational leadership in nursing, from expert clinician to influential leader* (pp. 225–231). New York, NY: Springer.

Masters, G., & the Camden Group. (2006). *Proposal to develop a strategic plan, presented to St. Francis Hospital, Inc.* Unpublished. Columbus, GA.

Moss, M. T. (2005). *The emotionally intelligent nurse leader*. San Francisco, CA: Jossey-Bass.

Naranjo-Gil, D. (2009). Strategic performance in hospital: The use of the balanced scorecard by nurse managers. *Health Care Management Review, 34*(2), 161–170.

Nelson, J. (2003). *Nurse environmental survey results*. Retrieved from nursingworld.org/Functional MenuCategories/MediaResources/mediaBackgrounders/The-Nurse-Work-Environment-2011-Health-Safety-Survey.pdf

Person, C. (2004). Patient care delivery. In *Relationship-based care: A model for transforming practice* (pp. 159–182). Minneapolis, MN: Creative Healthcare Management.

Peters, T. (1987). *Thriving on chaos* (p. 477). New York, NY: Harper & Row.

Roussel, L. (2013). *Management and leadership for nurse administrators*. Burlington, MA: Jones & Bartlett.

Rundio, A., & Wilson, V. (2013). *Nurse executive review and resource manual* (pp. 35–38). Silver Spring, MD: American Nurses Credentialing Center.

Smith-Pennington, S., & Simms, E. (2011). *Strategic planning and management: Management and leadership for nurse administrators* (6th ed., pp. 343–362). Sudbury, MA: Jones & Bartlett.

St. Francis Hospital Inc. (2006). *Strategic planning process*. Unpublished.

Studer, Q. (2003). *Hardwiring excellence* (pp. 184–206). Gulf Breeze, FL: Fire Starter.

Studer, Q. (2013, November 4). The power of priorities: How hospital leaders can regain control of their time. *Becker's Hospital Review*. Retrieved from http://www.beckershospitalreview.com/hospital-management-administration/the-power-of-priorities-how-hospital-leaders-can-regain-control-of-their-time.html

Wachter, R. M., & Pronovost, P. J. (2009). Balancing "no blame" with accountability in patient safety. *PSNet*. Retrieved from http://psnet.ahrq.gov/resources/resource/11854/balancing-no-blame-with-accountability-in-patient -safety

Yura, H., & Walsh, M. B. (1988). *The nursing process: Assessing, planning, implementing, evaluating* (5th ed., p. 1). Norwalk, CT: Appleton & Lange.

Zuckerman, A. M. (2011). Does the strategic plan require updating because of healthcare reform? *Healthcare Financial Management, 65*(2), 102, 104. Retrieved from https://www.hfma.org/control.aspx?id+2886

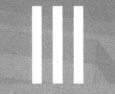

Leading Self
and Others

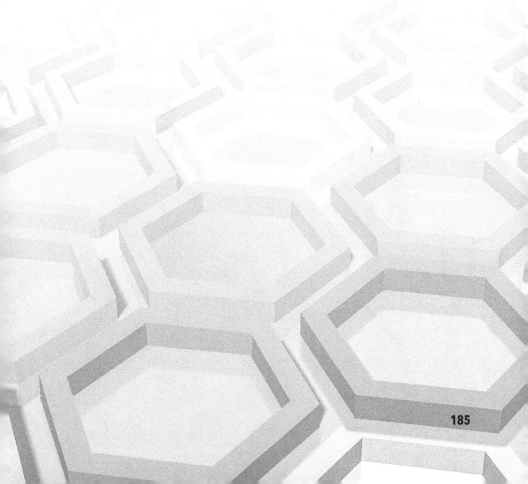

7

Focusing on Self
A Lifelong Journey

Uncertainty and turbulence in the work environment have been reported by nurses since the late 1990s (Webster & Cowart, 1999). O'Connor (2002) discussed the importance of self-care for nurses over a decade ago. In this chapter, the concept of self-leadership is explored. Nurse leaders are better poised to lead others more effectively once they have mastered leading themselves. The chapter begins with an overview of the Journey to Self-Leadership for Nurses, an innovation making up six integral dimensions of self. For the purposes of this chapter, these dimensions, which tend to overlap in real life, are meant to build on each other to lead to the overall outcome of self-leadership and include self-care, self-awareness, self-reflection, self and the art of listening, self and the art of communicating, and self and the art of collaborating. The boxes and tables reflect the information that Dr. Denise McNulty has presented during the past 20 years in her many successful workshops with health-care organizations.

THE JOURNEY TO SELF-LEADERSHIP

Nurses are called to lead others in academic and practice settings on a daily basis. To do so effectively, nurses need to be able to lead themselves, a process referred to as "self-leadership." Even while working within a team, nurses must possess self-leadership. The Journey to Self-Leadership for Nurses is presented as one tool to assist nurses in their growth and development (Fig. 7.1). It is depicted as a pyramid with six hierarchical dimensions. The goal of an individual's journey is to master each of the first six dimensions one step at a time with an ultimate goal of developing and mastering self-leadership. A considerable portion of this chapter is dedicated to the exploration of the first dimension, self-care, with a focus on mind, body, and spirit. Within the dimension of self-care, the concepts of self-healer, self-enrichment, and self-care plan are also examined.

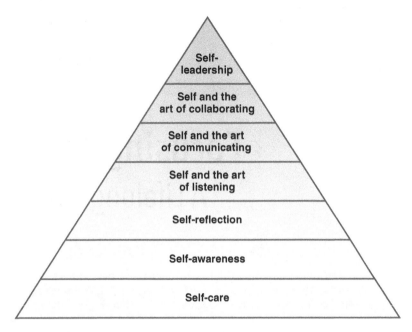

FIGURE 7.1 The Journey to Self-Leadership for Nurses. *(Courtesy of Denise McNulty)*

SELF-CARE

In the Journey to Self-Leadership for Nurses pyramid, self-care is positioned as the foundation to indicate the great significance that it plays. Nurses have a duty and a responsibility to take care of themselves. Iacono (2010) purports that every day there are multiple opportunities to find some balance and contribute to one's wellness by promoting self-care and making choices that are healthy and effective. According to Richards (2013a), the practice of self-care should be expected as part of the professional role of nursing. A 2015 qualitative study with 10 nursing professionals explored the meaning of self-care, attitudes, behaviors, and proposals that permeated self-care, as well as how self-care influences the work process and health of workers. The results of the study revealed that self-care was identified as an important factor in dealing with interpersonal relationships, whereas poor self-care was identified as leading to estrangement from work and potentially decreased quality of patient outcomes (Ferreira, Souza, Souza, Tavares, & Pires, 2015).

Changes in health care continue to demand decisions that compete for the priorities of the day. Resiliency has been identified in recent literature as a hallmark of successful nurse leaders. Resilience has been defined as the "process of adapting well to adversity, trauma, tragedy, threats, or significant sources of stress" (Cline, 2015, p. 117). Moreover, resilience is seen as a quality that can be learned (Dyess, Prestia, & Smith, 2015). Dr. Maureen Swick, the 2016 president of the American Organization of Nurse Executives (Brown, 2016), has also discussed self-care practices as an important part of resiliency.

Caring is at the heart of effective nursing leadership. Defined as tension between humanism and bureaucracy, caring is often learned by knowing oneself as caring (Newsom, 2010; Richards, 2013). Although many ways exist to define and explore self-care, here it is defined as caring for one's own mind, body, and spirit. Counselors consistently observe that when an individual's mind, body, and spirit are not in balance, the individual may express that he or she "does not feel right" but often does not know why. It may be that the nurse's mind, body, and spirit are not in harmony. The art of learning self-care through multiple pathways that integrate the mind, body, and spirit is a lifelong journey, yet one that must become routine (Richards, 2013a).

Mind

Maintaining emotional and mental wellness is vitally important for the nurse leader. Leaders encounter situations daily that require a calm, professional, and stable demeanor. If a leader's emotional and mental health is off balance, staff, patients, and coworkers may be negatively impacted. The ability to manage stress effectively is imperative for the nurse leader. The nurse's mental disposition and how he or she views stress is crucial in managing stress. What one nurse internalizes and experiences as stressful, another nurse may be able to compartmentalize, carefully managing his or her emotional state. Despite our best efforts, not everything is within our control. Adopting a mind-set that allows for and accepts limitations may help the nurse handle daily stress better.

Taking care of emotional and mental health requires a plan for managing stress that is effective for the individual nurse. Knowing oneself and knowing what strategies are effective for oneself is the first step. Box 7.1 highlights suggested strategies that nurses can use for their emotional and mental self-care. The leader has the power to change his or her perspective and to use positive energy when facing difficult circumstances.

BOX 7.1 Emotional and Mental Self-Care Strategies

- Limit exposure to toxic people.
- Get plenty of rest and at least 7 to 8 hours of uninterrupted sleep daily.
- Practice relaxation techniques (e.g., deep breathing).
- Take 1 hour at a time.
- Keep life as simple as possible.
- Practice giving yourself positive feedback (e.g., use positive self-talk; reflect on your accomplishments and achievements).
- Learn to laugh at yourself—be a little silly once in a while.
- Be an optimistic realist (the glass is half full, but sometimes in life reality gets in the way).
- Practice doing nothing once in a while.
- Enjoy some time alone (private time is very important for a mental rest).

Continued

BOX 7.1 Emotional and Mental Self-Care Strategies—cont'd

- Don't say yes when you want to say no.
- Screen your calls so that you can decide to whom and when you want to speak.
- Take a break from technology at home whenever possible (e.g., limit time on the computer and cell phone; turn off your text messaging service for a day or two).
- Do not stay in a job where you are not valued or appreciated.
- Spend time with friends who genuinely care.
- Stay emotionally connected with family.
- Keep home life and work life separate.
- Let go of situations out of your control.
- Take on a challenge that is meaningful and rewarding, such as a new position in a different specialty or a course in something totally unrelated to what you do.
- Be yourself and feel good about it.
- Find a trusted buddy to whom you can vent.
- Reconnect with an old friend.
- Use a journal to write down your thoughts, feelings, accomplishments, and special life experiences to remember and cherish.
- Have something other than work that you enjoy doing (all work and no play is not good for your mental health).
- Learn from past mistakes—experience is our best teacher.
- Forgive and forget.
- Always take a lunch or dinner break at work—you'll be happier, and your patients will benefit.
- Let go of any guilt; nurses are not perfect and we make mistakes—we're only human.
- Get a massage, a facial, or a pedicure.
- Find a quiet place to reflect.
- Take time off—stay home and rest or travel to a place that you enjoy.
- Let your home be your palace and a place for respite.
- Find a hobby that you would really enjoy (e.g., gardening, shell collecting).
- Lose yourself in a movie or a book—take a mental break and escape from reality for a moment.
- Take a hot bath with music in the background, and light a candle with your favorite scent.
- Prioritize what is most important to you (cherish family, friends, and health).
- Life is so short—treasure every minute and make the most of each day.

Body

Maintaining emotional and mental wellness is crucial for nurses, but maintaining physical wellness and engaging in self-care of the body is also essential. Self-care of mind and body goes hand in hand. Although nurses are educated to meet patients' basic needs, do they attend to their own basic needs? Leaders who are conscious of the need to establish boundaries and connect to their own self-care needs are better able to advocate for others, set priorities, and focus on making a difference (Dyess et al., 2015). Extended work hours have been shown to increase musculoskeletal disorders, bio-hazard exposures, and fatigue among nurses and may contribute to conditions such as depression, hypertension, diabetes, anxiety, and unhealthy behaviors such as smoking and alcohol use (Geiger-Brown & Trinkoff, 2010).

Nurses, as leaders, have a responsibility to use evidence in analyzing the effects of extended work hours and to model a work culture in which expectations support healthy, safe work environments (Lothschuetz Montgomery & Geiger-Brown, 2010). Nurses need to consider their own health and well-being first and foremost before considering the needs of others.

Box 7.2 includes recommended strategies for nurses that focus on physical wellness and self-care of the body.

BOX 7.2 Body Self-Care Strategies

- Take a walk at least once a day—wear a pedometer and walk 10,000 steps a day.
- When at work, take the stairs instead of the elevator.
- Engage in physical activity and have some fun with it (e.g., bike riding, swimming, yoga, spinning, weight-lifting, aerobic exercise, tai chi).
- Decrease your intake of fatty foods (stay away from fast foods and fried foods).
- Eat more fruits and vegetables.
- Increase your intake of wild salmon and avocados.
- Switch to whole wheat pasta, and try brown rice in place of white rice.
- Use olive oil to cook with in place of butter.
- Limit your intake of red meat to no more than one serving per week.
- Drink at least 6 to 8 glasses of water a day.
- Stay away from soda (even diet soda is unhealthy).
- Switch to decaffeinated tea or coffee, which is less problematic for your heart.
- Stop smoking.
- Get 8 hours of sleep.
- Wear comfortable shoes when at work.

Continued

BOX 7.2 Body Self-Care Strategies–cont'd

- Limit intake of sugar and white flour.

- Try switching to skim, 1%, or 2% milk (whole milk has too much fat).

- Avoid taking opiates, benzodiazepines, or pain medication for more than 2 weeks (if the need persists, speak to a health-care professional such as a physician or nurse practitioner).

- Avoid recreational use of illegal drugs, which often leads to problems and poor health.

- Limit your alcohol intake to within accepted levels to avoid medical problems and remember never to drink and drive.

- Always wear a seatbelt when driving, and do not text while driving.

- Consider taking a multivitamin if your diet lacks certain nutrients.

- See your primary care physician and dentist regularly

- Get some sun but be careful not to overdo exposure to sunlight (before 10 a.m. or after 3 p.m. is ideal).

- Remember to use the bathroom when on duty–do not hold urine.

- Take a lunch or dinner break at work–take time to refresh and recharge your battery.

- If you work full-time, 12-hour shifts, avoid that fourth shift–working more than 40 hours in a week can be too much.

Spirit

Being in tune with our emotional, mental, and physical wellness is vitally important for nurses, but nurses must not forget to practice self-care of the spirit. Richards, Sheen, and Mazzer (2014) define spiritual self-care as a reflection of one's connection with the world. Our beliefs shape our perceptions of our world and so serve either to nurture our souls or to deplete our spirits. What anchors an individual during uncertain times? What keeps a person steady when turmoil or tragedy occurs? Some find having a belief system or faith to be helpful in finding a sense of comfort and peace. It is important for nurses to get in touch with their spirituality. When nurses are fully in touch with their spirit, they may experience a sense of fulfillment and contentment.

Knowing what activities and practices feed the spirit is the key to spiritual self-care (Richards et al., 2014). Box 7.3 provides strategies that focus on self-care of spirit. In addition to these strategies, having a spiritual role model can also be very helpful. A spiritual role model is an individual who inspires and motivates others through his or her own good works and who helps others grow in their spiritual development. Reflective practices often assist the nurse leader in nurturing the spirit. Accepting the past and anticipating the future while finding meaning in leading others and appreciating humanity are important in caring for self (Dyess et al., 2015). Nurses deal with

BOX 7.3 Spirit Self-Care Strategies

- Take a walk in a park, garden, or field and get in touch with nature–ponder the beauty of every bird, butterfly, tree, flower, and scent.
- Spend time in prayer or meditation.
- Get involved in a worthwhile initiative or charity in the spirit of service and stewardship– giving of oneself does have its rewards.
- Visit a place where you feel a sense of comfort.
- Surround your home with items that reflect your spiritual beliefs.
- Listen to music.
- Consider talking to a priest, chaplain, pastor, or rabbi for spiritual direction.
- Be thankful for all of your blessings–gratitude helps to fill the soul.
- Forgive, forget, and move forward.
- Follow the Golden Rule: Do unto others as you would have them do unto you.
- Express love to those around you who mean the most to you.
- Keep a journal for inspirational moments that you would like to remember and reflect on.
- Respect your beliefs and have respect for others' beliefs.
- Leave a legacy of goodness, kindness, and caring.
- Spend some time by water (ocean, gulf, river, lake, pond, spring, or a stream).
- Read a book that nurtures self-care of the spirit and healing of the soul.
- Light a candle where there is darkness. Light represents hope and can help facilitate healing.
- If things are in despair in your workplace, find people who are the "lights" of hope and surround yourself with them.
- Try to think positive thoughts.

situations that involve illness; suffering; and, at times, death. These experiences can deplete a nurse's spirit. Actively nurturing their spirits, however, allows them to keep their hearts open to the abundance of life and all of the experiences, both positive and negative, in their work as healers (Richards et al., 2014). Self-care of the spirit is an integral part of nurses' self-care and a crucial part of their lifelong journey in the focus on self.

As nurses get in touch with their need for spiritual self-care, another important consideration in the focus on spirit is the "spirit" of nursing. Nurses take pride when they excel in the practice of nursing, but do nurses focus enough on the "spirit" of nursing? The spirit of nursing keeps nurses connected to their profession and inspires them much more than monetary rewards can ever do. It is important for nurse leaders to inspire and motivate themselves as well as other nurses and to always look for ways to ignite the spirit of nursing within their teams. When nurses have the spirit of nursing within them, they portray exuberance, compassion, and empathy in everything they do. It gives nurse leaders the courage, drive, passion, and stamina to persevere through difficult times in nursing and to carry the torch despite all odds.

Self as Healer

As healers, nurses have tremendous influence on creating a healthy and safe environment for patients (Richards et al., 2014). The healing presence of a nurse can be very therapeutic not only for the recipient of healing but also for the nurse who is providing healing. Being a healer can be very rewarding, but it can also be very draining. In order to heal others, nurses must first heal themselves. Healing oneself begins with embracing and practicing self-care of the mind, body, and spirit. Emulating wellness and disease-prevention habits can serve as the seed that germinates change in nurses, in their families, in their communities, in their patients, and eventually in the world (Richards et al., 2014).

Self-Enrichment

Another important component of self-care for the nurse is self-enrichment, the process of enriching one's mind and spirit with information and experiences to enhance growth. A wonderful way for nurses to immerse in self-enrichment outside of the workplace is to attend a retreat. Retreats can be educational and spiritual. Finding the time to attend a retreat may be difficult for some nurses, but it certainly can be worthwhile. Retreat programs usually focus on self-enrichment in a relaxed and tranquil setting to allow for introspective reflection.

Reading self-help books is another self-enrichment activity in which nurses can indulge. Other activities include taking classes; attending lectures; learning a new language; studying different cultures; investigating a new practice such as Reiki, yoga, or tai chi; and attending musical or theatrical performances. All of these activities can help to enrich the mind and spirit. Self-enrichment complements self-care and helps to foster personal growth.

Self-Care Plan

One way that nurses can formally make a commitment to self-care is to create an ideal self-care plan. The self-care plan needs to encompass mind, body, and spirit and can be viewed as "medicine" for a healthy life. It may not be something that nurses adhere to every day, but it gives nurses a concrete plan that they can turn to and use as a guide in beginning the journey of focusing on self. The self-care strategies listed in Boxes 7.1 through 7.3 can be used to formulate a self-care plan—start by selecting at least five strategies from each box (five strategies for mind self-care, five for body self-care, and five for spirit self-care). Although no set format exists for a self-care plan, a possible template to get the nurse leader started is provided in Box 7.4. Exploring what works best for self is part of one's unique self-care journey (Richards et al., 2014).

BOX 7.4 **Self-Care Plan for Nurses**

[Name]
[Date when my Self-Care Plan is initiated]

1. List five of my favorite strategies for self-care of my mind.

2. List five of my favorite strategies for self-care of my body.

3. List five of my favorite strategies for self-care of my spirit.

4. Who are my spiritual role models?

5. What activities would I enjoy engaging in for my own self-enrichment?

   I am making a commitment to myself to regularly practice the strategies I have listed on my self-care plan.

SELF-AWARENESS

Once the practice of self-care is mastered, the nurse may begin to explore the next dimension in the Journey to Self-Leadership, which is self-awareness, an essential quality of nurses as leaders. Oyeleye, Hanson, O'Connor, and Dunn (2013) purport that self-awareness is a key concept in psychological empowerment and important for a nurse's psychological well-being. Greater self-awareness increases the ability to manage and use emotions to respond more appropriately to one's own needs and those of others (Oyeleye et al., 2013). Self-awareness is an introspective process that entails getting in touch with one's own emotions, feelings, opinions, wants, and needs—getting to know who one is. It is continuous and evolving (Timmins, 2011). As with all dimensions in the self-leadership journey, progressing from self-care to self-awareness may not be a strictly linear process. Life circumstances may necessitate the need to refocus attention on self-care. For example, a nurse may find at different stages in this journey that he or she may be neglecting the practice of self-care and find the need to refocus on meeting his or her self-care needs. As stated earlier, self-care is the foundation of the self-leadership journey. Aspiring to higher-level dimensions such as self-awareness or self-reflection may be challenging if the nurse is not practicing self-care of the mind, body, and spirit. In fact, some call self-awareness the consciousness of one's values, strengths, and limitations (Horton-Deutsch & Sherwood, 2008). Regardless, this journey of self-discovery can be both exciting and enlightening.

Self-awareness also involves understanding how one comes across to others. A nurse leader needs to be aware of and monitor how others perceive him or her for example, in communication styles, mannerisms, and nonverbal behaviors. A nurse leader's actions can have positive and negative influences on the actions of others. Self-awareness, therefore, requires regular self-monitoring, and self-monitoring requires that the individual make an honest assessment of his or her behaviors and responses. Being honest with oneself is vital in the development of self-awareness. Honesty about oneself requires courage, confidence, and support from others who are trusted (Horton-Deutsch & Sherwood, 2008). Through self-awareness and self-monitoring of one's behaviors and responses, nurse leaders can use this insight and knowledge of self to enhance how they may react and respond to others in situations in the workplace and in their personal lives. Individuals who lack self-awareness may find it difficult to regulate their emotional expressions and their fears and to avoid impulsive behaviors when threatened or rejected (Jooste & Cairns, 2014).

According to Horton-Deutsch and Sherwood (2008), self-awareness is critical for therapeutic relationships with patients and accomplished nursing leadership. Through developing self-awareness, nurses become able to more fully engage in and lead in their work. Self-awareness is central to nurses' ability to integrate feelings with knowledge and experience. Horton-Deutsch and Sherwood (2008) further support that integrating awareness of self and others with the environment creates the openness necessary for authentically "being present." For nurses, being present means participating in an interpersonal encounter with a patient, who then experiences this "present-ness" (as opposed to just "presence") as a connection with one who is giving undivided attention to his or her needs and concerns (Drick, 2015). By considering feelings and attitudes, self-awareness makes use of the positive and deals with the negative aspects of situations, moving toward a more authentic way of being in caring relationships (Horton-Deutsch & Sherwood, 2008). For example, when a colleague says something potentially disrespectful or hurtful to a nurse who has mastered self-awareness, that nurse may pause and consider his or her thoughts and attitudes about what was said before reacting in a negative way. The self-aware nurse may also consider the positive aspects of the interaction in preparing to manage any negative feelings or consequences that may occur as a result of the interaction. Understanding one's moods and how one affects the nursing team provides an individual with the capacity to gain insight into one's basic behavioral inclinations and the way in which one interacts with other people (Jooste & Cairns, 2014). Actively practicing self-awareness can help nurse leaders in fostering and developing relationships with others while creating a healing presence and therapeutic environment in the workplace.

SELF-ACCOUNTABILITY

Self-awareness and self-accountability go hand-in-hand. Furthermore, it is an expectation of the nursing profession that nurses embrace and practice self-accountability: The American Nurses Association's (ANA) Nursing Scope and Standards of Practice states that registered nurses (RNs) are accountable for their professional actions to themselves, their health-care consumers, their peers, and ultimately to society (ANA, 2015). Nurses are also responsible for holding subordinates accountable for duties, performance, and actions. In using self-reflection to develop self-accountability, a nurse can achieve a level of growth and introspection that can be life changing. Examples of ways nurses can practice self-accountability in health care include regarding patient needs as the greatest importance; keeping up to date with regard to knowledge, skills, and competence; recognizing personal limits with regard to knowledge, skills, and competence; ensuring that nursing care is never compromised; and avoiding inappropriate delegation (Jooste & Cairns, 2014).

SELF-REFLECTION

As noted earlier, the Journey to Self-Leadership is not always linear, but it provides a framework to move within. Thus, once a nurse leader has awareness of self, he or she can progress to the next dimension in the Journey to Self-Leadership, which is self-reflection.

According to Horton-Deutsch and Sherwood (2008), reflection is about learning from experience, a critical aspect of knowledge development and a skill essential to leadership development. Reflection leads an individual to a fuller understanding of what one knows and increases one's potential for leadership. It also leads to understanding the ramifications of actions and responses. This is crucial not only in work life but also in personal life. In the workplace, nurses who are reflective leaders are mindful of past practices, past reactions of others, and the implications of these reactions. The nurse leader identifies patterns of behavior, interprets their meaning, and responds in a way that is growth producing for individuals and organizations (Horton-Deutsch & Sherwood, 2008). Self-reflection involves looking back over what transpired in practice with the goal of professional growth—it offers a creative way to recapture an experience for the purpose of developing professional practice and leadership (Horton-Deutsch & Sherwood, 2008). Self-reflection requires that nurses consider their thoughts, feelings, communication, behaviors, and actions. The practice of self-reflection requires taking the time to evaluate, examine, and understand. Box 7.5 provides three fundamental questions that can help a nurse move through a reflective process.

By actively engaging in self-reflection, a nurse leader can move toward more awareness and understanding of the experience of others. Self-reflection is crucial for nurse leaders to master in light of their need to work with others at all levels. A self-reflective nurse fosters the process of creating relationships with patients, families, and coworkers. Through the process of self-reflection and self-understanding, the aim is to better understand and become more aware of the experiences of self and others,

---

BOX 7.5 **Self-Reflection Questions**

What did I do?

What should I have done that I did not do?

How would I act differently next time?

Adapted from: Horton-Deutsch, S., & Sherwood, G. (2008). Reflection: An educational strategy to develop emotionally-competent nurse leaders. *Journal of Nursing Management, 16*, 946.

including what it means to be human. This process facilitates understanding of a broader context of human experience in caring for others and what it means to be a person in a world with accountability and responsibility to self and others. Self-reflection also helps individuals to identify personal beliefs and biases that are key in the process of developing relationships (Becker Hentz & Steen Lauterbach, 2005).

SELF AND THE ART OF LISTENING

The first three dimensions in the Journey to Self-Leadership focus primarily on growth and development as they pertain to the individual nurse. The next three dimensions broaden the nurse's horizons to include other people with whom the nurse interacts personally and professionally. Nurse leaders who have mastered these individual skills may then progress to the next dimension in the Journey to Self-Leadership, which is self and the art of listening. Listening is truly an art and a vital aspect of leadership and nursing practice. According to Denham et al. (2008), the art of listening is foundational to clinical practice. Listening is the oldest and conceivably most influential tool of healing (Browning & Waite, 2010).

Nurses, as leaders, need to continually work on enhancing their listening skills. The first step to enhancing listening skills is to practice listening to oneself. Nurses often have a sixth sense that they need to respect and tune in to. Listening to the inner self can be most useful in an individual's personal and professional life. Sometimes it is the inner voice that knows what is best. Listening to self takes practice in developing a sense of trust and belief in one's own insight and judgment.

Nurses not only need to listen to their minds, they need to listen to their bodies. As role models, nurse leaders should not only listen to what their own bodies are telling them, they should also listen to what the bodies of their subordinates are telling them. Nurses' bodies have a way of telling them what they can and cannot do any longer, and sometimes others may need to call a time-out for colleagues (Denham et al., 2008). This is where leadership comes into play. It is the responsibility of the nurse leader to look out for the team and to watch for signs and symptoms of potential burnout, fatigue, and distraction. These are all factors that can impede the ability of nurses to listen actively (Denham et al., 2008).

Listening to one's own mind and body is critical in the mastery of the art of listening, but another critical aspect of the art of listening is our ability to listen to others. Active listening is a demonstration of respect, empathy, and caring. The ability to listen with empathy is an essential skill for nurses to develop. When nurse leaders truly listen to their patients, students, and staff, they will learn much of what they need to know. If a nurse is listening and shows it, an individual may be more willing to tell his or her story. Patient stories contain critical information that leaders need to listen to. Nurses, as leaders, must realize how critical it is to allocate time to attend to patients' stories, for it is in their stories that patients reveal both the meanings they attach to their daily lives and the challenges they face in negotiating lives lived with mental and/or physical illness (Browning & Waite, 2010).

Listening supports the potential for healing and compassion (Browning & Waite, 2010). Professionals must have the courage to set aside their concerns and to be fully present for and attentive to the other (Browning & Waite, 2010). True active listening requires the listener to empty him- or herself of personal concerns, distractions, and preconceptions, which, in addition to courage, takes generosity and patience (Denham et al., 2008). Learning to listen deeply takes practice. When listening to another speak, the nurse should look into the eyes of the individual who is speaking, listen quietly while the individual is speaking, and concentrate intently on the content of what the individual is sharing. When practicing listening deeply, nurses may need to quietly remind themselves not to speak. Listening is a powerful agent of healing and a natural part of the repertoire of nursing; it is at its very heart (Browning & Waite, 2010). The art of listening is a skill that nurse leaders need to develop in order to communicate effectively with others, including their staff. Actively listening to staff is a behavior that helps nurses feel supported and requires leaders to be receptive to nurses' ideas. Leaders need to provide time and space to listen to staff experiences of care provision and any work-related problems they have (Timmins, 2011). Listening needs to occur in order for effective communication to occur.

SELF AND THE ART OF COMMUNICATING

Once a nurse leader feels confident in his or her development of the art of listening, the leader can progress to the next dimension in the Journey to Self-Leadership, which is self and the art of communicating. According to Timmins (2011), communication is a fundamental element of care at every level of nursing practice. It is important, therefore, for nurse leaders to create environments that promote and encourage good communication and help nurses develop their communication skills formally and informally. Nurses have a professional duty to maintain good communication skills. The absence of good communication can compromise patient safety and quality of care (Timmins, 2011).

Nurse leaders need exceptional communication skills because they serve as role models to their staff. Self-monitoring of communication skills is an important element for nurse leaders to consider in all aspects of their work, particularly when resolving conflicts and modeling good communication behaviors (Timmins, 2011). As discussed earlier in the self-awareness section of this chapter, nurse leaders need to be aware of their own communication styles and how others perceive them. The way in which nurse leaders communicate can affect others. Leaders in management positions are in relative positions of power, which may come across as intimidating to others (Timmins, 2011). Leaders need to continuously work on developing and refining their communication skills so that they can communicate with others in an effective and therapeutic manner.

Communication may come easily to some nurses, whereas others will admit to having difficulty communicating their thoughts, opinions, and feelings. One major barrier to communication is fear—fear of discomfort, fear of retribution, and fear of losing one's job (O'Keeffe & Saver, 2013). Fear can be paralyzing. When nurses work in an environment in which they fear retaliation for expressing their opinions, morale, satisfaction, and patient care can be negatively impacted. When nurses fear losing their jobs, they may develop a sense of insecurity and anxiety, which can result in nurses making poor decisions. When nurses make poor decisions, people's lives can be at stake. Patients are at the mercy of nurses' actions and decisions. Nurses, as professionals, have an obligation to learn how to cope with their fears and anxieties so that they can effectively manage their practice. Open and honest communication is one way to resolve fear. After making every attempt to openly communicate concerns, including following the chain of command when necessary, if a nurse feels that the resolution and outcome are not satisfactory, then the nurse may wish to consider transferring to another department within the organization or leaving the organization to pursue other options.

Every nurse should perform a self-assessment to see what his or her primary or dominant communication style is. There are four main communication styles that nurses tend to use: (1) passive, (2) passive-aggressive, (3) aggressive, and (4) assertive. To help nurses differentiate between the four communication styles, a scenario is provided in Box 7.6. Table 7.1 highlights characteristic behaviors of the four communication

---

BOX 7.6 Communication Scenario

An RN approaches her supervisor on a Friday to request the following Monday as a day off to be with her mother, who is scheduled to have surgery that day. However, the RN knows that the policy is to give at least 2 weeks' notice for a requested day off, and that the supervisor may not be able to grant the request.

Passive Response: After the supervisor declines the request for Monday off, the nurse politely thanks the supervisor, walks away, and feels sorry for herself, saying, "If anything happens to my mother, I'll blame myself for the rest of my life." The nurse goes home after work and continues to lament over the situation and starts to resent the supervisor for not approving her request.

Passive-Aggressive Response: After the supervisor declines the request for Monday off, the nurse politely thanks the supervisor, walks away, and feels sorry for herself. The nurse then shares what happened with other members of the team to try and get them to take her side, saying, "Can you believe the supervisor rejected my request after all that I do for her? I bring her an apple every day, I do whatever she asks me to do, and this is how she treats me? I hope none of you ever goes to lunch with her again. The supervisor is nothing but mean." The nurse then goes home and continues to lament over the situation. On Monday, the nurse calls in sick, saying that she has a migraine.

Aggressive Response: After the supervisor declines the request for Monday off, the nurse says to the supervisor, in a very angry tone, "Is that your final answer? After all I do for you, I bring you an apple every day, and this is how you show your appreciation? I cannot believe this." The nurse then slams the request form on the desk in front of the supervisor and says, "This is what I think of you!" The nurse then walks out of the supervisor's office and slams the door. One hour later, the supervisor reprimands the nurse and gives her a written disciplinary warning for insubordination.

Assertive Response: After the supervisor declines the request for Monday off, the nurse expresses her concern for her mother's health and requests that the supervisor kindly reconsider the request. The supervisor states that she understands the nurse's need to be with her mother, but there is no available coverage to grant the nurse the day off with such short notice. The supervisor reminds the nurse that Mondays are one of the busiest days of the week in the department because of work overflow from the weekend. After the supervisor declines the request again, the nurse thanks the supervisor for her consideration and time and then leaves the supervisor's office. The nurse returns to her unit and asks one of her coworkers who is off on Monday if she would be willing to switch a day with her and work for her on Monday. The nurse, in turn, would then work for her coworker on Tuesday. There would be no overtime incurred. The coworker agrees to work for the nurse, and the nurse expresses her thanks. The nurse returns to the supervisor's office and presents the above potential solution. The supervisor agrees with the suggested plan and approves the nurse's request for Monday off.

TABLE 7.1 **Characteristic Behaviors of Four Communication Styles**

Passive	Passive-Aggressive	Aggressive	Assertive
Dishonest, holds feelings in	Dishonest, holds feelings in but then brutally honest when expressing feelings	Brutally honest when expressing feelings at the expense of others	Tactful, sincere, direct, and honest when expressing feelings
Blames self	Blames self and others	Blames others for mistakes	Takes responsibility and accountability for self, behaviors, and actions
Avoids confrontation at all costs	Avoids confrontation initially but then provokes confrontation	Welcomes and provokes confrontation	Able to confront others appropriately and uses conflict-resolution skills to work through conflicts
Feels rights are always violated	Feels rights are violated but then violates rights of others	Violates rights of others–has no sense of boundaries	Respectful of others' rights and protects own rights
Wants to criticize but unable to verbally express criticism	Criticizes others but may do so quietly behind the scenes–will complain about something to any source other than to the direct source	Openly criticizes and ridicules others–can be judgmental	Does not criticize others or make judgments about others
Exhibits low self-esteem	Exhibits low self-esteem	Exhibits low self-esteem	Exhibits high self-esteem and confidence

Continued

TABLE 7.1 **Characteristic Behaviors of Four Communication Styles–cont'd**

Passive	Passive-Aggressive	Aggressive	Assertive
Often feels taken advantage of	Often feels taken advantage of but then also takes advantage of others	Takes advantage of others	Respectful of others' feelings and needs–does not violate those of others
Unable to express thoughts and feelings openly	At times, unable to express thoughts and feelings openly, but at other times expresses thoughts and feelings at the expense of others	Expresses thoughts and feelings at the expense of others	Able to openly express thoughts and feelings in a confident manner
Lacks confidence in self, has difficulty making decisions	Lacks confidence in self and has difficulty making decisions, but also can be boastful, arrogant, and domineering	Is boastful, arrogant, and domineering	Appears self-confident and self-assured without being boastful or domineering, able to make decisions
May have anger and hostility, but unable to express them	May have unexpressed anger and hostility at times, but then can present as angry, hostile, calculating, and manipulative	Presents as angry, hostile, demanding, calculating, and manipulative to get needs met	Presents in a calm manner without being angry and hostile

styles, from which it appears that the most optimal and effective style is assertive communication. Being assertive means expressing opinions, asking questions, and seeking clarification in an open, honest, direct, and professional manner while maintaining dignity and respect for others. Speaking directly to another, as opposed to going behind that person's back and speaking to others about that person, is the best way to communicate. Holding thoughts and opinions inside can lead the nurse to become stressed, angry, resentful, and perhaps hostile. When nurses do not express how they really feel, they may come across as "people pleasers," often saying yes to others when they really want to say no. In Chapter 8, developing assertive communication is presented as one of the key educational needs for nurses in their journey to psychological empowerment. Although nurses are highly educated professionals, they often admit to having a need for development of assertive communication skills.

In developing the art of communicating, nurse leaders should be mindful of their verbal and nonverbal communication. Both skills are important for effective communication in a nurse's personal life and professional life. Verbal communication pertains to the message being conveyed (what); voice tone, volume, and inflection (how); timing (when); and the intention, motive, and reason for the message (why). Once words are spoken, it is very difficult to take them back, so it is important that nurses always think before they speak.

Nonverbal communication pertains to eye contact, body language, posture, facial expression, positioning, and touch. Nonverbal communication can tell us a great deal about how a person is feeling. A nurse who exhibits poor eye contact, slumped posture, sad or angry facial expression, crossed arms while sitting, or an inability to receive or give touch can often give leaders clues about how that person may be feeling.

There are several verbal and nonverbal ways nurses can communicate. Nurses, as leaders, need to assess on a regular basis what the preferred communication method is for their staff (O'Keeffe & Saver, 2013). Some staff may prefer face-to-face communication, which would occur through rounding, staff meetings, change-of-shift report, and committee meetings. Other staff may prefer written communication, which could transpire through e-mails, bulletin board notices, and texting (O'Keeffe & Saver, 2013). Nurses may also choose to communicate by phone in conference calls. It would be beneficial for nurse leaders to use a variety of methods for sharing information with others in light of different communication styles and cultures, as well as generational differences. The ANA's Nursing Scope and Standards of Practice calls for RNs to communicate effectively in a variety of formats in all areas of practice (ANA, 2015).).

In the Journey to Self-Leadership, because listening is essential for effective communication, communication is essential for effective collaboration (O'Keeffe & Saver, 2013). As discussed earlier in this chapter, each dimension in the Journey to Self-Leadership builds on the prior dimensions; therefore, mastering the art of communicating is a skill that needs to be fully developed before nurses can effectively collaborate.

SELF AND THE ART OF COLLABORATING

Nurse leaders who have mastered the art of communicating can then progress to the next dimension in the Journey to Self-Leadership, which is self and the art of collaborating. Nurses provide direct care, education, and coordination of services, making them key players in the "collaboration wheel" of health care (O'Keeffe & Saver, 2013). Each health-care team member is a spoke in the wheel, and each spoke in the wheel is essential. It takes all spokes working together to make the wheel turn. Health-care environments are complex, dynamic, and stressful, requiring a team approach to care delivery that encourages effective interprofessional collaboration. Interprofessional collaboration promotes and optimizes active participation of all health-care professions in clinical decision making, acknowledging the contributions of all health-care professionals in the process (Rose, 2011). Collaboration is the process by which professionals relate to one another (O'Keeffe & Saver, 2013), work cooperatively, share responsibility, and make decisions jointly (Nair, 2012). The ANA (2010) defines collaboration as a professional health-care partnership grounded in a reciprocal and respectful recognition and acceptance of each partner's unique expertise, power, and sphere of influence and responsibilities, the commonality of goals, the mutual safeguarding of the legitimate interest of each party, and the advantages of such a relationship.

Collaboration implies interdependency as opposed to autonomy (Rose, 2011). Although nurses are encouraged to be autonomous in their practice, they need to work with every member of the team to ensure delivery of quality and safe patient care. When nurses do not collaborate with other members of the team or when other members of the team do not collaborate with nurses, service and the overall operation of an organization can be negatively impacted. Ineffective collaboration can contribute to team dysfunction, poor morale, poor decision making, increased patient harm, increased hospital length of stay, increased resource use, and increased employee turnover (Rose, 2011). Conversely, effective collaboration in health care is associated with decreased length of hospital stay, improved patient satisfaction, improved pain control, improved functioning in activities of daily living, and decreased mortality (O'Keeffe & Saver, 2013).

When using effective collaboration skills, nurses can be instrumental in fostering collaborative cultures within organizations. This includes both practice and academic settings. In health care, nurses need to ensure that they routinely collaborate with other nurses, with other disciplines, with patients, and with families to improve patient outcomes. In academia, nursing faculty need to collaborate with other faculty, students, parents, and community stakeholders to enhance student outcomes. The ANA's Nursing Scope and Standards of Practice requires that the RN collaborate with the health-care consumer, family, and others in the conduct of nursing practice (ANA, 2015).). Every member of a team in both the practice setting and academic setting can benefit from a culture that is collaborative.

Nurses can determine how effective they are at collaboration through self-assessment, such as answering the Team Player Self-Assessment Questionnaire (O'Daniel & Rosenstein, 2008), which can help guide nurses in assessing their skills as team players (Box 7.7). In addition to performing a self-assessment, nurses should also solicit feedback from others so that they have a full picture of their collaborative abilities (O'Keeffe & Saver, 2013).

SELF-LEADERSHIP

Once a nurse has mastered the art of collaborating, as well as the preceding dimensions in the journey, he or she has reached the goal of self-leadership. As noted earlier in this chapter, self-leadership is the process of influencing oneself to lead others. An effective leader has the ability to influence others while also possessing the ability to influence him- or herself. Learning how to influence oneself requires wisdom, introspection, motivation, and the ability to inspire oneself. Self-leadership radiates when leaders have developed a sense of who they are. These leaders know what they want and where they are going, and they have a sense of how to get there. In the Journey to Self-Leadership,

BOX 7.7 Team Player Self-Assessment Questionnaire

Am I a team player? If you can answer yes to most of these questions, you are well on your way to being an excellent team member and team player.

1. Do I value open communication with colleagues? Yes or no

2. Do I believe in a nonpunitive environment? Yes or no

3. Do I give clear direction? Yes or no

4. Do I request clarification when given ambiguous direction? Yes or no

5. Do I provide a respectful atmosphere for my colleagues? Yes or no

6. Do I share the responsibility for team successes? Yes or no

7. Do I balance member participation in a given task? Yes or no

8. Do I acknowledge and process conflict? Yes or no

9. Do I set clear specifications and expectations in respect to authority and accountability? Yes or no

10. Do I have a clear understanding of decision-making procedures? Yes or no

11. Do I communicate routinely and share information regularly? Yes or no

12. Do I enable others to access resources in the environment? Yes or no

13. Do I evaluate outcomes and adjust accordingly? Yes or no

Adapted from: O'Daniel, M., & Rosenstein, A. H. (2008). Professional communication and team collaboration. In R. G. Hughes (Ed.), *Patient safety and quality: An evidence-based handbook for nurses.* Baltimore, MD: Agency for Healthcare Research and Quality.

it is important for nurse leaders to value the importance of self-leadership and to recognize how self-leadership can impact every aspect of their lives.

In the workplace, individuals who practice self-leadership may have an advantage over other individuals who do not practice self-leadership. Self-led leaders take ownership of self and others. They assume accountability for their actions in the workplace. Self-leadership requires an individual to control personal actions, to be self-aware, and to employ personal strength, all of which are necessary for performing tasks (Jooste & Cairns, 2014). Nurses who exhibit self-leadership are assets to organizations.

CONCLUSION

Each dimension in the Journey to Self-Leadership plays a significant role in the growth and development of self-leadership. Leaders need to give themselves ample time to fully develop each of the dimensions so that they can attain self-leadership. Anything worthwhile in life takes work. Nurses may find that the Journey to Self-Leadership is well worth the effort and something that can lead to a sense of personal fulfillment and career satisfaction. Self-leadership is truly a lifelong journey requiring dedication and a sincere commitment to the development of self.

Nurses can be in a better position to effectively lead others once they have mastered leading themselves. The Journey to Self-Leadership for Nurses may help nurses to embrace and actively engage in self-care, self-awareness, self-accountability, self-reflection, the art of listening, the art of communicating, and the art of collaborating. The Journey to Self-Leadership can be an enlightening and life-changing experience for nurses. Focusing on and developing self is a continuous lifelong journey (Box 7.8).

BOX 7.8 Reflections for Self-Leaders

- If we do not look for something to be grateful for, we might obsess on the things missing from our lives.
- Adversity can help us grow and, at times, can even make us stronger.
- Adversity prepares us for what lies ahead.
- Adversity gives us compassion for others who are in pain.
- You cannot run a good race if you are constantly looking over your shoulder.
- As leaders, our goal should be to strive to be an emotionally healthy adult.
- Remember that an unforgiving spirit is destructive.
- Have realistic expectations of others and be the person that you expect others to be.
- You will touch a life and a life will touch yours.
- We may not always be able to control whether storms will come our way, but we may be able to control how we react.
- We should never assume that people quit their jobs for money or benefits—sometimes it is because of coworkers or their supervisor.

References

American Nurses Association. (2015). *Nursing: Scope and standards of practice* (3rd ed.). Silver Spring, MD: Nursesbooks.org.

Becker Hentz, P., & Steen Lauterbach, S. (2005). Becoming self-reflective: Caring for self and others. *International Journal for Human Caring, 9*(1), 24–28.

Brown, A. (2016). Leader to honor. *Nurse Leader, 14*(2), 99–102.

Browning, S., & Waite, R. (2010). The gift of listening: JUST listening strategies. *Nursing Forum, 45*(3), 150–158.

Cline, S. (2015). Nurse leader resilience. *Nursing Administration Quarterly, 39*(2), 117–122.

Denham, C. R., Dingman, J., Foley, M. E., Ford, D., Martins, B., O'Regan, P., & Salamendra, A. (2008). Are you listening . . . are you really listening? *Journal of Patient Safety, 4*(3), 148–161.

Douglas, K. (2010). When caring stops, staffing doesn't really matter. *Nursing Economic$, 28*(6), 415–419.

Drick, C. A. (2015). The essence of spirituality ~ coming alive in presence. *American Holistic Nurses Association Beginnings, 35*(5), 14–16.

Dyess, S., Prestia, A., & Smith, M. (2015). Support for caring and resiliency among successful nurse leaders. *Nursing Administration Quarterly, 39*(2), 104–116.

Ferreira, E., Souza, M., Souza, N., Tavares, K., & Pires, A. (2015). The importance of self-care for nursing professionals. *Cienc Cuid Saude, 14*(1), 978–985.

Geiger-Brown, J., & Trinkoff, A. M. (2010). Is it time to pull the plug on 12-hour shifts? Part 3. Harm reduction strategies if keeping 12-hour shifts. *Journal of Nursing Administration, 40*(9), 357–359.

Groff Paris, L., & Terhaar, M. (2010). Using Maslow's pyramid and the national database of nursing quality indicators to attain a healthier work environment. *The Online Journal of Issues in Nursing, 16*(1).

Horton-Deutsch, S., & Sherwood, G. (2008). Reflection: An educational strategy to develop emotionally-competent nurse leaders. *Journal of Nursing Management, 16*, 946–954.

Iacono, M. V. (2010). Nurses' self-care: A question of balance. *Journal of PeriAnesthesia Nursing, 25*(3), 174–176.

Jooste, K., & Cairns, L. (2014). Comparing nurse managers and nurses' perceptions of nurses' self-leadership during capacity building. *Journal of Nursing Management, 22*, 532–539.

Lothschuetz Montgomery, K., & Geiger-Brown, J. (2010). Is it time to pull the plug on 12-hour shifts? Part 2. Barriers to change and executive leadership strategies. *Journal of Nursing Administration, 40*(4), 147–149.

Nair, D. M., Fitzpatrick, J. J., McNulty, R., Click, E. R., & Glembocki, M. M. (2012). Frequency of nurse-physician collaborative behaviors in an acute care hospital. *Journal of Interprofessional Care, 26*(2), 115–120.

Newsom, R. (2010). Compassion fatigue: Nothing left to give. *Nursing Management, 41*(4), 43–45.

O'Connor, M. (2002). Nurse leader: Heal thyself. *Nursing Administration Quarterly, 16*(3), 69–77.

O'Daniel, M., & Rosenstein, A. H. (2008). Professional communication and team collaboration. In R. G. Hughes (Ed.), *Patient safety and quality: An evidence-based handbook for nurses.* Baltimore, MD: Agency for Healthcare Research and Quality.

O'Keeffe, M., & Saver, C. (2013). *Communication, collaboration, and you: Tools, tips, and techniques for nursing practice.* Silver Spring, MD: Nursesbooks.org.

Oyeleye, O., Hanson, P., O'Connor, N., & Dunn, D. (2013). Relationship of workplace incivility, stress, and burnout on nurses' turnover intentions and psychological empowerment. *Journal of Nursing Administration, 43*(10), 536–542.

Richards, K. (2013a). Self-care is a lifelong journey. *Nursing Economic$, 31*(4), 198–202.

Richards, K. (2013b). Wellpower: The foundation of innovation. *Nursing Economic$, 31*(2), 94–98.

Richards, K., Sheen, E., & Mazzer, M. C. (2014). *Self-care and you caring for the caregiver*. Silver Spring, MD: Nursesbooks.org.

Rose, L. (2011). Interprofessional collaboration in the ICU: How to define? *Nursing in Critical Care, 16*(1), 5–10.

Timmins, F. (2011). Managers' duty to maintain good workplace communications skills. *Nursing Management, 18*(3), 30–34.

Webster, J., & Cowart, P. (1999). An innovative professional nursing practice model. *Nursing Administration Quarterly, 23*(3), 11–16.

8

Empowering Nurses as Leaders

In the first few pages in Chapter 1, leadership is defined as "a process whereby an individual influences a group of individuals to achieve a common goal" (Northouse, 2014). Every nurse is a leader by virtue of the work that he or she does each and every day. It is essential that nurses feel empowered to be leaders so that they can be instrumental in making a difference in the lives of others. Nurses, as leaders, have a duty and an obligation to work on enhancing their own sense of empowerment so that they can effectively lead and empower others. If *structural empowerment* refers to power based on the employee's position in the organization, *psychological empowerment* consists of the fundamental personal convictions that employees have about their role in the organization (Knol & van Linge, 2009). Although both structural empowerment and psychological empowerment are important in the overall empowerment of nurses, this chapter focuses on nurses' enhancement of their sense of psychological empowerment.

Several studies have examined the positive effect of nurse empowerment on patient outcomes, yet information is limited in the existing literature on how to enhance nurses' sense of empowerment in the first place. Therefore, the beginning of this chapter focuses on strategies that nurse leaders can use to enhance their own sense of psychological empowerment as well as how nurse leaders can help other nurses to do the same. Several considerations are important in examining sense of empowerment as a leader, including emotional intelligence, resilience, mentoring, succession planning, coaching, precepting, and role development.

EMPOWERMENT OF NURSES AS A FACTOR IN PERFORMANCE

Evidence demonstrates a positive relationship between degree of nurse empowerment and improved patient care. Donahue, Piazza, Griffin, Dykes, and Fitzpatrick (2008) reported that nurses who perceive themselves to be empowered are more likely to use more effective work practices resulting in positive patient outcomes. Laschinger, Gilbert, Smith, and Leslie (2010) proposed that empowered nurses foster better health

209

outcomes. Improving nurses' sense of empowerment would seem to result in improved patient outcomes.

Conceptually, empowerment has been considered a process that leads to the experience of authority (Dimitriades & Kufidu, 2004). An empowered nurse can use this authority in positive ways in the professional working environment. An empowered nurse is self-confident, which allows for more freedom of action and benefits both patients and nursing staff (Kuokkanen & Leino-Kilpi, 2000). A leader who is empowered utilizes his or her experience and knowledge in making appropriate decisions that impact the organization and the followers. An empowered nurse leader is socially skilled and able to act under pressure and withstand criticism. An empowered nurse leader demonstrates successful professional performance and progress (Kuokkanen & Leino-Kilpi, 2001). All of these qualities can enhance the leader's effectiveness in addressing the needs of patients and employees in a health-care environment.

Although the literature defines nurse empowerment in many ways, Rao (2012) defines nurse empowerment as a state in which an individual nurse has assumed control over his or her practice, enabling him or her to fulfill professional nursing responsibilities within an organization successfully. This definition is particularly important to consider here because it specifically relates to the individual nurse. This implies that the individual nurse has some influence or control over his or her sense of empowerment. Other definitions are also considered throughout this chapter.

PSYCHOLOGICAL EMPOWERMENT

With the growing complexity and challenges of health-care delivery reform, nurses today more than ever need to feel psychologically empowered so that they can effectively manage their nursing practice and improve patient care. Because nurses are being called on to take an active role in leading health-care reform, it is essential that they become psychologically empowered to lead the way.

Spreitzer (2007) defined psychological empowerment as a set of psychological states that are necessary for individuals to feel a sense of control in relation to their work.

Evidence exists of a positive relationship between nurses' perceptions of power and the structure of the work environment and power in the organization (Faulkner & Laschinger, 2008). An organization that supports, values, and empowers nurses can only help to enhance a nurse's sense of empowerment. The literature also shows that an employee's perception of his or her work environment shapes feelings of empowerment and that structurally empowering conditions cannot be fully realized unless the individual is psychologically receptive (Faulkner & Laschinger, 2008). In social psychological theory, empowerment is seen as a process of personal growth and development in which empowerment originates within the individual and is concerned with the individual's reflection within the environment (Kuokkanen & Leino-Kilpi, 2001).

It is essential that individuals feel psychologically empowered in order to successfully perform in the workplace. Each nurse has a professional responsibility to assess his or her own empowerment and to find ways to enhance that empowerment to achieve the best outcomes for self, patients, and staff.

Assessing Nurses' Perceptions of Empowerment

As stated earlier, information in the literature on how to enhance nurses' sense of empowerment is scarce. However, before nurse leaders can begin to *enhance* their sense of empowerment, they must first *assess* their perception of their own empowerment to identify areas in need of improvement. As shown in Box 8.1,

---

BOX 8.1 Psychological Empowerment Instrument

Listed here are several self-orientations that people may have with regard to their work role. Using the following scale, please indicate the extent to which you agree or disagree that each one describes your self-orientation.

A. Very Strongly Disagree   **E.** Agree
B. Strongly Disagree   **F.** Strongly Agree
C. Disagree   **G.** Very Strongly Agree
D. Neutral

1. _____ I am confident about my ability to do my job.

2. _____ The work that I do is important to me.

3. _____ I have significant autonomy in determining how I do my job.

4. _____ My impact on what happens in my department is large.

5. _____ My job activities are personally meaningful to me.

6. _____ I have a great deal of control over what happens in my department.

7. _____ I can decide on my own how to go about doing my own work.

8. _____ I really care about what I do on my job.*

9. _____ My job is well within the scope of my abilities.*

10. _____ I have considerable opportunity for independence and freedom in how I do my job.

11. _____ I have mastered the skills necessary for my job.

12. _____ My opinion counts in departmental decision making.*

13. _____ The work I do is meaningful to me.

14. _____ I have significant influence over what happens in my department.

Continued

BOX 8.1   Psychological Empowerment Instrument–cont'd

15. _____ I am self-assured about my capabilities to perform my work activities.

16. _____ I have a chance to use personal initiative in carrying out my work.*

---

*Items that can be dropped to create a 12-item scale with three items per dimension. The 12-item version has been found to be highly reliable and valid.

The validation of the instrument is described in Spreitzer (1995, 1996). The instrument has been used successfully in more than 50 different studies in contexts ranging from nurses to low-wage service workers and manufacturing workers. The validity of the instrument is proven. Test-retest reliability has been shown to be strong, and validity estimates for the dimensions are typically about .80. More information on the empowerment profiles for different contexts and norm data for the empowerment dimensions can be found in Spreitzer and Quinn (2001).

References

Spreitzer, G. M. (1995). Psychological empowerment in the workplace: Dimensions, measurement, and validation. *Academy of Management Journal, 38*(5), 1442–1465.

Spreitzer, G. M. (1996). Social structural characteristics of psychological empowerment. *Academy of Management Journal, 39*(2), 483–504.

Spreitzer, G. M., & Quinn, R. E. (2001). *A company of leaders: Five disciplines for unleashing the power in your workforce.* San Francisco, CA: Jossey-Bass.

Gretchen Spreitzer's Psychological Empowerment Instrument is a useful tool for measuring psychological empowerment in the workplace. This tool has been found to be valid in health care (Spreitzer, 2007), particularly with nurses (Kraimer, Seibert, & Liden, 1999).

Spreitzer's measure taps the four empowerment dimensions of meaning, competence, self-determination, and impact (Dimitriades & Kufidu, 2004):

- *Meaning* involves a fit between the needs of one's work role and one's beliefs, values, and behaviors.
- *Competence* refers to self-efficacy specific to one's work, or a belief in one's capability to perform work activities with skill.
- *Self-determination* is a sense of choice in initiating and regulating one's actions.
- *Impact* is the degree to which one can influence strategic, administrative, or operating outcomes at work (Spreitzer 2007).

The instrument consists of 16 statements, the responses to which are rated on a seven-point Likert scale ranging from Very Strongly Disagree to Very Strongly Agree. Higher scores indicate higher degrees of psychological empowerment (Faulkner & Laschinger, 2008). Each dimension of empowerment is measured by four items (Laschinger, Finegan, Shamian & Wilk, 2001), as shown in Table 8.1. This instrument is in the public domain and available for nurses to access (University of Michigan, 2009).

TABLE 8.1 **Four Dimensions of Psychological Empowerment and Corresponding Questions on the Psychological Empowerment Instrument**

Four Dimensions of Psychological Empowerment	Corresponding Questions on the Psychological Empowerment Instrument for Each Dimension of Empowerment
Competence	Item numbers 1, 9, 11, and 15
Meaning	Item numbers 2, 5, 8, and 13
Impact	Item numbers 4, 6, 12, and 14
Self-determination	Item numbers 3, 7, 10, and 16

Using Professional Development to Enhance Nurses' Sense of Empowerment

Once a nurse has assessed his or her own degree of psychological empowerment, then he or she can begin working on enhancing it. According to Kuokkanen and Leino-Kilpi (2000), empowerment is associated with growth and development, processes that require critical introspection and changing patterns of activity. Educative efforts such as professional development and continuing education seminars and workshops enable employees to build knowledge, skills, and abilities, all of which can contribute to a greater sense of empowerment (Spreitzer, 2007).

Empowerment and professional development are remarkably synergistic. An empowered nurse assumes responsibility for and aspires to further training and progress in his or her work (Kuokkanen & Leino-Kilpi, 2001). Education, support, and information correlate positively with empowerment; furthermore, training and professional development for nursing staff can be used to improve nurses' empowerment (Kuokkanen & Leino-Kilpi, 2000, 2001). It is important to note that improving one's sense of empowerment is something that can be learned.

THE JOURNEY TO PSYCHOLOGICAL EMPOWERMENT

As stated earlier, this chapter's working definition of psychological empowerment is that it comprises the personal beliefs that an employee has about his or her role at work (Spreitzer, 2007). A comprehensive review of the literature clearly demonstrates that augmenting psychological empowerment is a skill that can be taught and learned. The Journey to Psychological Empowerment is a series of six professional seminars developed by Dr. Denise McNulty from more than 25 years of personal experience as a clinician, educator, and nurse leader. The seminar topics and content are specifically designed to provide an introspective focus on the nurse, as a leader, and his or her role in the workplace. Figure 8.1 shows the six seminars strategically arranged on a pyramid so that each seminar builds on the next sequentially, until they reach the apex—psychological empowerment. The Journey to Psychological Empowerment was designed as an intervention to enhance nurses' sense of their own psychological empowerment. The intervention was first tested with nurses in a private hospital in southwest Florida in partial fulfillment of the requirements for the doctor of nursing practice degree. The project was approved by the Duquesne University Institutional Review Board. Findings revealed that the intervention may have had a positive impact on nurses' psychological empowerment.

A formal research study was then conducted in a six-hospital health-care system in southwest Florida and approved by the health-care system's Institutional Review Committee. The Journey to Psychological Empowerment was offered to nurses employed by the health-care system. The effectiveness of the empowerment seminar in enhancing nurses' sense of psychological empowerment in the workplace was evaluated using a confidential survey. Dr. Gretchen Spreitzer's Psychological Empowerment Instrument was used to measure the study. A presurvey was conducted at the beginning of the empowerment seminar. Each instrument was assigned a number to protect the participants' identities. The nurses were invited to retake the instrument 3 months after attending the professional development seminar. A criterion to participate in

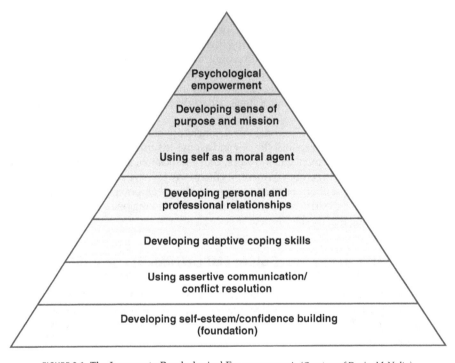

FIGURE 8.1 The Journey to Psychological Empowerment. *(Courtesy of Denise McNulty)*

the study was that participants be employed by the health-care system as an inpatient or outpatient registered nurse (RN) or licensed practical nurse. The following research question was asked: "What is the effectiveness of the Journey to Psychological Empowerment seminar on nurses' sense of psychological empowerment in the workplace?" During the time of the research study, 998 nurses attended the seminar, 780 nurses completed the presurvey (77% response), and 300 nurses completed the postsurvey (38% response). The data were analyzed using a paired sample t test. Findings revealed that the mean differences were statistically significant on all four dimensions of empowerment and the overall empowerment score ($p < 0.05$). Based on the findings of the study, the professional development seminar may have had a positive influence on nurses' psychological empowerment. The seminar may be an effective intervention in enhancing nurses' sense of empowerment, which may have implications for both practice and academic settings. The study was replicated in October 2015, with findings shown in Table 8.2.

Seminar 1: Developing Self-Esteem and Confidence Building

The first seminar topic is intentionally placed at the base of the pyramid to indicate the belief that self-esteem and confidence building are the foundation for nurses and nurse leaders and must be in place before moving up to the next level. Spreitzer asserts that self-esteem is positively related to psychological empowerment and that individuals

TABLE 8.2 **Research Study: The Effectiveness of Using the Journey to Empowerment Professional Development Seminar to Enhance Nurses' Sense of Empowerment Presurvey and Postsurvey Comparison**

	Presurvey Mean (n = 300) (Scale 1.0-7.0)	Postsurvey Mean (n = 300) (Scale 1.0-7.0)	Mean (paired) Difference
Competence	5.90	6.14	-.239
Meaning	6.12	6.26	-.149
Impact	4.27	4.49	-.223
Self-determination	5.06	5.35	-.295
Overall empowerment	5.34	5.56	-.225

with little self-esteem are not likely to see themselves as able to make a difference or influence their work and organizations (1995). According to Kuokkanen and Leino-Kilpi (2001), an empowered nurse possesses the high self-esteem that makes successful professional performance and progress possible. Individuals who feel good about themselves are confident, take pride in their work, and demonstrate respect and concern for patients and colleagues (Unal, 2012). A positive self-image and professional identity are prerequisites for a nurse to have a strong and therapeutic relationship with a patient (Unal, 2012). Thus, the literature clearly supports the need for nurses to have high self-esteem.

Seminar 2: Using Assertive Communication and Conflict Resolution

The second seminar topic in the Journey to Psychological Empowerment addresses the skill of using assertive communication and conflict resolution. According to Kuokkanen and Leino-Kilpi (2001), empowered nurses are socially skilled. Developing good interpersonal and counseling skills is essential for nurses working in any healthcare environment. Empowered nurses use assertive communication when interacting with coworkers, physicians, and patients.

It is important to differentiate between being assertive and being aggressive., however. Being empowered does not support being hostile or violent. *Assertiveness*, by contrast, is an interpersonal behavior that promotes equality in human relationships by assisting individuals to express their rights, thoughts, and feelings in a manner that neither denies nor demeans them and recognizes and respects the rights, thoughts, and feelings of others (Unal, 2012). Thus, assertiveness is a communication style that is considered an important skill for today's professional nurse and the key to successful relationships with patients, families, and colleagues (Unal, 2012).

Seminar 3: Developing Adaptive Coping Skills

The third seminar topic on the Journey to Psychological Empowerment is developing adaptive coping skills. No matter at what level or in what job a nurse works, some level of stress is inevitable; moreover, most individuals are simultaneously experiencing personal stress, making coping difficult at times. According to Lewis and Urmston (2000), a clear relationship exists between coping skills and empowerment. Worker powerlessness cultivates burnout—that is, the inability to function in any role, whether as a parent, spouse, student, or employee (Lewis & Urmston, 2000). An empowered nurse, by contrast, is able to act under pressure and withstand criticism (Kuokkanen & Leino-Kilpi, 2001).

Seminar 4: Developing Personal and Professional Relationships

The fourth seminar topic on the Journey to Psychological Empowerment is developing personal and professional relationships. According to Spreitzer (2007), employees who have developed better relationships with their leader, with their team members, and with customers report feeling more empowered. Effective teams and group support are reported to be essential features of professional support in practice and positive features in continuing professional education (Lewis & Urmston, 2000).

A powerful exercise is to ask nurses in the group to take turns reading a statement aloud from the "Building Healthy Professional Relationships" handout (Box 8.2).

Seminar 5: Using the Self as a Moral Agent

The fifth seminar topic on the Journey to Psychological Empowerment addresses the role of the nurse as it pertains to maintaining a practice that adheres to morals, principles, and ethics. Nurses are often placed in situations in which they need to make decisions that require consideration of doing the right thing for the right reason. According to the American Nurses Association (ANA) *Code of Ethics for Nurses*, the nurse promotes, advocates for, and protects the rights, health, and safety of the patient (2015). Nurses have a responsibility to serve the public in an ethical manner.

BOX 8.2 Building Healthy Professional Relationships

This set of tenets developed by Denise McNulty is intended to inspire nurses to be the best they can be in building healthy professional relationships.

- Try not to eat your young! Be welcoming to new nurses. Mentor them, show them what you know, and help them develop. Let's prove the article "Why Do Nurses Eat Their Young?" to be wrong.

- Support each other–do not be resentful, jealous, or envious of any nurse. Everyone on the team is important. Everyone has something valuable to offer.

- Do not bring others down with a negative attitude–if you do not like what you are doing, you need to make a change.

- Remember, it is healthier to be assertive rather than passive-aggressive. No one will ever respect you if you are passive-aggressive.

- Always take a lunch or dinner break. You will be happier, and your team members will benefit from you being happier.

- Whatever you do, wherever you go, always try to do the very best you can in your job. Go to your job with a good name, stay with a good name, and leave with a good name.

- Find a nurse mentor–someone you can learn from. Be a nurse mentor–to someone who can learn from you.

- Stay away from toxic people! Surround yourself with people who are good for you. You will find that if you do this, you will be happier and healthier.

- Be mindful of your boundaries with your nurse colleagues. Choose whom you entrust personal information to wisely.

- Continue to learn–knowledge is power!

- Do not get caught up with being liked or loved. If you are respected, that is all that matters!

Seminar 6: Developing a Sense of Purpose and Mission

The sixth and final seminar topic on the Journey to Psychological Empowerment presents important questions for every nurse to consider: Why does a nurse do what he or she does every day? What motivates a nurse to want to continue working in nursing? With all of the stress and, at times, uncertainty in the health-care environment, a nurse's sense of purpose and mission may often be the main force that keeps him or her engaged in the profession. What legacy do you want to leave when you retire from nursing? What legacy do you want to leave when you leave this world? What kind of nurse do you want to be remembered as?

At times, we work with nurses who appear to be struggling with finding a sense of purpose or direction, not only in their careers, but also in their lives. Helping nurses find meaning in their lives can only help improve their overall sense of empowerment and self-worth. The sixth level on the pyramid can perhaps be compared with Maslow's self-actualization. As self-esteem and confidence building are the foundation in a nurse's journey to psychological empowerment, finding a sense of purpose and mission is the final step in the journey. When a nurse finds a sense of purpose and mission, he or she may experience a greater sense of fulfillment from work as well as a healthier work-life balance. Indeed, finding that sense of purpose and mission in their work is something for which nurses often yearn. Therefore, nursing leaders must do everything they can to support a nurse in this journey, for it is truly the heart and soul of why nurses do what they do every day.

Completing the Journey

Upon completion of the Journey to Psychological Empowerment seminars, the nurse should retake the Psychological Empowerment Instrument to determine whether any improvement in self-perception of psychological empowerment has taken place. Additionally, nurse leaders may choose to assess their nurses' degree of empowerment and use the information to develop an alternative program or intervention other than the Journey to Psychological Empowerment if a need for improvement is identified.

Initiatives that focus on empowerment may have implications for enhancing nursing recruitment and retention in health-care organizations. As we continue to address attrition among nurses from the profession, an analysis of the perception of the power to change elements in the practice arena could be a major factor. Nursing leaders and educators may consider using empowerment-enhancing initiatives in orientation programs for new nurses and as an ongoing element of staff development and continuing education.

Every nurse should be encouraged to work on enhancing his or her own sense of empowerment. The Journey to Psychological Empowerment is one intervention that nurses can utilize to enhance psychological empowerment. Empowerment of self and others is truly a journey (see Leadership Applications in Practice 8.1 and 8.2 and Leadership Applications in Academics 8.1).

OTHER FACTORS THAT ENHANCE PSYCHOLOGICAL EMPOWERMENT

The topics that follow in this section—emotional intelligence, resilience, mentoring, succession planning, coaching, precepting, and role development—relate to and support psychological empowerment.

LEADERSHIP APPLICATIONS IN PRACTICE 8.1 One Team's Journey to Empowerment

At a private Florida hospital where she worked, the director of nursing observed high rates of nursing staff turnover, frequent call-outs from work lack of communication and teamwork between shifts, inability to resolve conflicts between patients and staff, and ineffective coping in response to stress in the workplace. The director had a hunch that the nurses did not feel empowered. She received approval from the hospital administration to conduct a quality improvement project to assess 31 nurses' sense of empowerment using Dr. Gretchen Spreitzer's Psychological Empowerment Instrument. The nurses were assigned an identification number that only a nursing Unit Secretary knew to keep the process anonymous.

Findings revealed that the nurses scored high in the dimensions of competence and meaning, but they scored low in the dimensions of self-determination and impact. The director invited her nurses to participate in the Journey to Psychological Empowerment seminars and served as facilitator for the sessions. At the end of the last session, the nurses retook the Psychological Empowerment Instrument, once again anonymously. A comparison of the results of the pre- and postassessments showed that the scores increased in each of the four dimensions. Moreover, the director observed several changes she believed to be the result of the nurses' participation in the journey seminars: decreases in patient and physician complaints, staff turnover, and call-outs from work and improvement in communication and teamwork between shifts. The nurses also appeared to be more engaged in their profession and expressed a desire to form a study group to prepare for their specialty certification examination.

Lessons Learned The nurse leader can be an integral part of effecting change and creating a healthier work environment for staff. It is important for a nurse leader to take the time to assess and evaluate what the underlying issues may be and then to develop a plan for improvement. It speaks volumes when nurse leaders take the time to express genuine care and concern for improving nurses' work environment.

LEADERSHIP APPLICATIONS IN PRACTICE 8.2 A Chief Nursing Officer Wants Her Nurses to Be More Empowered

A Chief Nursing Officer (CNO) for a large health-care system in Florida worked with her Director of Education to offer the Journey to Psychological Empowerment seminars to her nursing staff. The CNO insisted that her Nursing Leadership Team be the first group to attend the journey seminars so that they could subsequently help support and encourage nurses' attendance, and she herself attended the first seminar.

Afterward, the CNO stated that she wanted every one of her 3,600 nurses to attend the 1-day seminar. The CNO is to be commended for having a sincere desire to help enhance her nurses' sense of empowerment. She is a wonderful role model for nurses and a nurse executive who truly understands how important it is for nurses to feel empowered and to be empowered.

Lessons Learned It is important for a nurse executive to be a visionary and to be able to listen objectively to what his or her nurses need without feeling fearful or threatened. When a nurse leader has the support of his or her nurse executive, the nurse leader can accomplish great things.

LEADERSHIP APPLICATIONS IN ACADEMICS 8.1 **An Educator Welcomes the Journey on the West Coast**

A nurse educator, on staff at a large health-care system in California, viewed a webinar on the Journey to Psychological Empowerment and was inspired to offer the journey to her nurses. All six journey seminars were presented during 1-day sessions held on 5 consecutive days to allow as many nurses as possible to attend. In total, 500 nurses attended the journey seminars, and their responses were overwhelmingly positive. At the end of each day, nurses lined up to express their thanks and appreciation to the facilitator for teaching them how to improve their sense of empowerment.

The nurse educator is commended for identifying the need to provide a program for the nurses that focused on ways to enhance their empowerment. She also attended the seminar and was inspired to return to school for her doctor of nursing practice degree!

Lessons Learned The educator was astute in identifying that her nurses were in need of empowerment training. Nurse educators, as leaders, can be very instrumental in assessing the professional development needs of their nurses and staff. They usually know intuitively what is needed in the nursing work environment.

Emotional Intelligence

Emotional intelligence (EI), or the ability to effectively manage one's emotions (see Chapter 1), may enhance psychological empowerment and vice versa. Emotionally intelligent leaders may experience a strong sense of empowerment, which, in turn, may motivate and inspire them to empower others in the workplace. In the many difficult situations that their workday presents, leaders have an obligation to lead in a nonreactionary manner and to project a persona of emotional stability. Feather (2009) purports that a vital portion of the development of leaders in achieving success is to develop and enhance their level of EI.

Health-care leaders who are emotionally intelligent can improve the cultural "health" of their institutions at many levels, beginning with their own employees (Feather, 2009). Nurses in leadership positions have the vitally important responsibility of recognizing the precious resource they have in their nursing staff (Feather, 2009). The emotionally intelligent leader does not rush in to fix, cure, or control responses of staff members, but is empathetic to their concerns and allows them to express their feelings without judgment, pressure, or guilt (Feather, 2009). Through thoughtful, reflective, caring actions, emotionally intelligent leaders empower others to make decisions and solve problems.

Resilience

Resilience may be another factor that impacts psychological empowerment in a positive way. People who are resilient have the ability to "bounce back" in difficult times. To survive in the ever-changing and challenging world of health care, a nurse must not only feel empowered, he or she must also be resilient. Are people born resilient or is this something that can be learned? Life experience can be our best teacher, and adversity can make us stronger. According to Manzano Garcia and Ayala Calvo (2012), even experiences that are considered to be difficult, challenging, or negative are experiences we can learn from and that foster personal growth. Leaders may not be able to control all events, but how they view and respond to adversity can distinguish them as effective leaders. Grafton, Gillespie, and Henderson (2010) report that resilient leaders embrace adverse situations with optimism and use them to develop and grow, to restore and strengthen well-being.

Nurses need to be as mentally and emotionally prepared as possible for what lies ahead. Nursing is a profession that bears witness to tragedy and human adversity (East, Jackson, O'Brien, & Peters, 2010). Manzano Garcia and Ayala Calvo (2012) theorize that more resilient nurses display fewer signs of emotional exhaustion because, through exposure to difficult working situations and environments, they develop better coping mechanisms to deal with the concomitant stress. According to Grafton et al. (2010), resilience is not only a resource on which leaders can draw to cope more effectively during stressful and adverse situations, it can also reduce vulnerability to future stress. Resilient nurses, as leaders, rely on this component of empowerment when coping with challenging and adverse work situations.

One such coping mechanism is a technique that nurses can use as a form of "healthy" dissociation, or emotional detachment. This can be a very effective coping strategy for nurses as long as the emotional detachment does not devolve into emotional disconnection. For example, when working with patients who have psychiatric/mental health and/or substance abuse issues, nurses need to be able to offer care, concern, and support to their patients in an empathetic manner but also need to maintain a level of emotional detachment so that they do not become overwhelmed or emotionally absorbed in the patient's stress or crisis. The same could apply to nurses who work with patients in intensive care units, oncology, emergency settings, or in any crisis-oriented environment. To emotionally detach, the nurse should remain calm, taking slow, deep breaths and focusing on these breaths while listening to the patient who is stressed or in crisis. As the patient's emotions become more intense, the nurse should think of something else that is soothing and calming to remain present without absorbing the patient's anxiety. It must be done in such a way that the patient does not sense that the nurse is distracted or not attentively listening. If the patient senses that the nurse is not fully present during a crisis, trust and rapport with the patient could be compromised.

The active use of this strategy may help to prevent burnout and enhance resilience. Dean (2012) reports that burnout can cause nurses to withdraw emotionally from their patients, which is quite different from the purposeful and intentional use of emotional detachment as an adaptive coping mechanism. Under enormous work pressure, nurses may feel that they are not delivering the care they would like and are letting people down. If this goes on for an extended period, it could be destructive and lead to nurses shutting off and depersonalizing patients (Dean, 2012). This is not the goal of emotional detachment. The nurse continues to stay connected with the patient in a caring, empathetic manner, but the nurse does not become emotionally enmeshed in the patient's stress or crisis. Nurses who feel empowered may perhaps be viewed as more resilient than those nurses who do not feel empowered, which is yet another reason to support the need for nurses to improve their sense of empowerment.

Mentoring

One way to empower self and others is through mentoring. Every nurse leader should be a mentor and every nurse leader should have a mentor. Formal and informal mentoring has been associated with nurse leader development (McCloughen, O'Brien, & Jackson, 2009). Empowered nurses may be more receptive to being mentored by others and may show more of a willingness and a desire to mentor others. An empowered state of mind can be contagious—being mentored by someone who feels empowered may be empowering in and of itself.

Griffith (2012) reminds us that the ANA's Scope and Standards of Practice for nursing administrators lists mentoring as an essential component of the nurse administrator's managerial and leadership roles. Effective mentoring relationships have three necessary characteristics: (1) helping the mentee to acquire both the necessary competencies for the position as well as pertinent work relationships for his or her chosen career path; (2) a collaborative learning relationship in which mentors are committed to share knowledge and mentees are committed to learn from them; and (3) the recognition that the mentor–mentee relationship develops over time, evolves through phases, and is more than a casual relationship (Thompson, Wolf, & Sabatine, 2012). Attributes of mentors and mentees are highlighted in Table 8.3.

TABLE 8.3 **Attributes of Mentors and Mentees**

Attributes of Mentors	Attributes of Mentees
Altruistic	Willing to learn
Visionary	Willing to share
Available and challenging	Committed to their career
Competence	Eager to learn and develop
Personal confidence	Competent
Commitment to the development of others	Determination to succeed in the profession
Motivated	Strong self-identity and initiation
Possess time to devote to the mentoring experience and actively facilitate mentoring process	Motivated to participate in mentoring

TABLE 8.3 **Attributes of Mentors and Mentees–cont'd**

Attributes of Mentors	Attributes of Mentees
Strong self-esteem	Goal driven
Positive attitude and outlook	Determined
Champion their mentees' careers by unconditionally giving of themselves	Passion for nursing
Effective communication skills	Have the potential to succeed
Politically astute	Positive attitude
Well respected in the workplace	Possess effective communication skills
Hold a vision for the future	Willing to receive constructive feedback
Not interested in preserving the status quo	Able to work under the direction of another
Balance personal and professional responsibilities	Feel passionate about their profession
Highly knowledgeable in their field	Possess initiative
Willing to mentor	Have the ability to act responsibly
Motivated to mentor well	Have the ability to act independently
Interested in new challenges	Possess leadership potential

Adapted from: McCloughen, A., O'Brien, L., & Jackson, D. (2009). Esteemed connection: Creating a mentoring relationship for nurse leadership. *Nursing Inquiry, 16*, 326.

We also need to be mindful of the need to mentor diverse leaders who are representative of protected classes as well as the various intergenerational groups. With the increasing diversity of our nursing workforce, we need to mentor leaders who are diverse. It is imperative that if these nurses have an aptitude for leadership, they be recruited, trained, supported, mentored, and retained (Griffith, 2012). See Chapter 2 for additional information on workforce diversity.

Succession Planning

Another way nurses can empower self and others is through succession planning. A nurse leader engages in succession planning when he or she seeks out an individual(s) who may be groomed to assume the nurse leader's position and duties after the nurse leader moves on. Mentoring and succession planning go hand in hand insofar as mentoring is a key feature of any succession-planning program. This must be systematized so that experienced nurse leaders can begin preparing their replacements (Griffith, 2012). Continuous, focused leadership and succession planning are not optional (Robinson-Walker, 2013)—every nurse leader needs to develop a succession plan. According to Griffith (2012), the current and projected global nursing shortage and economic, political, and social factors affecting health-care delivery worldwide make effective succession planning an absolute necessity for the nursing profession.

We all work with exemplary nurses who serve as wonderful role models for other nurses. Experienced nurse leaders need to take these exemplars under their wing and train them as potential successors. Too often, when a nurse leader leaves a job, that position remains vacant for a protracted period of time, requiring an interim leader until a permanent replacement is hired. The practice of using interim leaders has pros and cons. One pro is that it gives an interim leader the opportunity to acquire a feel for the position and see whether it is something for which he or she would like to formally apply. Another pro is that it gives both administrators and staff a chance to assess the interim leader's ability to lead. However, a potential con is that sometimes the interim leader becomes so comfortable in the position that he or she does not want to let go of it and may attempt to sabotage efforts to find a replacement. Or, if the interim leader is not selected for the position and becomes angry, the interim may seek to undermine his or her replacement. These and other pitfalls of interim nursing leadership are described in Leadership Applications in Practice 8.3 and 8.4 and Leadership Applications in Academics 8.2.

To avoid pitfalls such as these, effective succession planning is essential to both the nursing academic and practice realms. In academia, effective succession planning is important in the face of the continuing nursing shortage and the aging of our nursing education leaders and doctorally prepared faculty (Griffith, 2012). In the practice arena, we have a nursing leadership crisis in the United States because of a large number of vacancies in nursing leadership positions, which is further complicated by the future uncertainty of and current challenges surrounding the nation's health-care system (Griffith, 2012). In addressing the related problem of effective succession planning, it is vital that the efforts of both academia and practice complement each other (Griffith, 2012). For example, nursing executives in the practice setting may encourage their master's-level and doctorally prepared nurses to consider teaching as adjunct or clinical faculty in the local nursing schools. This would give nurses in practice an opportunity to work part-time in academia, which

A nurse leader was hired to serve as a director of nursing in a specialty hospital, replacing the interim director of nursing who no longer wished to work in that position and had requested to serve the hospital in another role outside of nursing. When the new director of nursing came on board, however, the former director of nursing was not pleased and made her displeasure felt by interfering with nursing operations, acting as though she still had the responsibility for the nursing department, continuing to give directives to the nursing executive secretary (which opposed those of the new director of nursing), and creating confusion on the nursing units regarding to whom the nurses should be reporting.

The new director's assessment of this situation was that the former director still had a desire to maintain the status of being a director of nursing but without the responsibility that went with the position. Conflicts with the former director became so difficult that the new director requested a meeting with the hospital Chief Executive Officer (CEO), who scheduled a meeting with the two nurse leaders in an attempt to resolve the issue. Although the CEO respected the former director of nursing, he made it very clear that she was no longer the director and that she was to respect the new director for the position that she held. The former director became so angry that she picked up the chair she had been sitting in and carried it into the parking lot, resigned that day, and never returned to the hospital. The new director remained in her position and successfully led the nursing team in a positive direction.

Lessons Learned Working under a leader who "has your back" and who is supportive is vitally important for a nurse executive or any nursing leader. Having a good relationship with one's supervisor/direct report is key. Another lesson learned is to keep one's composure, maintain professionalism, and use EI when interacting with others.

A nurse leader was hired as the new CNO for a 100-bed hospital. Prior to the CNO coming on board, an interim director of nursing had served in the position for several months. During her interview for the position, the soon-to-be CNO asked the CEO how the interim director felt about stepping down from her position. The CEO shared that the interim director had no aspiration for remaining in the position but that she would like to remain as a supervisor. The CNO later confirmed this with the interim director herself but after coming on board discovered that although the former director did not wish to remain in the nurse executive position, she retained significant influence over several of her former employees with whom she had long-term relationships. The former director had strong opinions about how things should run and disagreed with several of the changes that the new CNO implemented. The former director also appeared to have the support of the other supervisors, who played the key roles of covering the facility and providing administrative oversight of the units in the CNO's absence. The charge nurses, staff nurses, and

Continued

supervisors reported directly to the CNO. The CNO attempted to make improvements in her department with a goal of improving patient care.

Despite a concerted effort to develop the leadership team in the facility, it became increasingly difficult for the CNO to be effective in her role given the undermining and negativity of the supervisors. The CNO went to the CEO for guidance on how to address the dysfunction, but the CEO appeared reluctant to become involved. Because of a mutual agreement to part ways, the CNO eventually left her position.

Lessons Learned Nurse leaders need to ask as many questions as possible during the interview process to fully assess the dynamics of an organization prior to joining a team. If an interim leader has been in place, during the interview process it is prudent to ask about the plan for the interim leader when he or she steps down from the position. Upon careful assessment, a new nursing leader may need to consider restructuring the current nursing management team.

Remember that adversity can make us stronger (some would say that everything happens for a reason). Because of the situation, after leaving the CNO position, the nurse leader was offered an opportunity to help design and implement a new nursing program for a university and was also recruited by a CNO to help begin the transformation of a culture in a large health-care system by empowering nurses and providing leadership development.

A nurse was hired to serve as an Associate Director for a college RN to bachelor of science in nursing (BSN) program. Although the leader had prior experience serving in executive positions in health care and prior teaching experience in academia, this was her first position as an academic leader. She was hired by the Associate Dean of Nursing, who functioned as the Nurse Administrator for the School of Nursing, and who announced her retirement 30 days later. The Associate Director agreed to serve as the interim Director/Nurse Administrator for the School of Nursing in addition to serving in her current role as Associate Director of the RN to BSN program.

Shortly after assuming her new responsibility, she discovered that the RN to BSN program was not accredited, despite students believing it to be so. She also was informed that the associate degree in nursing program's reaccreditation was under review and in need of a follow-up report. The interim director was unfamiliar with the accreditation process and had no formal mentor at the college who was familiar with nursing program accreditation, but the president of the college charged her with the responsibility of obtaining full accreditation within 6 months.

The interim director arranged for formal education to increase her knowledge of curriculum design, teaching strategies, evaluation methods, and accreditation standards. She rallied the

LEADERSHIP APPLICATIONS IN ACADEMICS 8.2 **Academic Leader Serves as an Interim–cont'd**

faculty and together they successfully achieved initial accreditation of the RN to BSN program from a national accrediting body. In addition, under the interim Director's leadership, the associate degree in nursing program received approval from a national accrediting body for successful completion of the follow-up report to maintain the program's reaccreditation.

Lessons Learned Hard work and determination have their own rewards. Experience is our best teacher and may help open doors to previously unimaginable new opportunities.

would help meet faculty recruitment needs. Griffith (2012) purports that effective succession planning can offer a means of providing health-care organizations and nursing education programs with a ready supply of capable, qualified nurse leaders. These leaders need to be ready to move into vacant positions as soon as openings occur to help prevent disruption in the functioning of an organization (Griffith, 2012). According to Robinson-Walker (2013), the future of the health-care enterprise in the United States rests with the leaders who are "in training" now. These nurses are learning from their leaders every day. Nurse leaders need to be mindful of how they are leading, how they are living, and how they are developing and influencing those around them (Robinson-Walker, 2013).

Nurses who are empowered can be instrumental in promoting succession planning within their work environments. As discussed in an earlier section of this chapter, empowered nurses are confident and self-assured, do not fear being replaced, and are not threatened by qualified talent. They understand the importance of succession planning and how essential this is for the nursing profession and further empower themselves by practicing it.

Coaching

Nurses, as leaders, may use coaching as a strategy to empower self and others. Although coaching might seem synonymous with mentoring, Griffith (2012) reminds us that there is a significant distinction. Mentoring is self-selected and can be a gradual long-term commitment, whereas coaching is performance related to a goal of developing specific skills (Griffith, 2012). If mentors provide specific advice and opinions about actions to take and skills to develop, the coach works with the nurse to put that advice into action (Thompson et al., 2012). Coaching takes various forms, but for the purposes of this chapter, only managerial coaching and executive coaching are covered.

Managerial Coaching

Managerial coaching is a form of coaching that can be used in both practice and academic settings. The literature shows a paradigm shift in managerial coaching from a process of control and prescription that focused on telling people what they needed to do to improve performance to an interpersonal relationship intended to empower and promote self-efficacy (Batson & Yoder, 2012).

As shown in Table 8.4, managerial coaching requires both facilitating and empowering attributes (Batson & Yoder, 2012). Facilitating attributes deal with the practical side of coaching whereas empowering attributes promote psychological empowerment and development of self-efficacy. Nurse leaders should also consider which managerial behaviors are conducive to developing a coaching relationship as well as those that would impede coaching, as shown in Table 8.5 (Batson & Yoder, 2012).

TABLE 8.4 Managerial Coaching Attributes

Facilitating Attributes	Empowering Attributes
Developing an interpersonal relationship of mutual trust and respect	Role modeling
Setting clear expectations for performance	Promoting a sense of positive accountability for actions
Providing and soliciting feedback	Removing obstacles
Setting goals	Challenging/broadening perspectives
Providing training and/or resources	

Adapted from: Batson, V. D., & Yoder, L. H. (2012). Managerial coaching: A concept analysis. *Journal of Advanced Nursing*, *68*(7), 1658.

TABLE 8.5 Managerial Coaching Behaviors

Managerial Behaviors Conducive to Coaching	Managerial Behaviors That Impede Coaching
Providing genuine feedback	Being too authoritarian and directive

TABLE 8.5 **Managerial Coaching Behaviors–cont'd**

Managerial Behaviors Conducive to Coaching	Managerial Behaviors That Impede Coaching
Demonstrating caring through support and encouragement	Not being available or approachable
Demonstrating a demeanor of approachability and availability	Being unclear
Communicating using a balance of active listening and reflective questioning	Being too intense and emotional
	Failing to assess the situation from the employee's perspective to validate feedback

Adapted from: Batson, V. D., & Yoder, L. H. (2012). Managerial coaching: A concept analysis. *Journal of Advanced Nursing,* *68*(7), 1658.

Executive Coaching

Inherent in the role of nurse leaders is providing managerial coaching for subordinates, but who provides coaching for the nurse leader? Executive coaching is an organizational intervention focused at the individual level (Savage, 2001). It can be a useful modality for nurse leaders and should be included as part of every leader's professional development plan. Even experienced leaders may find themselves in work situations in which they require additional support and guidance.

Some organizations may provide the services of an internal executive coach who is available to the organization's leaders on a full-time, part-time, or contractual basis. Although convenient, using an internal executive coach might have some downsides, such as issues dealing with confidentiality— for example, will the executive coach be sharing meeting/discussion content with senior management? Another consideration is the potential bias of the executive coach—where does his or her loyalty lie among the management hierarchy?

Using an external executive coach is another option. One advantage of using someone who is outside of the organization is that a leader can insist on maintaining confidentiality as part of the agreement for services. In addition, no one in the nurse leader's organization should know about the leader securing the services of a coach unless the leader him- or herself chooses to disclose that information. Furthermore, an outside executive coach can provide an objective view because he or she is not employed by or has no affiliation with the organization (which the nurse leader should verify prior to formalizing an agreement). Box 8.3 provides questions a nurse leader

BOX 8.3 **Questions to Ask When Choosing an Executive Coach**

- Do I feel comfortable enough to "let my hair down" with this person?
- Do I feel certain that this coach will maintain confidentiality?
- Does this coach possess the necessary expertise to provide appropriate support through the change process?
- Does this coach understand organizational politics well enough to effectively counsel me?
- Does this coach possess the skills to push back and challenge me in ways that I can hear and accept?

Adapted from: Savage, C. M. (2001). Executive coaching: Professional self-care for nursing. *Nursing Economic$*, *19*(4), 178.

can ask a potential executive coach (Savage, 2001). Answering yes to these questions may indicate a good match between a leader and a potential coach.

Nurses who feel empowered may be more receptive to receiving coaching, viewing it as an opportunity for growth and further development rather than as a probationary measure to address underperformance. These nurses may also be more apt to seek out a coach as compared with nurses who do not feel empowered (see Leadership Applications in Practice 8.5).

LEADERSHIP APPLICATIONS IN PRACTICE 8.5 **One Leader's Experience With an Executive Coach**

A Director of Mental Health and Detox served in an acute care hospital in Philadelphia, where a new Vice President of Nursing was hired. The vice president met with the director on a Friday and announced that effective the following Monday, Maternal and Child Health and Pediatrics would be added to the director's jurisdiction. With this restructuring, the director's span of control would now include nine cost centers and 150 employees, but the promotion was a promotion in title only, as a salary increase did not accompany the increase in responsibilities. The Maternal/Child Health area included Labor and Delivery, Well-Baby Nursery, Level II Neonatal Intensive Care Unit, Postpartum, Pediatrics, an Obstetrics/Gynecology clinic, and a small Medical-Surgical unit.

The director felt that she needed some guidance to handle all of this new responsibility but was reluctant to seek it from the new vice president. She met with an executive coach outside of the organization for only one $500 session, but that session changed the director's entire career, carrying the coach's advice with her in every management position she held for the next 20 years. This advice consisted of scheduling 30-minute meetings with every one of her new employees in the first few weeks of her new assignment. The goal of each meeting was to allow employees to

---

**LEADERSHIP APPLICATIONS IN PRACTICE 8.5 One Leader's Experience With
an Executive Coach–cont'd**

---

share their backgrounds in nursing, details about their current positions, what they liked about their units, and what opportunities for improvement they had identified. The director then shared her vision with each employee and welcomed him or her to her team. Information shared during the meetings was kept confidential. The director summarized information that was shared and devised themes that represented the most significant problems in the department. The information was utilized to develop a restructuring proposal that contained an action plan for improvement. The director has successfully used this one-to-one approach in every leadership position she has since held in health care.

Lessons Learned Due to the hospital's restructuring of nursing units, which resulted in a downsizing, the director made a conscious decision not to ask for an increase in salary as she viewed the promotion in title and responsibility as a career opportunity. These types of career decisions need to be carefully considered by nurse leaders prior to accepting new assignments. Securing the services of an executive coach may prove to be most beneficial for nurse leaders. It can be very worthwhile for one's future.

Precepting

Precepting is vital to the learning experience of the nursing student and new graduate as another way for nurses, as leaders, to empower self and others. Precepting is very different from mentoring in that the preceptor role is to guide student nurses and new graduate nurses from the theory of nursing to the application of nursing theory, functioning as a role model, and teaching clinical skills and clinical thinking, whereas the role of a mentor is focused more on supporting, inspiring, and nurturing rather than on the transfer of practical clinical skills or formal evaluation of clinical performance (Omansky, 2010; Yonge, Billay, Myrick, & Luhanga, 2007). A mentorship is voluntary and can occur at any point in a nurse's career. Another important differentiating factor is that mentees can select their mentors for a long-term relationship, but with the preceptorship relationship, preceptees and preceptors may not be involved in the selection process, and the relationship is usually short term.

The following are considerations for nurse leaders to be mindful of regarding preceptors:

- The preceptor needs a clear definition of his or her role and expectations for that role.
- The preceptor should be given a preceptor orientation.
- The preceptor needs to know what learning outcomes are expected from the experience.
- The preceptor should be given a manual or list of written guidelines, if possible.
- The preceptor should know beforehand what compensation, if any, will be provided for precepting.

- The preceptor's liability should be determined beforehand and made clear to the preceptor.
- The preceptor's workload should be kept manageable to prevent role overload.
- The preceptor needs support from both management and coworkers.

Another consideration is the selection of a preceptor; not every nurse is a suitable candidate for precepting nursing students and new graduates. Clinically competent nurses may not be prepared to function as preceptors with clinical teaching and evaluation competencies (Luhanga, Dickieson, & Mossey, 2010). A preceptor should be a positive role model who has the patience and willingness to precept students and new nurses. A preceptor should be someone who enjoys teaching others and who can motivate and inspire others. Nurses need to be adequately prepared for the preceptor role regardless of their years of clinical experience.

Serving as a preceptor confers several benefits, including personal satisfaction, personal growth, competence development, teaching opportunities, enhancement of knowledge base, mutual learning, support for the nursing profession, and staying up to date clinically (Carlson, Pilhammar, & Wann-Hansson, 2010; Luhanga et al., 2010). Precepting can be a very positive experience for both the preceptor and the preceptee.

Empowered nurses may be reasonably viewed as empowering preceptors. Empowered nurses are considered by their colleagues to be individuals who have the desire to share their knowledge with others. They take great pride in having an active role in the growth and development of other nurses. Nurse leaders can have a tremendous influence on the success of the preceptor–preceptee relationship. It is important that nurse leaders ensure that preceptees and preceptors have a positive experience and that they are afforded every opportunity to excel in the preceptor-preceptee relationship.

Role Development of Self and Others

Dr. Ester Buchholz reminds us in one of her famous quotes: "Others inspire us, information feeds us, practice improves our performance, but we need quiet time to figure things out, to emerge with new discoveries, to unearth original answers."

Nurses may find role development to be very empowering. Nurse leaders must embrace the need for role development of self as they move into their various professional roles. Nurse leaders also need to be mindful of the need to support and engage in the role development of others—students, nursing graduates, nursing staff, educators, nursing leaders, and advanced practice registered nurses (APRNs)—in both the practice and academic environments.

A key component of the leadership role is the desire for lifelong learning. All nurses, regardless of their position and specialty, need to engage in lifelong learning, according to one of the Institute of Medicine's (IOM) *Future of Nursing Report (2010)* recommendations. The ANA's (2015) Nursing *Scope and Standards of Practice* states that RNs need to demonstrate a commitment to lifelong learning and lists lifelong learning as one of the ANA's required educational competencies for RNs. As we are reminded by O'Connor (2011), ensuring that nurses are provided with opportunities for learning is an organizational obligation.

An excellent example of a regional effort that has been instrumental in supporting role development of nurses as leaders is the Southwest Florida Future of Nursing Task

Force, with its goal of increasing the opportunities for nurses in that area to engage in lifelong learning (Morrison & McNulty, 2012). The Southwest Florida Future of Nursing Task Force also aligns initiatives with the IOM's recommendation that nurses are prepared and enabled to lead change to advance health.

Nurse Leader Role Development

Nurses may develop in a number of professional roles, but for the purposes of this chapter, the focus here is on the development of a nurse as a leader, educator, and clinician. As mentioned, nurse leaders in practice have a duty and an obligation to continuously develop in their roles and to assist both their experienced nursing staff and new nurse graduates in their role development.

According to O'Connor (2011), two areas of preparation that are foundational for nurse leaders to be successful in reaching and achieving roles in high-level positions within an organization include formal education and experience in nursing. Nurse leaders in both the practice and academic environments should consider the following strategies in the further development of their education and, thus, their roles:

- Pursuing advanced education
- Maintaining skills and competencies as outlined by the American Organization of Nurse Executives (AONE)
- Networking with other nurse leaders
- Subscribing to nursing administration journals
- Remaining current in the latest innovations in nursing and health care
- Attending leadership development programs
- Finding a mentor
- Joining professional nursing associations such as AONE
- Reflecting to achieve balance personally and professionally

Just as formal education is vitally important, experience is also a prerequisite for being a successful leader. If nurse leaders in the practice setting have no experience in clinical practice, gaining credibility with nurses and other members of the multidisciplinary team may be difficult (O'Connor, 2011).

Academic leaders likewise have a responsibility to provide professional role development for new educators and to assist students in their role development as they learn their roles as aspiring nurses. Academic leaders should have prior teaching experience so that they can relate to their faculty's and their faculty's students' world, which is the classroom.

Educator Role Development

Faculty members have a vital role in the development of nursing students as future leaders. Leadership development must begin in the schools of nursing, where faculty members, as leaders, can serve as role models for nursing students. Students can also develop their leadership skills through clinical experiences with preceptors; through the classroom in discussions, assignments, presentations, and case studies; and through completion of a leadership practicum. Nursing faculty can be instrumental in promoting nursing leadership as a career track for those students whom they identify as having the potential to serve in future leadership roles. A formal mentoring program for new educators should also be in place so that they can benefit from the knowledge and experience of the seasoned educators. An orientation program for faculty is additionally very important. Janzen (2010) purports that in response to the shortage of qualified faculty, nurses who are expert practitioners are being recruited into clinical faculty roles. Although these nurses have significant experience in the clinical setting, they are considered novice clinical nurse educators.

Therefore, faculty at all program levels and every status (full-time, adjunct, and clinical) should continuously work on developing their roles as nurse educators. This also applies to staff development educators in practice settings. Educators should be familiar with the National League for Nursing (NLN) Core Competencies of Nurse Educators, which provide a comprehensive framework for preparing new nurse educators, implementing the nurse educator role, evaluating nurse educator practice, and advancing faculty scholarship and lifelong professional development (Kalb, 2008). Engaging in lifelong learning for nurse educators includes advancing their education and participating in continuing education and professional development.

Additionally, nurse educators should have experience in and knowledge of various teaching strategies, evaluation methods, curriculum design, and the role of the educator. Experience in online, blended, and traditional face-to-face classroom formats would be beneficial. Maintaining active membership in the NLN and/or other professional nursing education associations would also be useful for nurse educator role development. Regardless of their academic preparation, nursing faculty should be current in nursing practice,, system trends, and interventions designed to change health outcomes. Faculty must be up to date on the latest innovations in health care in order to meet the demand for highly educated nurses who are knowledgeable and equipped to lead the way in transforming health care in the United States.

Clinician Role Development

Just as some nurses may need role development as leaders and/or educators, other nurses may need development in their role as clinicians. Nurses who serve as clinicians are leaders in patient care, which is part of their everyday nursing practice. Whether a clinician as a frontline clinical nurse leader or an APRN, each clinician has a responsibility to continuously work on developing his or her role. Clinical nurses should consider the following strategies in achieving role development:

- Pursuing advanced education
- Maintaining skills and competencies as outlined in the professional nurse practice act and the ANA standards for each clinical specialty in which the nurse practices
- Networking with other clinicians
- Subscribing to and reading professional nursing peer-reviewed journals
- Remaining current in the latest innovations in nursing and health care
- Attending leadership development programs
- Finding a mentor
- Joining professional nursing associations such as the ANA
- Reflecting to achieve balance personally and professionally

APRNs (nurse practitioners, clinical nurse specialists, nurse midwives, and certified registered nurse anesthetists) are considered experts in their field, having a solid clinical foundation in addition to mastery of their clinical specialty. This requires that each APRN continuously works on developing his or her role by pursuing advanced education in order to meet the demands of tomorrow's patients. In 2004, the American Association of Colleges of Nursing required nursing programs to adopt the doctor of nursing practice (DNP) degree as minimal educational preparation for APRNs (Acorn, Lamarche, & Edwards, 2009). In 2015, a DNP degree became a requirement to enter practice as a new APRN in the United States (Acorn et al., 2009). With the advent of the DNP degree, the options for nurses who are considering a terminal degree are even greater and provide opportunities to earn a practice-focused doctorate. The DNP nurse is prepared for a career in delivering services and translating scientific and theoretical knowledge into the solution of practice problems (Edwardson, 2010). The goal of DNP programs is to equip nursing practitioners at the highest level of practice with knowledge together with the skills and resolution to apply that knowledge to the solution of health system problems (Edwardson, 2010). DNP programs emphasize scholarly practice, evaluation of health-care outcomes, practice improvement, and leadership in establishing clinical excellence (Acorn et al., 2009).

CONCLUSION

Nurse leaders have a duty and an obligation to work on enhancing their own sense of empowerment so that they can effectively lead and empower others. With the growing complexity and challenges of health-care delivery reform, nurses need to feel psychologically empowered to manage their nursing practice and improve patient care. The Journey to Psychological Empowerment is one intervention that may be used to enhance nurses' sense of empowerment. When examining our sense of empowerment as leaders, considering our development and levels of EI and resilience is also important, as is mentoring, succession planning, coaching, precepting, and role development. Because evidence shows that nurses who feel empowered may have an advantage in their growth and development as compared with nurses who do not feel empowered, the need for nurses to work on enhancing their sense of empowerment is clear. Empowerment of self and others is truly a journey.

References

Acorn, S., Lamarche, K., & Edwards, M. (2009). Practice doctorates in nursing: Developing nursing leaders. *Nursing Leadership, 22*(2), 85–91.

American Nurses Association. (2015). *Code of ethics for nurses with interpretive statements.* Silver Spring, MD: Author.

American Nurses Association. (2015). *Nursing scope and standards of practice.* Silver Spring, MD: Author.

Batson, V. D., & Yoder, L. H. (2012). Managerial coaching: A concept analysis. *Journal of Advanced Nursing, 68*(7), 1658–1669.

Carlson, E., Pilhammar, E., & Wann-Hansson, C. (2010). Time to precept: Supportive and limiting conditions for precepting nurses. *Journal of Advanced Nursing, 66*(2), 432–441.

Dean, E. (2012). Building resilience. *Nursing Standard, 26*(32), 16–18.

Dimitriades, Z., & Kufidu, S. (2004). Individual, job, organizational and contextual correlates of employment empowerment: Some Greek evidence. *Electronic Journal of Business Ethics and Organization Studies, 9*(2). Retrieved from https://jyx.jyu.fi/dspace/handle/123456789/25365

Donahue, M. O., Piazza, I. M., Griffin, M. Q., Dykes, P. C., & Fitzpatrick, J. J. (2008). The relationship between nurses' perceptions of empowerment and patient satisfaction. *Applied Nursing Research, 21*, 2–7.

East, L., Jackson, D., O'Brien, L., & Peters, K. (2010). Storytelling: An approach that can help to develop resilience. *Nurse Researcher, 17*(3), 17–25.

Edwardson, S. (2010). Doctor of philosophy and doctor of nursing practice as complementary degrees. *Journal of Professional Nursing, 26*(3), 137–140.

Faulkner, J., & Laschinger, H. (2008). The effects of structural and psychological empowerment on perceived respect in acute care nurses. *Journal of Nursing Management, 16*, 214–221.

Feather, R. (2009). Emotional intelligence in relation to nursing leadership: Does it matter? *Journal of Nursing Management, 17*, 376–382.

Grafton, E., Gillespie, B., & Henderson, S. (2010). Resilience: The power within. *Oncology Nursing Forum, 37*(6), 698–705.

Griffith, M. B. (2012). Effective succession planning in nursing: A review of the literature. *Journal of Nursing Management, 20*, 900–911.

Institute of Medicine. (2010).). *The future of nursing: Leading change, advancing health.* Washington, DC: National Academies Press. Retrieved from http://www.iom.edu/Reports/2010/The-Future-of-Nursing-Leading-Change-Advancing-Health.aspx

Janzen, K. J. (2010). Alice through the looking glass: The influence of self and student understanding on role actualization among novice clinical nurse educators. *Journal of Continuing Education in Nursing, 41*(11), 517–523.

Kalb, K. A. (2008). Core competencies of nurse educators: Inspiring excellence in nurse educator practice. *Nursing Education Perspectives, 29*(4), 217–219.

Knol, J., & van Linge, R. (2009). Innovative behaviour: The effect of structural and psychological empowerment on nurses. *Journal of Advanced Nursing, 65*(2), 359–370.

Kraimer, M. L., Seibert, S. E., & Liden, R. C. (1999). Psychological empowerment as a multidimensional construct: A test of construct validity. *Educational and Psychological Measurement, 59*(1), 127–142.

Kuokkanen, L., & Leino-Kilpi, H. (2000). Power and empowerment in nursing: Three theoretical approaches. *Journal of Advanced Nursing, 31*(1), 235–241.

Kuokkanen, L., & Leino-Kilpi, H. (2001). The qualities of an empowered nurse and the factors involved. *Journal of Nursing Management, 9*, 273–280.

Laschinger, H., Gilbert, S., Smith, L., & Leslie, K. (2010). Towards a comprehensive theory of nurse/patient empowerment: Applying Kanter's empowerment theory to patient care. *Journal of Nursing Management, 18*, 4–13.

Laschinger, H. K. S., Finegan, J., Shamian, J., & Wilk, P. (2001). Impact of structural and psychological empowerment on job strain in nursing work settings. *Journal of Nursing Administration, 31*(5), 260–272.

Lewis, M., & Urmston, J. (2000). Flogging the dead horse: The myth of nursing empowerment? *Journal of Nursing Management, 8*, 209–213.

Luhanga, F. L., Dickieson, P., & Mossey, S. D. (2010). Preceptor preparation: An investment in the future generation of nurses. *International Journal of Nursing Education Scholarship, 7*(1), Article 38, 1–18

Manzano Garcia, G., & Ayala Calvo, J. C. (2012). Emotional exhaustion of nursing staff: Influence of emotional annoyance and resilience. *International Nursing Review, 59*, 101–107.

McCloughen, A., O'Brien, L., & Jackson, D. (2009). Esteemed connection: Creating a mentoring relationship for nurse leadership. *Nursing Inquiry, 16*, 326–336.

Morrison, T. L., & McNulty, D. M. (2012). Response from the southwest Florida nursing community supporting the future of nursing. *Journal of Nursing Administration, 42*(1), 52–57.

O'Connor, M. (2011). Beyond the classroom nurse leader preparation and practices. *Nursing Administration Quarterly, 35*(4), 333–337.

Northouse, P. (2014). *Leadership: Theory and practice* (6th ed.). Thousand Oaks, CA: Sage.

Omansky, G. L. (2010). Staff nurses' experiences as preceptors and mentors: An integrative review. *Journal of Nursing Management, 18,* 697–703.

Rao, A. (2012). The contemporary construction of nurse empowerment. *Journal of Nursing Scholarship, 44*(4), 396–402.

Robinson-Walker, C. (2013). Succession planning: Moving the dial from "should" to "must." *Nursing Administration Quarterly, 37*(1), 37–43.

Savage, C. M. (2001). Executive coaching: Professional self-care for nursing. *Nursing Economic$, 19*(4), 178–182.

Spreitzer, G. (2007). Taking stock: A review of more than twenty years of research on empowerment at work. In C. Cooper & J. Barling (Eds.), *The handbook of organizational behavior.* Thousand Oaks, CA: Sage.

Spreitzer, G. M. (1995). Psychological empowerment in the workplace: Dimensions, measurement, and validation. *Academy of Management Journal, 38*(5), 1442–1465.

Thompson, R., Wolf, D. M., & Sabatine, J. M. (2012). Mentoring and coaching a model guiding professional nurses to executive success. *Journal of Nursing Administration, 42*(11), 536–541.

Unal, S. (2012). Evaluating the effect of self-awareness and communication techniques on nurses' assertiveness and self-esteem. *Contemporary Nurse, 43*(1), 90–98.

University of Michigan. (2014). Gretchen Spreitzer. Retrieved from http://webuser.bus.umich.edu/spreitzer/

Yonge, O., Billay, D., Myrick, F., & Luhanga, F. (2007). Preceptorship and mentorship: Not merely a matter of semantics. *International Journal of Nursing Education Scholarship, 4*(1), Article 19, 1–13.

9

Creating a Culture of Excellence

It goes without saying that nurses, as leaders, experience many challenges in their day-to-day work lives and throughout their careers, as does everyone. How to effectively address these challenges to create a culture of excellence is the focus of this final chapter.

Chapter 8 discussed how important it is for nurses to enhance their own sense of psychological empowerment. Nurses, as leaders, have a professional obligation to empower others. Empowered nurses can weather storms and are usually fairly skilled in managing challenges that come their way. Managing challenges and potential barriers is an essential skill for nurse leaders in transforming a culture to one of excellence. The previous chapter makes a great segue into this final chapter, which explores several challenges that leaders may encounter in the professional work environment. Strategies for addressing these challenges are also discussed. Topics include (but are not limited to) conflict resolution, crisis management, supervising, delegating, and networking. In addition, the Journey to a Culture of Excellence is introduced as an innovation that may be useful to nurse leaders in addressing leadership challenges and transforming cultures within their organizations. Finally, assessing how well a department leader is functioning is addressed.

CONFLICT RESOLUTION

Dealing with conflicts in the workplace setting is not always a leader's favorite duty, but it is certainly an inevitable one, and being skilled in conflict resolution is vital. Regulatory agencies such as The Joint Commission require that hospitals' governing bodies provide a system for resolving conflicts among individuals working in a hospital (Morreim, 2015). Conflicts can arise between staff, between leaders, between employees and leaders, between employees and patients' families, and even between employees and patients. Conflicts in academia may occur between staff, between faculty, between faculty and leaders, and between faculty and students. Interpersonal conflict is inevitable in the workplace and has many costs including moral distress, burnout, absenteeism, and turnover (Pines et al., 2014). Not everyone who is engaged in a conflict is being "difficult," but it may be helpful to first look at conflict resolution when someone behaving in a difficult way is in the mix (Box 9.1). Certain external factors might also contribute to difficult behavior (Box 9.2). Although human resources departments can be helpful in resolving conflicts, Morreim (2015) argues that some situations may be better addressed by carefully facilitated conversations in a safe space rather than by invoking mechanisms that may feel, or actually be, more punitive than problem-solving. Addressing tensions through well-constructed conflict resolution processes can lead to stronger relationships and improved quality and satisfaction (Morreim, 2015).

BOX 9.1 Examples of "Difficult" Behavior

Know-it-all-ism	Dishonesty
Complaining	Playing the victim
Negativity	Insecurity
Overt aggression	People pleasing
Narcissism	Defensiveness
Argumentativeness	Attention seeking
Faultfinding	Arrogance
Being overly competitive	"It's my way or the highway" attitude

BOX 9.2 Reasons People May Present as Being Difficult

Personal issues	Life stress
Pain	Peer pressure
Fatigue	Low self-esteem
Not being heard	Guilt
Needs not being met	Anger
Substance abuse	Feeling threatened/fearful
Behavioral disorders	Unrealistic demands
Job stress	Political pressure

Dealing With Difficult People

A difficult person can negatively affect people who work in the organization and even customers of the organization. Nurse leaders need to be mindful that a difficult person may present in a positive way to the boss but negatively to his or her coworkers. Various approaches that nurse leaders can use to resolve conflicts with a difficult person, depending on the nature of the conflict, include the following:

1. Neutralize any response made to the person, even when he or she is attempting to trigger an emotional reaction.
2. Refrain from using labels such as "arrogant" or "stupid" and focus on the person's behavior. Explain how his or her behavior is negatively affecting others.
3. Ask for a commitment from the person to stop the behavior.
4. Handle confrontations privately and remain calm.
5. Listen, empathize, and show respect: the difficult person may need some attention paid to his or her problem.
6. Do not take it personally if the difficult person expresses anger or frustration.
7. Avoid blame or anything that would further antagonize the difficult person.
8. Disarm anger with kindness, and remember to control your body language.

If all of the approaches fail, and the conflict continues, consider bringing in a third-party mediator. Organizations should consider retaining the services of an individual, inside or outside the organization, with conflict resolution skills who can help implement a conflict resolution process and perhaps even manage conflicts when needed (Morreim, 2015).

CRISIS MANAGEMENT

Leaders need to be skilled in managing crises—like conflict resolution, crisis management is another one of those duties that can be difficult for leaders to address, but for which effective leadership is essential. Although people may view crisis situations very differently—what one views as a crisis, another sees as just a normal event in the workday—typically a crisis is a situation affecting an individual, team, or organization that is perceived to be out of control and creating higher-than-ordinary stress. As nurses, we tend to be fairly skilled in helping patients manage a crisis, but we may not always feel skilled or comfortable in managing a crisis within a team or within an organization.

The ability to be resilient (see Chapter 8) always comes into play during a crisis, whether in practice or in academia. For example, in academia, a crisis might concern allegations of sexual misconduct between a faculty member and a student. In the practice world, nurses could argue that crises occur on a daily basis, but one example is when a patient jumped out of a hospital window in a successful suicide attempt. Although each crisis scenario may be different, the overall strategies that are usually the most effective in any crisis situation include the following:

1. Remain calm.
2. Take a step back and carefully consider all options prior to executing any one of them.

3. Listen to all parties who are involved in the situation in order to get to the heart of the issue.
4. Execute an action plan that is based on evidence and a careful assessment.
5. Be decisive and confident in executing actions that are directed at de-escalating the crisis so that healing can begin.
6. Evaluate and follow up to determine whether the action plan was effective.

In addition to experiencing crisis situations involving patients, nurse leaders may also experience work-related crises such as those involving staffing. When a leader receives a call in the middle of the night that staff are threatening to walk out, this is a potential crisis for the leader and for the institution.

SUPERVISING OTHERS

As discussed, conflicts, difficult people, and crises are inevitable challenges that leaders must manage in order to create cultures of excellence in organizations. Another challenge that is crucial to successful culture transformation is the ability to effectively supervise others. Regardless of a nurse leader's formal title (director, manager, supervisor, clinical coordinator), for the purposes of this chapter the supervisory aspects of a nurse leader's role are referred to as "supervising." It is often assumed that nurse leaders know how to effectively supervise others and they are comfortable with this important task. The reality is that not all leaders are good at supervising people, and not all leaders (by title) are good leaders. Supervising is one of the managerial tasks that often requires making difficult decisions. Although supervising can be very rewarding, it can also be quite challenging. Humans are not always predictable creatures. Nurses, as leaders, deal with people who have different personalities as well as differences in age, levels of experience, educational backgrounds, and cultures. They have an obligation to treat all subordinates with respect, dignity, and fairness. How people are treated in the workplace setting can impact their feelings of self-worth as well as their morale and sense of satisfaction with their work. It can also affect their personal life if they carry those feelings with them even after leaving work. Nurse leaders have a responsibility to serve as positive role models when supervising others. According to a German proverb, "When you walk your talk, people listen," meaning *do* as you *say*. This and other "leadership pearls" are given in Box 9.3.

Healthy Versus Unhealthy Work Environments

The goal of every nurse leader should be to refrain at all costs from portraying a supervising style that may be viewed as toxic, meaning "poisonous" or "harmful" (Chu, 2014). Toxic leadership fosters a toxic work environment. Nurse leaders may have worked with individuals who appear dysfunctional and they may have worked in environments that could be assessed as being dysfunctional. Individual dysfunction may be positively addressed with such interventions as employee assistance counseling, coaching, continuing education, professional development seminars, and leadership development programs and initiatives.

Toxic leadership and toxic work environments may be more difficult to turn around. Toxic individuals can "spread" their toxicity to other team members, which may contaminate the work environment. These individuals may be very challenging

BOX 9.3 **Leadership Pearls**

1. Leaders may not always be liked, but it's most important that they are respected.

2. Leaders need to "walk the talk" (align their actions with their words).

3. Leaders genuinely care about the well-being of others.

4. Leaders are always fair and consistent. Everyone should be held accountable to the same rules–no one should be viewed as "untouchable."

5. Leaders should be visible–especially evenings, nights, and weekends. The "after-hours" shifts sometimes feel neglected.

6. Leaders should remain calm under pressure, even when they feel otherwise.

7. Leaders should never give the impression that staff are replaceable.

8. Leaders hire the right people for the right jobs and allow them to do their jobs.

9. Leaders surround themselves with quality people–they all advance together.

10. Leaders are not threatened by talented individuals or high performers.

11. Leaders know their boundaries–they are always professional and serve as role models.

12. Leaders are not afraid of losing their jobs–fear is paralyzing.

13. Leaders trust their employees rather than micromanaging.

14. Leaders feel empowered and empower others.

and difficult for leaders to supervise. If the culture of an organization dictates that leaders should do everything possible to turn someone around, then a leader may be held accountable to coach the toxic individual (setting limits and expectations for behavior) and may place the individual on a corrective action plan for improvement within a stated time frame. A leader who shows compassion for a toxic individual may, at times, create a positive outcome. Chu (2014) purports that when nurses feel that their bosses are willing to listen to them and empathize with their negative emotions, the strength that arises from this compassion could moderate the toxicity of their emotions. If the toxic individual continues to display toxic behaviors, then the leader may need to make a difficult decision to terminate the individual's employment. If leaders cannot cope with toxic behaviors in a constructive way, the harmful effects they have on individuals, such as lowering self-confidence, hope, and self-esteem, can threaten work morale and performance, eventually harming the organization (Chu, 2014).

Nurse leaders need to maintain the health of their work environments. Boxes 9.4 and 9.5 describe characteristics of healthy and unhealthy work environments.

Tomey (2009) argues that there is a correlation between healthy workplace environments and healthy patients and the well-being of personnel. A healthy work environment is crucial to job satisfaction, best practices, and retention (Ritter, 2011). Healthy places of work enable nurses to achieve personal satisfaction while meeting organizational objectives (Moore, Leahy, Sublett, & Lanig, 2013). Organizations with unhealthy workforces may have a cost burden from high rates of absenteeism, presence at work but inadequate work performance, loss of productivity, work-related accidents, high levels of stress, and high incidence of health-related litigation (Tomey, 2009). Positive management initiatives can help foster healthy staff-focused work environments (Box 9.6). It is imperative for nurse leaders to promote and implement as many positive initiatives as possible so that their staff may enjoy a healthy work environment. Leaders who are proactive in this effort understand that this is a crucial element in creating cultures of excellence.

BOX 9.4 Characteristics of a Healthy Work Environment

Valued employees	Sense of community
Standardized processes	Strategic planning that reflects the mission, vision, and goals of the organization
Staff empowerment	
Strong leadership	

Adapted from: Ritter, D. (2011). The relationship between healthy work environments and retention of nurses in a hospital setting. *Journal of Nursing Management, 19,* 27.

BOX 9.5 Characteristics of a Healthy Work Environment

Poor communication	Lack of vision or leadership
Abusive behavior	Lack of trust
Disrespect	Conflict with values, mission, and goals
Resistance to change	Loss of understanding of core business

Adapted from: Ritter, D. (2011). The relationship between healthy work environments and retention of nurses in a hospital setting. *Journal of Nursing Management, 19,* 27.

BOX 9.6 **Positive Management Initiatives That Foster Healthy Work Environments**

Shared organizational goals	Participation and empowerment strategies
Learning opportunities	Employee health and well-being programs
Career development	Job satisfaction
Reward schemes	Open management styles
Autonomy	

Adapted from: Tomey, A. M. (2009). Nursing leadership and management effects work environments. *Journal of Nursing Management, 17*, 15.

Horizontal Violence

Working in toxic environments is neither pleasant nor healthy for any employee. Although nurses are sometimes subject to incivility and violence from physicians and other health-care providers, staff, patients, visitors, and suppliers, nurses often are most concerned about aggression from their colleagues (Tomey, 2009). This may include physical aggression, bullying, intimidation, passive-aggressive behavior, antagonism, criticism, sexual innuendo, gossiping, scapegoating, undermining, and withholding information (Tomey, 2009). Horizontal violence (see Chapter 2) has been correlated with decreased morale, job satisfaction, and job performance (Tomey, 2009). Many nurses work in unhealthy settings where disruptive nurse relationships have become the norm. Poor nurse-to-nurse relationships have grave consequences for nurses, the nursing profession, and health-care organizations, including poor work performance, absenteeism, and rapid job turnover. Nurse-to-nurse relationships are a key component in the health of a work setting (Moore et al., 2013). In supervising others, nurses, as leaders, need to take action to decrease toxicity in workplaces (Box 9.7).

BOX 9.7 **Strategies to Decrease Workplace Toxicity**

Role-modeling professional behaviors	Using conflict resolution
Validating assumptions and perceptions before drawing conclusions	Rewarding nurses for supporting one another
Using open communication	Nurturing a culture of recognition
Socializing new staff members	Having a policy of zero tolerance for violence

Adapted from: Tomey, A. M. (2009). Nursing leadership and management effects work environments. *Journal of Nursing Management, 17*, 15.

Abusive supervision is another toxic situation that nurses may encounter, which may include verbal and nonverbal behaviors. To be considered abusive, the behaviors must be willfully hostile to hurt subordinate feelings and the exposure to the abuse continues, rather than being an isolated incident (Estes, 2013). Abusive supervision differs from nurse bullying in that it is exclusively hierarchical, whereas bullying is more horizontal (nurse to nurse) (Estes, 2013). In addition to horizontal bullying (employees against employees), the ANA Position Statement on Incivility, Bullying, and Workplace Violence (2015) refers to two other types of bullying—top down (employers against employees) and bottom up (employees against employers). Regardless of what type of bullying an individual encounters, it is important that nurses be able to effectively identify and address these types of behaviors in the workplace. Several workplace abuse constructs found in the literature that leaders need to be aware of are listed in Box 9.8.

Although nurses at all levels have been reported as perpetrators of unhealthy nurse-to-nurse relations, nurses in management positions are key perpetrators of abusive behaviors (Moore et al., 2013). Abusive supervision can result in subordinate problem drinking, family problems, lower self-esteem, and lower organizational commitment (Estes, 2013). When an employee works under the supervision of a leader who is abusive, he or she may be reluctant to report the abuse for fear of retribution or retaliation (Rodwell, Brunetto, Demir, Shacklock, & Farr-Wharton, 2014). This can be a very real concern for the employee. As an example, *retribution* occurred when a supervisor learned that one of her nurses submitted a transfer to another department, which resulted in the supervisor preventing the nurse's transfer by providing a poor reference to the other department manager because the leader did not want the nurse to leave. As an example, *retaliation* occurred when a supervisor learned that a staff nurse utilized the chain of command to report the supervisor's abusive behavior, which resulted in the supervisor denying the staff nurse's requests for vacation time, micromanaging the nurse's every step on the unit, and changing the staff nurse's schedule without any discussion. It is imperative that nurse leaders ensure that the work environment is structured so that employees are empowered to be successful without fear of retribution (Macauley, 2015).

When supervising, nurse leaders need to hold others accountable for their actions, and they need to hold themselves accountable as well. Leaders have an obligation to staff never to abuse their authority and position by abusing others. Carolyn Jarvis

---

BOX 9.8 **Workplace Abuse Constructs**

Abusive managerial behavior	Brutal bosses
Petty tyranny in organizations	Workplace bullying
Verbal abuse	Supervisory undermining
Workplace mistreatment	Employee-abusive organizations

Adapted from: Estes, B. C. (2013). Abusive supervision and nursing performance. *Nursing Forum, 48*(1), 3.

reminds us of this in the following quote: "The character of a nurse is just as important as the knowledge he or she possesses."

DELEGATING

Dwight D. Eisenhower famously said, "Leadership is the art of getting someone else to do something you want done because he wants to do it." Delegating tasks and projects to staff provides opportunities for learning, sharing ideas, and working collectively (Curtis, de Vries, & Sheerin, 2011). Yet nurses at all levels will often report that one of their most difficult tasks is delegation—when to delegate, how to delegate, and to whom to delegate. However, delegation becomes much easier when the nurse feels empowered to delegate. It is important that the organization supports appropriate use of delegation and that the nurse feels comfortable that appropriate use of delegation falls within his or her role as a nurse. A disconnect on either end, organizationally or individually, could negatively impact the use of delegation in a professional nursing work setting. The word "appropriate" is purposefully included here because there are nurse leaders who abuse their authority with "overdelegating," thereby giving the impression that they believe themselves to be above the duties of a nurse. These nurse leaders manage from control towers and are often referred to as "clipboard leaders." Conversely, there are nurses who believe that if they want something done right, they need to do it themselves. These leaders present as martyrs and convey a lack of trust in the employees to get the job done. Then there are leaders who micromanage their employees, which also can give the impression that the leader does not trust the employees to do their job.

Thus, every leader should learn the art of appropriate delegation, to develop a sense of when it is time to step in and do the job (or help to do the job) him- or herself as well as when he or she should ask for help in order to get the job done. How leaders communicate when delegating is also important. Nurse leaders need to use assertive communication when delegating (see Chapter 5). Leaders who master the appropriate use of delegation can serve as role models for their nurses. When delegation is accompanied by trust, respect, and a mutual exchange of information and ideas, it creates an environment of team cohesiveness and strengthens outcomes beneficial for the patient and for the institution (Saccomano & Pinto-Zipp, 2011). As discussed in Chapter 8, nurse leaders need to empower others, and one strategy to do this is through delegation (Curtis et al., 2011). Leaders need to allow staff to use their skills in problem-solving and making decisions.

Delegation From Employees

Nurse employees may also find themselves at some point in their careers in situations where they need to delegate to others. Whereas some staff nurses may be born with the ability to intuitively delegate and lead, most must learn these skills through educational experiences. It is imperative that nurse educators provide a base from which new nurses can develop and advance delegation skills to facilitate transition into the workforce. The process of delegating requires the registered nurse (RN) to remain accountable for the task. Unfortunately, RNs are often poorly prepared to perform delegation activities and may not have the level of confidence needed to delegate.

According to Saccomano and Pinto-Zipp (2011), when an RN needs to delegate but has little or no training in and development of leadership or delegation skills, the nurse assumes great personal risk. Nurse leaders need to ensure that their nurses are provided with the appropriate training and educational opportunities to develop and enhance delegation skills. Leaders may consider offering in-service training for their nurses on enhancing delegation skills and professional development seminars on using assertive communication to delegate appropriately. An adequately trained team working cohesively together will be able to overcome delegation difficulties, such as what, when, and to whom to delegate (Saccomano & Pinto-Zipp, 2011).

NETWORKING

Another leadership challenge for some nurse leaders is networking; however, it can be effectively utilized as they become comfortable with the process of networking. There are many different venues for networking in nursing, both formally and informally and both inside and outside of the workplace. Informal networks are important in knowledge-intensive sectors where people use personal relationships to find information necessary to do their jobs (Downey, Parslow, & Smart, 2011). Knol and Van Linge (2009) purport that networking may be important for gaining informal power and that space should be created for this within organizations.

Networking Opportunities for Nurses

Nurses, as leaders, are in key positions to engage in networking activities. The first step is to be open minded and flexible, seizing every opportunity that presents the potential for networking. Joining and actively participating in professional nursing associations is one example of an external networking opportunity. Nurses can get involved on a national, state, or local level. Serving in volunteer leadership positions within professional nursing associations is a wonderful way not only to give back to the nursing profession but a way to get actively involved in networking with professional colleagues. For example, serving in a volunteer leadership position for a state nurses association can be instrumental in fostering relationships with nursing colleagues throughout that state. Associations provide many opportunities for leadership development through nationally elected offices, committees, task forces, leadership specialty assemblies, state councils, and local chapters (Strech & Wyatt, 2013). Another external networking opportunity is participation in action coalitions and community initiatives. Serving as a volunteer on community advisory boards is an excellent way for nurse leaders to network within their communities. Becoming involved politically to advocate for changes in legislation that impact health care and professional nursing licensure and scope of practice issues can enhance a nurse leader's visibility in the community. There are also networking opportunities for nurse leaders within organizations in which they are employed. Nurses can gain wider support networks within their employing organizations by, for example, joining workplace committees (McDonald, Vickers, Mohan, Wilkes, & Jackson, 2010). Nurse leaders can network with other nurse leaders in their organizations by meeting for lunch, attending conferences, and participating in social activities after business hours. Nurse leaders can also use social media as a way to network with colleagues. Social media is an easy-to-use and efficient way for nurses to connect with others (Simpson, 2014).

Networking provides many benefits to nurse leaders, including opportunities to find new positions, obtain references for future positions, find mentors, learn about opportunities that support scholarship and service, and stay connected with professional colleagues. Networking can be particularly beneficial in situations in which nurse leaders desire to promote a new program or initiative within an organization. The support of other leaders, physicians, or staff within an organization can be very useful to the nurse leader in this effort.

THE JOURNEY TO A CULTURE OF EXCELLENCE

Brian Tracy reminds us in his quote that: "Excellence is not a destination; it is a continuous journey that never ends." The chapters in this unit have so far addressed the individual nurse leader in his or her leadership journey and pursuit of individual excellence. Here, the focus is on both an individual's and an organization's pursuit of a culture of excellence. Most health-care organizations probably strive for organizational excellence, but in order to achieve it, first they need to develop a *culture* of excellence. When an organization has truly developed a culture of excellence, it can be "felt" within the walls of the organization. The Journey to a Culture of Excellence, shown in Figure 9.1, can assist health-care organizations to achieve organizational excellence. Similar to the design of the Journey to Psychological Empowerment (see Chapter 8), the Journey to a Culture of Excellence was created by Dr. Denise McNulty for individual teams in health-care organizations as a pyramid with four sequential levels, or steps, which need to be achieved and instilled in an organization in order to create a culture of excellence. Each level on the pyramid builds on the one below it. The team must integrate one level proceeding to the

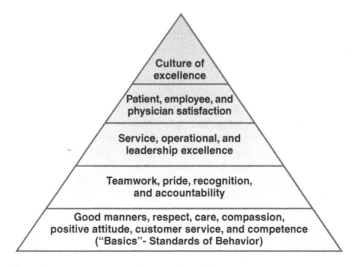

FIGURE 9.1 The Journey to a Culture of Excellence. *(Courtesy of Denise McNulty)*

next. The overall goal is to have every team in an organization complete the journey so that the entire organization moves in the same direction. Every organization is made up of multiple teams. In order for an organization to improve its overall culture, every team in the organization should make the journey. If every team is successful in developing a culture of excellence within their unit or department, over time, the overall organization may achieve a culture of excellence. It truly is a journey.

It is also important to note that no matter where a team or organization is in the Journey to a Culture of Excellence, assertive and effective communication at all levels is essential. Collaboration with every individual and team in the organization must occur at each level in the journey and must be continuous and pervasive throughout the organization.

The Pyramid Foundation

The first level of the pyramid is referred to as the "standards of behavior" and includes good manners, respect, care, compassion, positive attitude, customer service, and competence. The standards-of-behavior level is viewed as the most important level on the pyramid and the very foundation upon which the other levels of the pyramid are built. The foundation of the pyramid comprises the very "basic" qualities that team members need to possess before they can move into the next level in their journey to developing a culture of excellence. Teams lacking a core group of employees who possess these standards of behavior may find their attempts to achieve organizational excellence most challenging. Several of the behaviors may be influenced by an individual's upbringing. Not every individual is fortunate enough to have these standards of behavior instilled during childhood. The basic premise of the standards of behavior supports the Golden Rule—"Do unto others as you would have them do unto you." This seems most appropriate for practical use in healthcare environments where the public expects people to exhibit these behaviors in the workplace.

For nurse leaders, the standards of behavior really come into play during recruitment of new employees. Conducting behavioral interviews can be one way to assess an individual for his or her ability to meet the basics or standards of behavior. Some standards of behavior, such as competence and customer service, can be learned at any age through education and training, role modeling, mentoring, and coaching, but there are some qualities that are very difficult to impart, especially in the workplace setting. In health care, it is so important that employees exhibit care and compassion. When someone is compassionate, he or she shows an empathetic response to another's distress and suffering. According to Bramley and Matiti (2014), compassion is a fundamental part of nursing care that unites people in difficult times and is a foundation to building the human relationships that can promote both physical and mental health. Nurses can develop their knowledge and skills in providing compassionate care through nursing education, hearing the stories of others, vignettes, role playing, and learning about the impact of uncompassionate actions (Bramley & Matiti, 2014). Most leaders do not have the time to dedicate to "parenting" their employees. Therefore, it is essential that leaders have an effective interview process in place to appropriately screen applicants for these behaviors. Selecting and then hiring employees who are a good fit for the organization is extremely important in enhancing the culture. The standards of behavior should be included in the employee performance appraisal so that employees can be evaluated on how well they consistently and appropriately exhibit these behaviors. Once a nurse leader is confident that all of his or her team members consistently and genuinely exhibit good manners, respect, care, compassion, a positive attitude, customer service skills, and competence in their work, the leader can begin to move the team to the second level.

Pyramid Level Two

The second level in the Journey to a Culture of Excellence includes teamwork, pride, recognition, and accountability. This is a key level in the journey because it builds on the individual team members' attainment of and adherence to the basics or standards of behavior described in the first level. The second level demands ongoing commitment and dedication on the part of the leader to guide the team on this step of the journey, as it requires leader engagement with the team members to foster a sense of teamwork and pride. This level in the journey pertains to both leader and employee engagement. Although teamwork, pride, recognition, and accountability are all equally important to leader and employee engagement, teamwork will be addressed first.

In Chapter 7, one section focused on self and the art of collaboration. In this chapter, the focus is on teamwork as it relates to interprofessional collaboration. Teamwork depends on strong interprofessional collaborative relationships. There is ample evidence in the literature to support the importance of teamwork and interprofessional collaboration. In practice settings, collaboration is an essential aspect for ensuring quality health care and the work unit is the main environment where collaborative patient-centered care is provided. High-functioning interprofessional collaborative care is required for patients to have positive outcomes and for achievement of high scores on patient satisfaction surveys (Galletta, Portoghese, Battistelli, & Leiter, 2013). In the Institute of Medicine's *Future of Nursing: Leading Change, Advancing Health* report (2010), interdisciplinary partnership between nurses and other health-care professionals and nursing leadership were underscored as opportunities to advance nursing and improve the quality of health care. The Quality and Safety Education for Nurses project identified safety competencies for nursing education to include teamwork and collaboration, whereas the American Nurses Credentialing Center stated that nurses should incorporate interprofessional collaborative practice within their plan of care (Lomax & White, 2015). Ma, Shang, and Bott (2015) purport that creating an environment of strong collaboration among care providers and nursing leadership can help hospitals maintain a competitive nursing workforce supporting high quality of care. Participation in collaborative teams provides safe, high-quality, and accountable care.

Team-building initiatives would be most helpful at this level in the journey. For example, a leader may initiate a contest for his or her department as a competition with other departments for patient satisfaction scores in an effort to build team spirit. A leader could secure the services of an internal or external consultant to offer team-building workshops or perhaps conduct an off-site retreat for nurses, physicians, and other health-care providers to help build comradery, improve communication and teamwork, and discuss goals and strategic planning for the future.

Teamwork requires open-mindedness and a willingness to value differences and interact genuinely (Lomax & White, 2015). It is vitally important for team success that the nurse leader sets the example, as a role model, in collaborating with others through shared problem-solving and decision making. In order to gain buy-in from the staff at this level in the journey, it is important that the leader serve as a positive role model and team player who collaborates well with others.

As discussed earlier, leader engagement is crucial in this level in the journey in that leader engagement is a prerequisite to employee engagement. The second level in the Journey to a Culture of Excellence concentrates the greatest amount of work for employee engagement. Macauley (2015) believes that employee engagement often starts with a nursing leader and that nursing leaders have significant impact on the way employees feel about their career and their organization. Greater employee engagement can lead to a higher quality of individual participation and teamwork, which then can lead to higher growth, productivity, and revenue for an organization (Macauley, 2015). Teamwork goes hand in hand with recognition, pride, and accountability. Recognition and reward are important components in developing a high level of engagement in the workplace (Macauley, 2015). Rewarding and recognizing team members can help develop a sense of pride among individual team members and in the team as a whole. Although there are various ways to reward and recognize employees, it is important for leaders to remember that not all employees are motivated by the same method(s) of reward and recognition. One employee may value a simple "thank you," whereas another employee may be more motivated by a gift card or public recognition at a staff meeting for a job well done. The leader should actively recognize team member accomplishments as well as hold all team members accountable for shortcomings.

Chapter 7 addressed accountability of oneself in the self-awareness section. Each team member, including the nurse leader, needs to maintain accountability for his or her own actions. In this chapter, accountability is more team focused, wherein leaders ensure that they consistently hold team members accountable, while team members hold one another accountable. A team that successfully achieves this level in the journey is one in which teamwork, pride, recognition, and accountability come together. Once the leader and the team feel that they consistently exhibit teamwork, pride, recognition, and accountability, they can move to the third level in the journey.

Pyramid Level Three

The third level includes service excellence, operational excellence, and leadership excellence. Leadership has an indisputable role in the achievement of cultural change, and successful cultural change is an indicator of successful leadership (Boomer & McCormack, 2010). Excellence is achieved when employees feel valued, physicians feel the organization is of the highest quality, and patients feel that the service is extraordinary (Studer, 2003). The organization consistently exceeds expectations. In order to achieve and maintain excellence in service, operations, and leadership, there must be a commitment in the organization for excellence from top management to the staff in the trenches.

Quality and consistent leadership both at the departmental level and at the executive level is absolutely essential in order for organizations to be successful at this level on the pyramid. As an example of an organization's commitment to leadership excellence, consider a chief executive officer and his senior leadership team who initiated a leadership institute that was composed of a series of monthly 1-hour sessions during which all leaders in the organization came together to learn and share best practices. Topics focused on inspiring and motivating leaders, as well as determining how leaders can inspire the workforce to enhance service and operational excellence. The initiative was like a wave of positive energy that flowed throughout the entire organization. This can be applied to both practice and academic settings. In order for this to occur, organizations must ensure that all leaders in the organization "get it." In other words, leaders need to exemplify excellence in how they manage and treat their employees, in how they treat customers, in the services they provide to customers, and in the quality of the overall operation of their departments.

In an organization, each leader needs to exemplify excellence in his or her own area(s) for which he or she is held accountable. If each department within an organization demonstrates excellence in leadership, service, and operations, then the entire organization benefits. Transforming cultures requires a concerted effort on each team member's part in order to make this happen. It needs to occur both at the individual departmental level and at the organizational level. In organizations that aspire to embark on this journey, the chief executive of the organization at the helm sets the tone for a commitment to excellence, while each leader in the organization carries out that commitment in each and every area of the organization. Achieving success in the third level requires a concerted effort on everyone's part. As stated earlier, changing the culture of an organization takes time, but those organizations that commit to excellence will remain intact, whereas others will likely fold. Achieving excellence in service and operations is extremely important, but the critical element is excellence in leadership.

Quality and consistent leadership both at the departmental level and at the executive level is absolutely essential in order for organizations to be successful at this level on the pyramid. Once the organization has achieved excellence in service, operations, and leadership, it can move to the fourth and final level on the pyramid.

Pyramid Level Four

The fourth level includes patient satisfaction, employee satisfaction, and physician satisfaction, which together add up to successful health care. With respect to employee satisfaction, the formula addresses employees at all levels in the organization (both patient care and nonpatient care). Box 9.9 highlights several proven effective patient satisfaction initiatives.

Patient satisfaction initiatives can be beneficial in enhancing the patient experience, but regardless of the particular initiative, all spring from a common foundation: If leaders take care of their employees, the patients will be well cared for. Box 9.10 highlights several employee satisfaction initiatives.

In addition to the initiatives listed in Box 9.10, leaders may also want to offer programs that focus on self-care (see Chapter 7) and improving the health and well-being of their employees. The need for self-care and ongoing stress management for nurses is essential (Gerard, 2012). Although it is important to work on enhancing employee satisfaction at all levels in the organization, experienced health-care professionals may attest to the fact that if leaders make a concerted effort to improve the satisfaction of their nurses, the patients benefit in a positive way. Satisfied nurses provide safer and

BOX 9.9 **Patient Satisfaction Initiatives**

Rounding on patients

Service recovery program

Enhancing the "patient experience"

Meeting patients' basic needs

Get well cards postdischarge

Follow-up discharge phone calls

Patient satisfaction survey

BOX 9.10 **Employee Satisfaction Initiatives**

Rounding on employees

Reward and recognition program

Team-building program

Meeting employees' basic needs

Thank-you notes for employees

Employee satisfaction committee

Managing up (at all levels)

Employee satisfaction survey

higher quality patient care, and they strive for higher patient satisfaction (Macauley, 2015). Most physicians would admit that the satisfaction of their patients is of the utmost importance to them; therefore, if their patients are satisfied, the physicians probably are also.

Thus, in striving to create a culture of excellence, visualize a "cycle" of satisfaction: Satisfied nurses = Satisfied patients = Satisfied physicians in a continuous bidirectional loop. The satisfaction of nurses in any organization is an important factor for leaders to consider. Just as nurse leaders need to care for their nurses and staff, nurse executives have an obligation to care for their nurse leaders. Nurse leaders who are in positions as directors, managers, supervisors, and coordinators are considered "middle management." This can be one of the most challenging positions to serve in because they are expected to satisfy their subordinates and at the same time they must satisfy upper management. When supervising nurse leaders, nurse executives need to be mindful of this, and they should make a concerted effort to take care of their nurse leaders.

In the big picture, nurse leaders need to be satisfied before there can be a level of satisfaction from other levels. Although each party is interdependent, the nurse leader can have a powerful impact on how this all plays out. Thus, to take the cycle a step further for best practice in achieving success, consider: Satisfied leaders = Satisfied employees = Satisfied patients = Satisfied physicians. This formula implies that leaders are the key members of the team and employers and organizations need to be cognizant of them when considering employee satisfaction. Again, although each party is interdependent, the message here is that the nurse leader can be a powerful force in how this all works. In health care, a satisfied leader can have a tremendous positive impact on the satisfaction of his or her staff, patients, and physicians. Macauley (2015) suggests that nursing leaders play an integral role in employee and patient satisfaction. In academic settings, a satisfied academic nursing leader can have a major positive influence on nursing faculty and staff, which then transmits to the students as the primary customer. In organizations in which there is a true culture of excellence, leaders take care of their staff, staff take care of their patients, and physicians are satisfied that their patients are well cared for. Box 9.11 highlights several physician satisfaction initiatives.

LEADER ASSESSMENT

One way to assess how a leader of a department(s) is performing is to take a look at three measures—employee satisfaction, patient satisfaction, and employee turnover. Employee satisfaction can be assessed by using an outside vendor that specializes in employee satisfaction surveys. This is usually anonymous and can provide leaders with valuable information about their employees' satisfaction in the workplace. Patient satisfaction can also be assessed by using the services of an outside vendor. As addressed in Chapter 4, in the United States, assessing patient satisfaction in health-care organizations is required for reimbursement (Weigand, 2013).

Human resource departments in health-care organizations usually monitor employee turnover percentages. According to Galletta et al. (2013), nurse leaders play a main role in preventing excessive turnover among nurses. Although employee turnover in some circumstances may be welcomed, excessive turnover may compromise team cohesion and quality of care. Voluntary nursing turnover is an issue of critical importance and one that is considered a serious problem that has an impact on many levels (Galletta et al., 2013). This may also provide an indication of the level of the leader's own satisfaction in his or her role. Low levels of employee and patient satisfaction and high rates of employee turnover may be an indication of a disconnect between the leader and the staff or an indication of ineffective leadership. Employee satisfaction impacts patient satisfaction. Ineffective leadership and leader dissatisfaction will likewise negatively impact employee satisfaction. If a leader is ineffective or dissatisfied, the leader's supervisor should intervene by providing leadership coaching and ample opportunities for the leader to receive additional training and mentoring. It may be necessary to create an action plan with the leader with a specified time frame for improvement.

BOX 9.11 Physician Satisfaction Initiatives

Rounding on physicians and other providers	Physician leadership institute
Reward and recognition program	Physician forums
Meeting physicians' basic needs	Physician satisfaction survey
Thank-you notes for physicians	

CONCLUSION

Nurses, as leaders, experience many challenges in their workday and throughout their careers. In order to manage these challenges, leaders need to be able to master essential skills in conflict resolution, crisis management, supervising, delegating, and networking in the professional work environment. In a leader's own personal leadership journey, he or she should always strive for excellence. Individuals as well as organizations may have a desire to pursue excellence. In order for organizations to achieve organizational excellence, they need to develop a culture of excellence. The Journey to a Culture of Excellence is one innovation that may assist health-care organizations in doing so. As Lao Tzu once wrote, "A journey of a thousand miles begins with a single step." Closing this chapter are six real-life patient satisfaction stories (Leadership Applications 9.1 through 9.6) that exemplify the heart and soul of service excellence and lessons learned.

LEADERSHIP APPLICATIONS IN PRACTICE 9.1 **A Patient's Story Can Reveal What's in the Heart**

A nurse leader responded to a complaint from an elderly patient who was in the VIP suite for medical treatment. The nurse leader visited with the patient and asked the patient how she could be of help. The patient complained that she did not like the whole wheat toast she was being served and went on to say that she was very wealthy. She reported that she had a Jaguar with her own personal driver, a butler, a maid, and a full-time caregiver. Finally, the patient stated that she could buy anything she wanted. The nurse did not understand why the patient felt she needed to elaborate about her wealth. The patient went on to say that she felt "the nurse" was far wealthier than she because she did not have the one thing she wanted most— the love of her daughter, who had not spoken to her in 14 years. After spending time with the patient and listening to her story, the nurse leader had a better understanding of why this patient appeared so upset about being served whole wheat toast. It was not only about the whole wheat toast—the patient wanted to share about the tremendous loss she was experiencing in not having the love of her daughter.

The patient was so grateful to the nurse leader for taking the time to listen to her, she wrote a letter to the chief executive officer of the organization praising the nurse leader and the team.

Lessons Learned When we take the time to really listen to the patient, we can learn about his or her emotional pain. This vignette portrays a nurse leader's intervention in resolving a customer service issue but even more important was the special moment between a nurse and a patient. The nurse leader exhibited several standards of behavior in the Journey to a Culture of Excellence (care, compassion, respect, customer service). The nurse also utilized service recovery to help turn a difficult situation around.

Leadership Applications in Practice 9.2 **A Complaint Can Be a Gift**

An oncology nurse in an acute care hospital was caring for an angry 70-year-old male patient. The nurse was losing patience and could not understand why he was being so difficult. She called her nurse leader for assistance, who entered the patient's room and observed him yelling at his wife. The patient addressed the nurse leader in a loud voice, asking, "What do you want? Leave me alone!" The nurse leader honored the patient's wish and left the patient's room.

She returned the next morning to see how the patient was doing. After stating, "You came back," the patient began to complain about his floor not being cleaned. "See, I left a red pen on the floor to show you that my floor was never cleaned because the red pen is still there." He went on to say that he never received his sandwich. He then complained that he did not know the results of the ultrasound of his arm. The nurse leader immediately took care of his concerns—made sure his floor was cleaned, went to the kitchen to pick up his sandwich, and made sure that the patient spoke with his physician regarding the results of his ultrasound. After all the service complaints were addressed, the patient then broke down in tears, saying, "My doctor gave me 2 months to live. I have lung cancer, nurse, and I can't handle it. I'm afraid." The nurse leader then realized why the patient was so angry and distressed. She encouraged the patient to cherish the time he had left with his wife and make the most of each day. The nurse leader communicated this to the rest of the team so that they could understand why this patient presented so angrily.

Lessons Learned In this vignette, we learn that complaints can be a gift. The leader exhibited several of the standards of behavior in the Journey to a Culture of Excellence (compassion, respect, positive attitude, customer service). The leader also used this experience with the patient as an opportunity to coach her team. Patients may present as angry and complain about service issues, but perhaps their real concern may be much deeper than what it appears to be. This patient was afraid to die. We can learn a great deal from our patients. Our experiences with our patients can be some of our very best educational opportunities in helping us grow.

Leadership Applications in Practice 9.3 **It's Not Always About the Soft-Boiled Egg**

A nurse leader in an acute care hospital was presented with a situation in which a patient's husband became extremely agitated and was verbally abusive to staff. The patient was dying of cancer, and the husband was upset because his wife could not get a soft-boiled egg. Each time he ordered her a soft-boiled egg, it arrived hard boiled. The staff who were assigned to the patient could not understand why the husband was so angry over an egg, as the patient was not even able to tolerate fluids. The staff kept insisting that the egg was soft boiled (thinking that it was). The nurse leader asked the executive chef to visit with the patient. The chef explained to the husband that because of the possibility of salmonella poisoning, the facility did not serve soft-boiled eggs. The nurses were unaware of this. The husband seemed to be satisfied with the explanation from the chef.

The next day, the nurse leader arrived at work and decided to stop by to check on the husband and the patient before heading to her office, but the room was empty. The patient had

Continued

LEADERSHIP APPLICATIONS IN PRACTICE 9.3 **It's Not Always About the Soft-Boiled Egg–cont'd**

---

died during the night. Several days later, the husband contacted the nurse leader to apologize for his anger toward the staff: "I knew my wife was dying, and I did not want to lose her," he said. "The only thing that I felt that I could do to help her was to order her something that she really enjoyed–a soft-boiled egg." The nurse leader realized that the husband's anger was not really about a soft-boiled egg but rather losing his beloved wife. The nurse leader used this example as a teaching opportunity to share with her team at their morning huddle.

Lessons Learned As leaders, when we are presented with difficult patient and family situations, we may not always be able to determine why their reactions may appear to us as exaggerated or unrealistic. Many factors that upset patients and families may be seemingly unrelated to the immediate situation. This vignette reminds us that people handle difficult situations in different ways. The leader demonstrated several standards of behavior in the Journey to a Culture of Excellence (care, compassion, customer service). The leader also appropriately enacted service recovery by asking the chef to come and speak with the patient's husband. Communication at all levels is essential. The chef is a part of the patient care services team. Leaders need to remember to include each member of the team in the plan and delivery of patient care and to encourage their staff to do this on a consistent basis.

LEADERSHIP APPLICATIONS IN PRACTICE 9.4 **A Leader Holds Herself Accountable for the Team**

A patient in her 40s was on a medical-surgical unit in an acute care hospital. The patient had a tracheostomy and could not speak. She rang the call bell to ask for assistance. The unit secretary who took the call said to the patient through the intercom, "If you do not speak up, I cannot help you." When the staff member did not hear a response from the patient, she asked, "What is it that you need? I cannot hear you." The patient later described this incident to her husband in writing, and he was irate.

The next day, the patient developed a medical complication that necessitated a "code blue." The patient survived. The nurse leader was notified and apologized to the husband for the staff member's insensitivity to his wife's needs. The nurse leader took responsibility for the situation and felt that she was accountable for not educating the ancillary staff on how to handle such situations. The story was shared with all staff on the unit as a teaching example that clearly illustrates why it is so important that staff know their patients and communicate with all members of the team.

Lessons Learned Rather than reprimanding the staff member, the nurse leader made a decision to use this example to educate and coach her team on the importance of communicating patient needs and conditions to all members of the team. Although the staff member who answered the call was a unit secretary, the unit secretary is part of the patient care services team and needs to be informed about a patient's special needs. This can negatively

---

LEADERSHIP APPLICATIONS IN PRACTICE 9.4   A Leader Holds Herself Accountable for the Team–cont'd

---

impact patient satisfaction if staff do not know how to respond to a patient's needs. The nurse leader exhibited several standards of behavior in the Journey to a Culture of Excellence (care, compassion, respect, customer service, competence). The nurse leader also served as a role model for staff in taking ownership and holding herself accountable, as well as holding her team accountable (the second level in the Journey to a Culture of Excellence).

As discussed throughout this chapter, employees and leaders need to exhibit the "basics"–standards of behavior in the first level and the qualities listed in the second and third levels–before an organization can achieve overall satisfaction. This team has some work to do in their journey to establishing a culture of excellence. From this example, we may deduce that the nurse leader appears to have an understanding of where improvement is needed and is using her leadership skills to implement change.

LEADERSHIP APPLICATIONS IN PRACTICE 9.5   Intensive Care Nurses Learn That a Book Cannot Be Judged by Its Cover

---

Several intensive care nurses were complaining about a patient's daughter who was not responding to their attempts to reach her about her mother's condition. The patient was in critical condition and on a ventilator. The nurse who was working with the patient left several messages for the daughter but received no response from her. Several days later, the patient's daughter arrived from out of state and shared with the nurse leader that she did receive the messages from the nurses but chose not to return their calls. The daughter went on to say, "That woman is a patient to *you*, but she is *my* mother. She used to beat my sister and me and lock us in a closet for days. I am here to pay respect to her because she is my mother and I want to see that she is buried properly, but I will never forget what she did." The nurse leader asked the daughter whether she would meet with the nurses so that she could share from a family member's perspective how important it is to show compassion for family members as well as patients.

The meeting between the daughter and the nurses had a meaningful impact. The daughter shared how grateful she was to the nurse leader for allowing her to speak with the nurses. The nurses understood why the daughter did not return their calls. They learned a great lesson that day–do not judge others for their actions, which might stem from personal circumstances.

Lessons Learned   The nurse leader served as a positive role model for the staff and took the initiative to involve the daughter in the patient's care by providing her with an opportunity to help educate nurses regarding how they can be more helpful to families. This was a very positive approach to help rectify the situation and one way to hold the nurses accountable for their actions. The nurse leader exhibited several standards of behavior in the Journey to a Culture of Excellence (respect, care, compassion, competence) and exhibited exceptional leadership skills (leadership excellence) in fostering patient (family) satisfaction. This vignette is an excellent example of how effective leadership can be instrumental in promoting a culture that supports excellence.

LEADERSHIP APPLICATIONS IN PRACTICE 9.6 **Sometimes It's the Little Things That Matter Most to Patients**

A nurse leader in an urgent care center was making rounds one day and received a request for Ivory soap from a blind patient. The smell of that particular soap reminded her of being washed by her mother as a child. Because soap bars were no longer used by the hospital, the nurse leader asked the vice president of nursing for permission to grant the patient's request. The patient was very happy that the nurse leader was able to obtain the soap for her. The successful event led to further discussions about a possible need for changing policy to allow for the use of Ivory soap for patient care. A task force was formed with a focus on meeting patients' basic needs.

Lessons Learned Sometimes it really is the little things that matter most to patients. Health-care environments are so high-tech today that, at times, nurses may forget the importance of attending to the small requests and basic needs of patients. The nurse leader exhibited several of the standards of behavior in the Journey to a Culture of Excellence (care, compassion, respect, customer service). The nurse leader advocated for the patient by asking her supervisor for permission to grant the patient's request. This is an excellent example of a leader who serves as a wonderful role model for other nurses and staff and someone who puts patient satisfaction as a top priority. The patient's request also resulted in the formation of a task force to make improvements in this area.

References

American Nurses Association. (2015). *Position Statement on Incivility, Bullying, and Workplace Violence.* Retrieved from https://www.nursingworld.org.

Boomer, C. A., & McCormack, B. (2010). Creating the conditions for growth: A collaborative practice development program for clinical nurse leaders. *Journal of Nursing Management, 18,* 633–644.

Bramley, L., & Matiti, M. (2014). How does it really feel to be in my shoes? Patients' experiences of compassion within nursing care and their perceptions of developing compassionate nurses. *Journal of Clinical Nursing, 23,* 2790–2799.

Chu, L. (2014). Mediating toxic emotions in the workplace—the impact of abusive supervision. *Journal of Nursing Management, 22,* 953–963.

Curtis, E. A., de Vries, J., & Sheerin, F. K. (2011). Developing leadership in nursing: The impact of education and training. *British Journal of Nursing, 20*(6), 344–348.

Downey, M., Parslow, S., & Smart, M. (2011). The hidden treasure in nursing leadership: Informal leaders. *Journal of Nursing Management, 19,* 517–521.

Estes, B. C. (2013). Abusive supervision and nursing performance. *Nursing Forum, 48*(1), 3–16.

Galletta, M., Portoghese, I., Battistelli, A., & Leiter, M. P. (2013). The roles of unit leadership and nurse-physician collaboration on nursing turnover intention. *Journal of Advanced Nursing, 69*(8), 1771–1784.

Gerard, B. (2012). Healthcare reform begins with caring for ourselves. *Beginnings, 32*(4), 8.

Institute of Medicine. (2010). *The future of nursing: Leading change, advancing health.* Washington, DC: National Academies Press.

Knol, J., & Van Linge, R. (2009). Innovative behavior: The effect of structural and psychological empowerment on nurses. *Journal of Advanced Nursing, 65*(2), 359–370.

Lomax, S. W., & White, D. (2015). Interprofessional collaborative care skills for the frontline nurses. *Nursing Clinics of North America, 50*(1), 59–73.

Longo, J. (2011). Acts of caring nurses caring for nurses. *Holistic Nursing Practice, 25*(1), 8–16.

Ma, C., Shang, J., & Bott, M. J. (2015). Linking unit collaboration and nursing leadership to nurse outcomes and quality of care. *Journal of Nursing Administration, 45*(9), 435–442.

Macauley, K. (2015). Employee engagement: how to motivate your team? *Journal of Trauma Nursing, 22*(6), 298–300.

McDonald, G., Vickers, M. H., Mohan, S., Wilkes, L., & Jackson, D. (2010). Workplace conversations: Building and maintaining collaborative capital. *Contemporary Nurse, 36*(1–2), 96–105.

Moore, L., Leahy, C., Sublett, C., & Lanig, H. (2013). Understanding nurse-to-nurse relationships and their impact on work environments. *MEDSURG Nursing, 22*(3), 172–179.

Morreim, H. (2015, Winter). Conflict resolution in the clinical setting: A story beyond bioethics mediation. *Journal of Law, Medicine & Ethics*, 843–856.

Pines, E. W., Rauschhumber, M. L., Cook, J. D., Norgan, G. H., Canchola, L., Richardson, C., & Jones, M. E. (2014). Enhancing resilience, empowerment, and conflict management among baccalaureate students. *Nurse Educator, 39*(2), 85–90.

Ritter, D. (2011). The relationship between healthy work environments and retention of nurses in a hospital setting. *Journal of Nursing Management, 19*, 27–32.

Rodwell, J., Brunetto, Y., Demir, D., Shacklock, K., & Farr-Wharton, R. (2014). Abusive supervision and links to nurse intentions to quit. *Journal of Nursing Scholarship, 46*(5), 357–365.

Saccomano, S. J., & Pinto-Zipp, G. (2011). Registered nurse leadership style and confidence in delegation. *Journal of Nursing Management, 19*, 522–533.

Simpson, R. L. (2014). Social media creates significant risks for nursing. *Nursing Administration Quarterly, 38*(1), 96–98.

Strech, S., & Wyatt, D. A. (2013). Partnering to lead change: Nurses' role in the redesign of health care. *AORN Journal, 98*(3), 260–266.

Studer, Q. (2003). *Hardwiring excellence*. Gulf Breeze, FL: Fire Starter.

Tomey, A. M. (2009). Nursing leadership and management effects work environments. *Journal of Nursing Management, 17*, 15–25.

Weigand, L. (2013). Customer service: The nursing bundle. *Journal of Emergency Nursing, 39*(5), 454–455.

Index

Note: Page numbers followed by "b," "f," and "t" indicate boxes, figures, and tables, respectively.